CW01496223

HEALING THE SOUL

Volume two

The Archetype and the Psyche

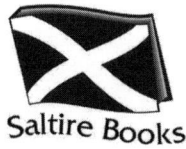

Saltire Books   *Saltire Books Limited, Glasgow, Scotland*

HEALING THE SOUL

Volume two

The Archetype and the Psyche

DAVID LILLEY
MBChB, FFHom, LLCO

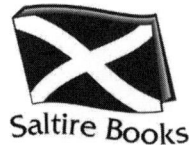
Saltire Books   *Saltire Books Limited, Glasgow, Scotland*

Published by Saltire Books Ltd

18–20 Main Street, Busby, Glasgow G76 8DU, Scotland
books@saltirebooks.com   www.saltirebooks.com

Cover, Design, Layout and Text © Saltire Books Ltd 2018

 is a registered trademark

First published in 2018

Typeset by Type Study, Scarborough, UK in 9¼ on 13½ Stone Serif
Printed and bound in the UK by TJ International Ltd, Padstow, Cornwall

ISBN 978-1-908127-09-9

For Saltire
Project Development: Lee Kayne
Editorial: Steven Kayne
Designer: Phil Barker
Indexer: Laurence Errington

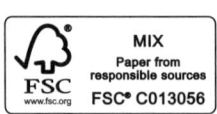

CONTENTS

part two   THE PSYCHE

*This book is dedicated to my beloved wife Paddy,
whose support, patience and understanding have
made it possible*

ABOUT THE AUTHOR

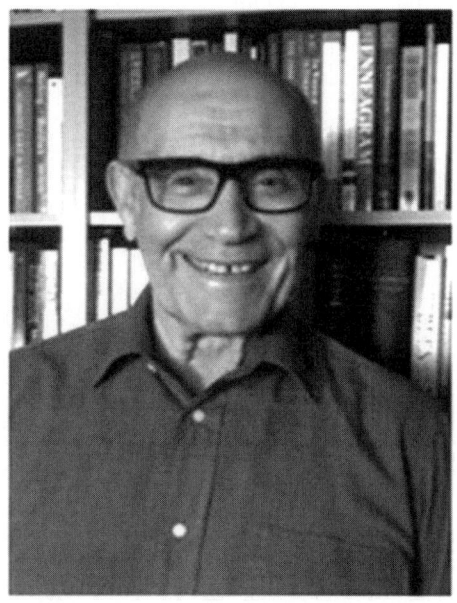

David Lilley was born into a homeopathic family in Leeds, Yorkshire, England, in 1940. His father, William Henry Lilley, was a renowned psychic healer and also a homeopathic practitioner and chiropractor. In 1949, the family emigrated to South Africa. David studied medicine at the University of Pretoria, qualifying in 1962. He spent three years at the Royal London Homeopathic Hospital and obtained his MFHom qualification in 1965. The following year, he completed his training in osteopathy at the London College of Osteopathy.

Returning to South Africa, he joined his father and has practiced as a homeopath and osteopath for the past 52 years. In 1995, he founded the South African Faculty of Homeopathy to provide homeopathic education for medical doctors and acted as dean until 2012.

Since 1999, David has lectured widely in the UK and also internationally. In his lectures, he weaves together homeopathic art and science, analytical psychology, mythology, symbolism, chakra and colour theory, natural science and spiritual philosophy to provide a rich tapestry of perennial wisdom and knowledge.

In December 2007, David retired from private practice in Pretoria and moved to Cape Town where he currently conducts a small select practice and is devoting his time to writing and lecturing. He has published two titles to date: *Healing the Soul – Volume 1 The Lives of Samuel Hahnemann and William Lilley* (2014, reprinted 2018) and *The Wolf* (2017) both of which were greeted with considerable acclaim.

ACKNOWLEDGEMENTS

In writing this book, which ventures into the intangible realm of the psyche and the mysterious, mythical world of dreams, I am indebted to the two masters of the mind, Sigmund Freud and Carl Gustav Jung for providing me with the tools to do so. I am further indebted to Anthony Stevens the distinguished Jungian analyst, psychiatrist and author whose writings have made Jung's work so much more accessible; to Michael White for his insightful biography of Isaac Newton; to Almaas for his spiritual teachings of the Enneagram; and to Mario Schiess, the German born playwright, director and producer based in Pretoria, who was both patient and friend and a passionate Jungian. It was Mario, who first focussed my attention on Jung's thinking and, in the late-1980s, intuitively analysed two profound archetypal dreams that I experienced synchronistically at an important transitional point in my life. The first, revealing the inevitable certainty of the path I must follow and the second, the imminence of the Great Mother Goddess in my life – both, continue to influence and direct me. Finally, I owe so much to the guidance and friendship of my publisher, Steven Kayne of Saltire Books, whose unerring vision and timing has ensured the safe birth of each of my books.

The use of capitals in the text e.g. Universe, Cosmos, Universal or Supreme Intelligence, Divinity, Self, Spirit – and Wolf, Dog, Cat, denotes universality or archetypal status. For instance, wolf indicates the animal, whereas, Wolf denotes the archetype or the homeopathic remedy: Lac lupinum. The same distinction is used when describing the functions of gods e.g. Hermes the messenger god is descriptive of Hermes, the personage, whereas, Hermes, Messenger of the Gods is an archetypal designation; another example is: Apollo, the sun god and Apollo, God of the Sun. When considering the elements of the psyche, I use capitals for the Id, which is universal. However, I always give the Shadow a capital because of personal preference and to make it stand out in the text. The Self, being synonymous with the Spirit, which in turn is synonymous with the indwelling Divinity within us all, is written in capitals, which aptly differentiates it from the soul that is working towards becoming the Self. I have adhered to the original Greek spelling of names taken from Greek mythology, rather than their Roman and modern derivatives: e.g. Herakles (Hercules), Kerberos (Cerberus) and Hephaistos (Hephaestus).

INTRODUCTION

The Soul's Journey continues . . .

In the first volume of *Healing the Soul*, I brought together the science and art of homeopathy and the science and art of spiritual healing to lay a foundation for further concepts essential to 'healing' at the deepest level: the soul/ego-self dimension. Since 'illness', like any life experience, has positive and beneficent intent, and is a healing process, destined and designed to facilitate the journey of the soul towards Self-realisation (individuation), treatment that honours the 'illness' and its objective, by faithfully matching its every nuance, hastens it towards consummation, releasing the soul from the necessity of the 'illness' and steering it towards a higher, less ego-distorted expression of itself. Homeopathy provides the means to achieve this ideal. It is a healing paradigm that restores psychic balance and harmony and reinstates the soul as sovereign of the psyche: a transformation indispensable to both cure and individuation.

Hom / of / balance / Obsoul of psyche

Physician and patient are companions travelling the same sacred path. Cast in the role of guide and mentor, the physician needs to be conversant with the terrain traversed on the journey towards transcendence; aware of the milestones and signposts that mark the way; recognise the cues and prompts of synchronicity; and interpret the parable within a narrative and the myth within a dream. The physician, like our noble sibling, the wolf, needs to be psychically keened to all dimensions, able to conduct souls through all boundaries and spheres of existence. This calls for a different kind of thinking and a different kind of perception. It is for this purpose that *Healing the Soul* is written.

Through its pages, we enter the realm of the archetype in which symbols, images, metaphors, dreams and myths become real; for behind the external appearance of things, a more radiant beauty, a greater wisdom and a higher reality exists, whose ineffable essence can only be comprehended in symbolic form. Myth and symbol possess the power to reveal deeper meaning with clarity and richness; bringing together aspects of the conscious and the unconscious, the rational and the intuitive – providing a portal into a finer dimension.

On examining the significance of symbols, we discover that they can be compared to homeopathic remedies. They direct us to something beyond themselves, to that which would otherwise remain unknown, intangible and indefinable. The symbol is the portal to a spiritual realm; its energy is continuous with its ethereal counterpart and inseparable from that which it symbolises. The potentised remedy is the portal to a mysterious archetypal world of healing power with which it is confluent. In contemplating a physical image or a remedy archetype, we are in the presence of its invisible essence, for it is the epiphany of a hidden force. Every object and every remedy is a unique revelation of the mystical and expresses specific archetypal attributes, intimating another more potent reality that informs and energises it.

By revisiting the fantasy world of our childhood, returning to the time when we still dwelt in the realm of the archetype and recapturing its magic and mystery, this faculty can be reawakened. The homeopath needs to have the intuitive, imaginative and uncluttered mind of a shaman to walk with confidence in the hallowed halls of fable and fantasy where the inner mysteries of life are revealed.

The two major remedies presented in Part 1, Graphites and Silicea, have been considered in totally different ways to demonstrate analysis of the archetype by application of the *doctrine of signatures* (Graphites) and by *personality profiling* (Silicea). Both methods are rewarding: encouraging lateral thinking, archetypal thinking and dream thinking and aiding memory and understanding while installing the archetype 'deep in the homeopathic muscle.'

The plight of conventional medicine

It is of great concern that despite the remarkable advances of conventional Western medicine, it has failed to develop a healing system of therapy. The benefits this medical paradigm has delivered through high technology, sophisticated diagnostic methods, refined surgery and a formidable arsenal of chemical substances capable of combating infection, palliating and controlling symptoms and modifying body functions and chemistry, have not been attended by a commensurate ability to heal the sick. Healing calls for the restoration of a patient's health to an on-going state of vigour, strength, resistance, comfort and balance experienced physically, intellectually and emotionally, independent of chemical support. Disappearance

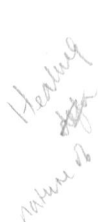

of symptoms and signs through the intervention of drugs elaborated by orthodox pharmaceutical research is achieved through synthetic suppression, control or substitution and not through encouraging and enhancing the body's own defensive and restorative powers: functions that are essential for healing. Drug action, despite bringing symptomatic relief and altering body chemistry, inevitably results in the energy of the disease being displaced inwards, disturbing the economy at a deeper and potentially more damaging level. This repressed energy will be transferred to future generations, steadily increasing the complexity and intensity of the disease continuum.

Of greater concern than the failure to elaborate a healing therapeutic model is the complacency of the medical orthodoxy that has arisen from the measurable success of its superficial, mechanistic methods. Born of this, comes an arrogant unwillingness to recognise the limitations of the conventional model or to accept that there could be valid alternatives. This dismissive attitude, which in recent years has hardened to open hostility against alternative forms of medicine, is a serious obstacle to medical progress.

The therapeutic horizon of conventional medicine is restricted and set by the parameters of Newtonian physics, which asserts that matter is the ground of all existence and that life springs from the confluence of chance events and evolves through random mutations in genetic material without purposeful design and without necessarily leading to the emergence of higher forms. In keeping with this scientific perspective, conventional medicine, no matter the personal persuasion of individuals within its ranks, has no concept of the existence of the human soul or of a spiritual dimension pervading and informing the material realm. Without these perceptions, the dominant school lacks insight into the true nature of the patient and lacks the means to penetrate the mystery of disease causation. Although the notion of psychosomatic disease is not foreign to the orthodox medical mind, the deep significance of this phenomenon escapes conventional thinking, which is aligned with the anomalous doctrine of an inverted hierarchy in which matter gives birth to mind and to subjective consciousness. In such a hierarchy, emotions are biologically driven and controlled by a constellation of interacting brain systems amongst which the amygdala (memory brain) is crucial. The pivotal role of emotions in disturbed function and pathology is lost in their association with conditioned behaviour and patterns of physiological activity ruled by a plethora of hormones and neurotransmitters such as dopamine, noradrenaline, acetylcholine, serotonin, vasopressin, oxytocin and cortisol. With earthbound vision, science concludes that we are what we are because of genetic influences, our neuronal complexity and what our holding environment feeds into us.

In Shakespeare's great tragedy, *Hamlet*, Hamlet's mother Gertrude exhorts her son to cease his mourning for his father with these words:

> Good Hamlet, cast thy nighted colour off. Do not for ever with thy vailéd lids seek for thy noble father in the dust.[1]

Paraphrasing the Danish queen, conventional medicine should be beseeched in like manner:

> Do not forever with thy blinkered vision seek for the cause and cure of disease in the realm of matter.[1]

The fruitless searching for the origins of disease at cellular level focuses medical vision on the dust of life rather than its essence. Unable to assimilate the concept of the spiritual nature of the creation and of life and to incorporate this special knowledge into its science, the orthodoxy remains blind to the subtle source of the diseases that confront them; a source that lies at the level of the soul and its incessant engagement with the disruptive activities of the ego-self. Misdirected focus on the material effects of disease is indicative of the vast gulf separating chemistry-based 'scientific' medicine from the healing paradigm of 'soul' medicine.

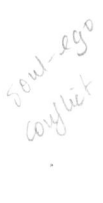

Given the imponderable nature of the soul and the ego-self-disease that afflicts it, the chemical tools of modern medicine, however they may modify the effects of disease, are incapable of influencing the soul-ego conflict that lies at its root. Striving to counter an unseen enemy, unfathomable to ordinary medical investigative diagnosis, with primitive weapons that influence only the chemico-physical level of life, is the plight of orthodox medicine. Compounding this limitation is the inability of the average medical mind, accustomed to using powerful, Newtonian, molecular medicine, to perceive the healing potential of gentle, homeopathic, non-molecular, quantum medicine. Only medicine that is imponderable can address the imponderable nature of disease at the causative level.

A higher and deeper perspective

In part one of *Healing the Soul* (volume 1)[2], I considered the founding of homeopathic science by recounting the life of Samuel Hahnemann and other early pioneers and presented the fundamental principles upon which this healing science is based. In part two, my father's remarkable life revealed the interpenetrating unity of spirit and matter and postulated that healing the body, in its entirety, necessitates healing the soul.

To complement this knowledge and give it practical application, it is necessary to fathom the complexities of the human psyche and to recognise the dysfunctional strategies of compensation and survival employed by the ego-based soul that feels abandoned, isolated and exposed in a seemingly hostile, alien environment, fraught with danger, not governed by law and devoid of higher purpose. The consequence of this profound misconception is 'dis-ease', which, with its attendant, dysfunctional responses to the challenges of life, becomes disease.

As with all evolutionary processes, the origin of disease must have commenced with slight and almost imperceptible changes, which, over generations, mounted incrementally until a critical point was reached when normal function was disturbed: an imbalance that finally manifested in physical change. Since disease, even when seemingly precipitated by impingements from without, is primarily soul-based, it must have begun with disruptions in thinking and feeling that gradually lead to disturbance of function followed, eventually, by changes in structure that became pathological. Over tens of thousands of years, disease must have followed a specific path that gradually diversified into the protean forms of acute and chronic disease that afflict humanity today. This proposes an unbroken continuum of disease that over generations matured from simple, superficial beginnings into deep-seated complexity. By tracing this morbid evolution in the light of Hahnemann's theory of the origin of chronic diseases, it is possible to clinically recognise and unravel disease relationships and intelligently address their presentation therapeutically.

origins of disease

The Soul Dimension

For the clinical encounter between physician and patient to have the deepest relevance and consequence, both participants need to be aware of their own spirit nature and the spiritual purpose of life. Only then can the exchange be conducted on a plane sufficiently profound to achieve the required resolution demanded by the emotional and physical ailments of the patient and the circumstances that provide their background. Regardless of the demands of the physical state of the patient, other than in acute and emergency situations, *healing needs to be achieved at soul level.*

The physician should never regard the sick being as merely a physical mechanism to be tuned, adjusted, modified or mended, or consider the disturbed emotional inner-world of the patient to be solely due to conditioning and chemical imbalance. Nor should the physician ever imagine that the disappearance of symptoms brought about by chemical or surgical

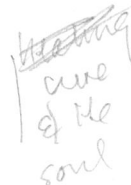

Healing cure of the soul

intervention constitutes cure or be satisfied when such an outcome is achieved. Regardless of appearances, the underlying dysfunction responsible for the symptoms and signs of ill-health is still present and will be acting detrimentally upon the constitution of the patient at a deeper level than before. Sometimes, the consequences of suppression may be so remote that they are not recognised for what they are, and, in some instances, may only be witnessed in following generations.

The physician, who would heal at the deepest level needs to fully appreciate the complex nature of the person seeking their help. This viewpoint is of signal importance in the treatment of chronic conditions and for conducting *constitutional or archetypal healing.* Similarly, it is essential for the person wishing to embark on such deep, searching therapy to be conscious of the complexity of their own psyche and to know that this is the major cause of the emotional and physical difficulties they are contending with. Such awareness permits them to play a more definite and participatory role in their own healing and to grant the process sufficient time to evolve and achieve success.

Individuation – Self-realisation

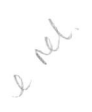

Both physician and patient need to be cognisant of the purpose of life and of the dynamics that exist between the incarnated soul and the ego-self the soul constructs in defence of its fears and lack of basic trust.

The human being is not merely a sentient assemblage of molecules and cells, but an immortal Spirit; a multi-dimensional being: divine in essence and potential; eternal and imperishable: a soul in transit!

At physical birth, this immaculate Spirit-being, a flame of the fire of Divinity (Supreme, Universal Consciousness), veiled by the attributes of its soul/ego-self complex, descends from a greater Reality and incarnates into the physical arena of the relative dimension: this Earth school.

The purpose of this momentous descent is the individuation or Self-realisation of the soul (true-self): a sacred quest consummated by traversing *the hero path* that ultimately leads to the merging of the soul with its Divinity: its own Essence or Self.

In 1949, using the idiom of myth, Joseph Campbell, the renowned American mythologist and author, defined *The Hero Path* in imagery that inspires and directs:

We have only to follow the thread of the hero path.
And where we had thought to find an abomination
we shall find a God.
And where we had thought to slay another
we shall slay ourselves.
Where we had thought to travel outwards
we shall come to the centre of our own existence.
And where we had thought to be alone
we shall be with all the world.[3]

The *'slaying' of ourselves* is the *'slaying' of the ego-self* (false-self): casting off
the ego-based perspectives built up over lifetimes, overthrowing the ego-
self's usurped dominion of the psyche, asserting the sovereignty of the soul
and realising the perfection of the Spirit-self by mastering the paradoxes
and polarities of mortal existence.

Life exposes the soul to a subtle and seductive illusion (*Maya*) fraught
with temptations, distractions, obstacles and pitfalls, but replete with
opportunities for growth and enlightenment.

Despite all circumstances and events that inform us differently, the
universe into which the soul incarnates is perfectly ordered and harmonious, governed by a Universal Intelligence that is everywhere present
(omnipresent), all-powerful (omnipotent), all-knowing (omniscient), wise
and loving; always acting with beneficent intent.

Nothing happens by chance; there is no such thing as coincidence, no
good or bad luck: nothing is random or arbitrary. All happenings, all situations and all circumstances are essential and have meaning; all are defined
by and subject to law: a law that is perfect, harmonious, just, wise and
loving. Every incident, no matter how dire and painful, has positive
purpose, design and intent. The Universe is consciously, caringly and
lovingly interacting with each individual soul in every instant – every
'Now' – providing it with circumstances (its entire holding environment)
perfectly tailored for its spiritual unfoldment.

As Shakespeare's *Hamlet* affirmed to Horatio:

There is a special providence in the fall of a sparrow. If it be now, 'tis not to come;
if it be not to come, it will be now; if it be not now, yet it will come: the readiness
is all. Since no man has ought of what he leaves, what is to leave betimes? Let
be.[4]

A profound truth is imbedded in these few lines. The *"readiness is all"* signifies that most precious state of being: living with *basic trust*; not faith, not
belief, not hope – *trust*! Hope is always for tomorrow, an ego-based wish
that tomorrow will be better than today; faith is the belief that that hope
will be realised; trust, however, is the abiding consciousness that, come

what may, *all is well*. *'Let be'* is the act of surrender to the trust that what providence unfolds is correct and necessary, and, above all, perfect, wise and loving. *'Let be'* is neither acceptance nor resignation, which merely constitute passive submission. *'Let be'* is active, willing, positive and creative participation in life's dispensation. Through trust and right-action, we put our shoulder and commitment to the wheel of life's unfolding.

We are not born before our time, nor shall we die before our time. In life, we move through an ever-evolving and unfolding web of perfectly designed events to which we respond with our inalienable *freedom of choice*. In the context of every moment, life is unfolding immaculately on behalf of and for the benefit of the soul. Like an alert, attentive, caring sheepdog, the Universe manoeuvres in each instant of 'Now', responding appropriately to every nuance of thought, emotion and action of its beloved; ever-prompting and urging the developing soul towards spiritual maturity and individuation (realisation of the divine Self).

In the simplest terms, the goal of the entire Creation is the spiritual unfolding of the individual soul. From the perspective of each soul, the entire Creation has been created and is still being created, in every instant, every 'Now', for the express purpose of its individuation. For each soul, only the Creation and itself exists and the Creation is its Source, its Essence and its goal. For the Creation, the existence of each and every soul is as critical to the continued order of the universe as are all the galaxies in the heavens.

The individual is a combination of *endowed traits* derived from the soul and *inherited traits* derived from the body. The soul is the immortal aspect of the individual that bonds with its physical vehicle at conception, animates it at the quickening, is tested and seasoned by the events of life, and at physical death, discards the body, leaves the earth plane and returns to the spirit dimension from which it descended. The soul unconsciously bears the accumulated memory and experience of its temporary sojourns on the physical plane and harbours the residual attributes of the ego-self that veil the divine perfection of the Spirit that is the soul's Essence.

The ego-self (ego, ego-personality, false-self) represents that part of the soul that requires healing.

The soul's morality, born of many lives on the material plane, is encapsulated in the conscience, which pricks and stings the soul into opposing the self-serving manipulations and rationalisations of the ego-self that deviate the soul from the path of healing and enlightenment.

The soul incarnates into the world through a multifaceted vehicle – the body/mind/emotion complex – which, be it advantaged or disadvantaged, is specially fashioned (customised) to temper and test the indwelling soul.

Divine providence

Nothing is by chance; all is orchestrated and tailored to urge and prompt the soul along its journey towards the realisation of the Self.

The situations and circumstances that condition and challenge the soul and the constellation of significant others with whom it consorts through life, are in perfect keeping with the character and nature of the ego-self and, therefore, with the soul's need for healing. All those who play a role in the soul's life experience, and all happenings that impinge upon the soul, are indispensable to the fulfilment of the soul's journey.

Life is a divine prescription for the healing of the soul: a sacred dispensation, urging the soul to banish the usurper ego-self from the psyche, assume its sovereignty and merge with its Divinity. Oft times, the ego-enslaved soul may require trauma or tragedy to jolt it out of complacency or somnolence and urge it to commence its sacred journey.

Synchronicity

defn

What we perceive as *meaningful coincidence* happens because of *synchronicity*: the concept that a governing, intelligent, purposeful dynamic elaborates the whole of human experience and world events. Seemingly random happenings are expressions of this deeper order: a creative tide that urges individual and collective ascent through sublimation. Each of us is imbedded in an ordered, dynamic framework, which has our spiritual awakening as its focus and concern. *Spiritual awakening, soul healing and dismantling of the ego-self are inseparable.*

healing of ego self

I experienced a touching example of synchronicity some twenty years ago. One summer afternoon in our garden in Pretoria, I was relaxing and reading in the shade of the trees that surround the 'magic' circle where Dr Letari used to visit us.[i] My preoccupation with my book was suddenly interrupted by my focus shifting to the incessant, high-pitched shrilling of the cicadas in the tree above me. It was a hot, sunny day and they had been active all morning, but for some reason, although I was habituated and usually indifferent to their clamour, at that moment they claimed my attention. The thought dropped into my mind that the soliciting 'song' the males emit was akin to the awful *tinnitus*, or ringing in the ears, which is so frequently met in practice and proves so difficult to relieve or cure. The most common cause of tinnitus is noise-induced hearing loss caused by

---

[i] Lejan Tari Singh ('Dr Letari') was a Brahman, physician seer, who, from my earliest years, opened my eyes to the magnificence of the Creation and tutored me in the mysteries of life. His influence on my father's healing work and my practice of homeopathy are covered at length in the first volume of *Healing the Soul*.[2]

exposure of the ear to immoderate volumes of sound. The correspondence between the noise generated by the cicada and human tinnitus is strengthened by the fact that although only the male cicada is responsible for the distinctive sound, both sexes possess *tympana*, membranous structures that vibrate to sound waves: the insect's equivalent of eardrums. The volume of sound generated by the male when calling is capable of distorting and disabling his own tympana. The homeopathic significance of this is at once apparent; pursuing the 'like cures like' principle, *Cicada* should prove a valuable remedy for the treatment of tinnitus and loss of hearing, especially when caused by acoustic trauma.

On the spur of the moment, I resolved to catch one of the noisy insects with the intention of macerating and triturating it into homeopathic potency and then testing its efficacy clinically. Although, they like hanging upside down on the underside of tree branches, at the approach of a likely predator, the cicadas quickly manoeuvre themselves onto the upper surface and out of sight. To make matters worse, despite the noise they generate, they are difficult to locate because they all chirp in unison; the pitch of the sound carries well and comes to the ear from every possible direction. I was thinking of getting a ladder to improve my chances when I was called away, and later, when free to pursue my intention, the light was failing, and the insects had fallen silent.

The following morning, I was abruptly awakened by our ten-year-old tabby cat, Matata, leaping onto the bed and then onto me with a very live and intact cicada in her mouth, which she proudly deposited on my chest. She was a great ratter and often presented her trophies to us, but had never shown any interest in insects, unlike her sister Snookums, who loved playing with crickets and chasing flies. I was deeply moved by this clear evidence of the interest and participation of the Cosmos in my life. I knew I had received a gift from a subtler dimension. Forthwith, I put the cicada into rectified spirits and the following day handed it to my laboratory staff to be triturated through the lower six decimal attenuations and then potentised to the 200th centesimal potency. The pharmacist who monitored the procedure was very interested to know what the insect remedy was likely to be good for. I explained to him. Intrigued, he told me that his wife, who was in her early seventies, suffered from a distressing level of tinnitus and asked if she might try it out for me. I agreed and gave her a 200th potency once per day and asked her to continue in this way until she noticed a change. Within two weeks, she experienced a lessening in the intensity of the noise. This was an indication to reduce the frequency of the dosage. She successfully continued with treatment until the level of unwanted sound was reduced to a fraction of what it had been. Probably due to her age, this proved to be as much as could be achieved but was a huge relief to her and important to me, because the improvement held. The remedy derived from the cicada, *Platypleura*, is worth trying out for any case of tinnitus, but is particularly successful when the affliction is induced by injury to the ear due to excess noise, e.g. gunshot or the use of in-ear head-phones set at excessive volume.

As simple as this anecdote is, it demonstrates a profound truth that we exist in a living, thinking, feeling and caring Cosmos that is ever alert to our needs and activities and intimately involved in our lives at every level. Conscious awareness and focus on this imminence will be rewarded by evidence of its action and proof that no happening is random or arbitrary. Synchronicity must be regarded as an inherent and pervasive dynamic, which underlies and evidences the meaning in our lives.

With the knowledge that every life experience is structured and tailored to facilitate the spiritual awakening and spiritual unfolding or *individuation* of the patient, the homeopathic physician knows that the Cosmos is already prescribing for their patient.

The divine prescription is revealed in the patient's ego-based 'disease'; their emotional, intellectual and physical constitution; their relationships, especially those most intimate, significant and influential; and the circum-stances, situations and events that impinge on them.

Some vital premises derive from this knowledge.

- *Individuation is the path of Self-attainment traversed through healing the soul.*
- *The life experience is a divine prescription uniquely designed for the healing and individuation of the soul.*
- *The individuation of the soul is opposed by the nature and attributes of the ego-self.*
- *The ego-self is the disease from which the soul suffers.*
- *The part of the psyche that requires healing is the ego-self (ego-personality).*

Therefore, the nature of the ego-self – its emotions, fears, feelings, desires, tendencies, habits, attributes, attitudes, perceptions, prejudices, prefer-ences, beliefs and values – together with the nature of the holding-environ-ment that conditions the ego-self, give the physician a template that must be matched in selecting the most similar homeopathic prescription.

Unity – Non-duality

Critical to understanding life and its purpose is the spiritual perception that *All is One* – the Creator, the created and the creation are one – the entire

Cosmos is one – all nature is one – and we are all part of that Oneness and inseparable from it. The Creation is a complex and complete system with all parts totally integrated, interdependent and in touch.

The Absolute Oneness, the eternal, immutable Reality, Essence or Being (God), constantly unfolds into a multiplicity of ever-changing forms, which are never separate or discrete, but always connected to Being (to the Source and Essence), to its unfoldment and to one another. Despite multiplicity, there is no duality. There is total Unity. Duality and separateness are an illusion of ego-consciousness. Without duality, the whole of physical reality is witnessed as being imbued with the Essential Dimension and is therefore experienced as being one with the ultimate Reality. The Absolute is not only the source and cause of everything; everything (including ourselves, all energy and matter) is the Absolute, and represents the omnipresence, omnipotence and omniscience of the Universal Intelligence (God). We are not separate or disconnected from Being, nor are we separate from others or from our environment. All souls are connected to one another and to their Source or Origin. The only boundaries are those constructed by the ego-mind. The ego-based perception of separate identity is a delusion. We are each an inseparable part of the Whole. Although each of us is a unique, individual expression of Being, we remain at the same time inseparable from the totality of the Universe and our boundaries are spiritually porous and transparent.

The wholeness of the universe is expressed in ever-repeated patterns throughout nature. The entire system, visible and invisible, is governed by vast rhythms and cycles – *a wondrous dance of Creation* – all permeated with the truth, perfection, wisdom and love of a Universal Consciousness.

The dynamic Unity of the living, loving Cosmos is the ultimate Truth of existence.

Reincarnation

In the face of this Unity and the cycles that characterise it, witnessed in the heavens, in the seasons and in the tides, it is puzzling that with the exception of contemporary followers of Kabbalah and the Rosicrucian Order, the three orthodox Middle Eastern religions, Judaism, Christianity and Islam have failed to incorporate the concept of reincarnation, or rebirth, in their religious doctrines: the understanding that the soul develops spiritually through experience gained in many lifetimes spent on the material plane. Central to the canon of all these religions is the teaching that the goal of the soul is the achievement of spiritual excellence or perfection, culminating in Self-realisation and mergence with God. Implicit to this teaching is the belief that such transcendence is within the moral capacity of every soul. Rejection of reincarnation places the burden for this profound transformation, from an ego-based to a soul-based being, on the vagaries of a single lifetime. This expectation is absurd, at odds with sincere self-appraisal and the moral evaluation of those best known to us. We might as illogically expect a schoolchild to achieve university graduation after a single year of study.

The belief that *"you only live once"* has been foisted upon the laity by a patriarchal, religious hierarchy that profits by holding the devotee captive with the promise of redemption through faith and observance. A one-chance-only scenario and the threat of retribution for the lapsed and the reprobate apply coercive urgency. This indoctrination is reinforced through ceremony, ritual and scripture and the glorification and worship of exalted beings believed to possess the power to intercede on behalf of the observant. A sense of difference and exclusivity is cultivated: only those who follow the faith are worthy and chosen – only they can attain salvation, all others are outside the fold: lesser beings deserving of dehumanisation, scapegoating and victimisation. Distinction is stressed by dietary restrictions, uniformity of dress and various formalities of behaviour and worship. Pious self-righteousness, fundamentalism and fanaticism can take hold. The seeds for division, bigotry, hatred and conflict are sown, often harvested in persecution, terrorism and genocide. The twenty-first century bears witness to this.

My Catholic schooling sought to burden me with original sin, my Methodist origins threatened me with hellfire and eternal torment; both gave me but one life to achieve paradise. In addition to these irrationalities, I was persuaded that despite the subversive autonomy of a predatory, satanic force, loose and pervasive in the world, bent on the downfall of humanity, the creation was presided over by an all-powerful, loving God, painted simultaneously as harsh, implacable and jealously possessive of his power and worship. The God of the three Abrahamic religions is overbearingly masculine, a God to fear rather than love. How often do we hear the unctuous intonation of the trinitarian formula: '*In the name of the Father, the Son and the Holy Spirit*' and never '*In the name of the Mother, the Daughter and the Vital Force?*' The insidious effect of this programming, through doctrine and an ever-repeated mantra, emphasised by a poignant, symbolic gesture performed with pontifical solemnity cannot be overestimated.

We all create our own reality in response to imprinting, conditioning, belief, experience and habitual thinking, hence, through ego-perception. Some, assimilate programming with little analysis or modification; others, magnify or mitigate their impressions through ego-based filters. Instilled during the highly impressionable, formative years of childhood, religious doctrines repress the innate curiosity and discriminatory powers of the soul and nurture the distorted values, prejudices, conceits and fears of the ego-self. Unquestioning belief, indoctrinated from the earliest years, at one extreme induces somnolence of the soul and at the other provides a fertile ground for radicalisation and exploitation by fanatical extremists.

Religious doctrine shares much with conventional medicine: the former is guilty of suppressing the soul with bonds of superstition and prejudice; the latter suppresses disease with bonds of technology and chemistry. Both empower the ego-self at the expense of the soul; thus, both contribute to the soul's disease and the suffering of humanity.

Obscured by dogma and superstition, the ineffable beauty of the Perennial Truth lying at the heart of all religions is only glimpsed or is lost in a revolt against implausible doctrines. In a patriarchal, materialistic world, agnosticism and atheism often result: stealthy co-conspirators of the ego-self, quelling conscience, empathy and altruism and providing cold comfort when heartache and tragedy ensue. For those who remain devoted to the faith, reality is distorted and the ground for hypocrisy, self-righteousness, religious prejudice and fundamentalism is laid down.

I emphasise the difficulties that stem from religion and superstition because they are deeply influential in the dysfunctional emotional life of many. Apart from the weight of original sin, still a substantial concept in many communities, patriarchal authority is indoctrinated, insidiously favouring male dominance and encouraging the inequality and abuse that contributes to so much domestic unhappiness and consequent disease. On a broader front, evidence of the militancy that religion can arouse when married to nationalism and political ends has become increasingly evident in today's world: it fosters ethnic cleansing, terrorism and ideological war. This apart, the fallacies of religious doctrine construct a deeply imprinted system of delusional thinking that obscures Reality and is difficult to modify or erase. Life observed through distorted, ego-based filters creates stresses that contribute to disease. This sequence confirms the importance of recognising a patient's singular delusion or misconception – their wrong believing, wrong-perceiving, wrong-imagining, wrong-thinking and wrong assumptions – in case analysis and remedy choice. Religious conviction, distinct from spiritual insight, constitutes one of the major delusions confronted in practice and signals the importance of certain repertory rubrics: *Delusions, imaginations: religious – Religious affections, general – Doubtful: soul's salvation*, etc.

Given that every incarnated soul has the same spiritual goal, reincarnation is the only just explanation for the stark contrasts in opportunity afforded each ego/soul complex by its innate nature, its aptitudes and the circumstances that impinge upon it. It is inconceivable that the prodigious genius evidenced in the arts, literature and music and in the advances of science and technology, could be the product of beings living but a single life. Study of the greatest minds, points to the presence of innate talents present from birth; often blooming in the face of significant obstacles and disadvantages. Observation of our own children, reveals character traits and talents unexplained by inheritance or conditioning: indications of their coming into life with previous life history and previous life-experience; bearing both gifts and baggage from the past. The immortality of the soul predicts and demands not only survival after death, but also life before birth.

The dynamics of the living universe are expressed through vast and eternal cycles. The concept of reincarnation is in harmony with this natural phenomenon; the delusion of a single life conflicts with it. Just as the seasons pass before us in stately procession, so life has its spring, its summer, its autumn and its winter, each season blessing the soul with invaluable experience. At the end of a cycle, the soul withdraws from the physical dimension and for a time resides in its natural state, a spirit dimension with which it is in harmony. After a shorter or longer sojourn in the domain of spirit, the time comes for the soul to reincarnate onto the earth plane, thus, heralding a new spring, and, depending on the soul's destiny, another summer, another autumn and another winter of experience. The soul transitions from a finer dimension into one more dense: a dimension in which polarity and paradox prevail, affording the developing soul, through freedom of choice, the opportunity to gain sovereignty of the psyche and expel the perennial usurper: the delinquent ego-self, whose selfishness, materialism, conceit, self-justification and rationalising over lifetimes have held the soul captive in its own domain. This wondrous hero journey, primed with diverse challenges perfectly fashioned to persuade, urge and direct the soul towards freedom, independence and individuation, also gives the soul occasion to enrich the material plane with its unique talents.

The descent enfolds the immortal soul with its destiny, placing it unerringly in a holding environment ideal for the soul's mission on the earth plane: nothing that transpires in the soul's life-experience is fruitless or fortuitous! All is perfect, wise, beneficent and loving – all is ordained – *all is well*!

David Lilley
Fresnaye, Cape Town
March 2018

Key concepts

Like its companion, this volume of *Healing the Soul* comprises two books in one: the first part deals with *the archetype* and the second part with *the psyche*. For ease of understanding, the following brief definitions will prepare the reader for the larger text. These abstract concepts are open to contrasting opinions and my perspectives may differ from accepted theory, even Jungian, but these definitions provide a reliable foundation for understanding my use of the terms in this text.

The Self is synonymous with the Spirit: the Divinity at the core of every soul: it is the soul's True Nature or Essence. Union with the Self is the goal of the hero's journey.

The Psyche represents the totality of the human mind, incorporating both the conscious and unconscious aspects. It pertains to the totality of all psychic processes and the soul/ego-self/emotion/mind complex that gives rise to these processes. Unlike the soul, the psyche is transpersonal; it has no face, destiny or existence of its own; it is not synonymous with either the Spirit or the soul; it is an all-embracing definition for psychological processes and psychic structures, not an entity. It is an energy field, a dynamic territory that the soul needs to hold dominion over to achieve union with the Self.

The Soul is not equated with the personality, which it far transcends, or the Spirit, which is its goal. The soul is who we really are, the immortal traveller on a mystic journey in search of the 'Holy Grail' of Self-enlightenment: the realisation of our Divinity. Through many life times, the soul is destined to confront and contend with the ego-self; a pseudo-self, which, through the fear and doubts of the soul, has usurped its position and identity, shrouding its pristine purity with layers of compensatory personality, denying it expression. The arduous journey of the soul is an inward one towards its own radiance; a goal achieved by casting off the obscuring structures of the ego-self to reveal the effulgent glory of Spirit.

The Ego-self (ego or ego-personality) is the adversary confronting the soul on its journey of attainment. It is the false-self, masquerading as the soul; it is the usurper that takes control of the psyche and prevents the soul from realising its goal. The ego-self represses anything it finds threatening to its self-preservation into the Shadow, and then projects what it has repressed onto others and hates them for it. The ego-self is the cause of all misery, suffering and disease.

The Anima is the feminine principle within man.

The Animus is the masculine principle within woman.

The Persona is the social face or mask that the ego-self dons when interacting with the outside world; it is designed to impress, please and influence others, ease social exchange, facilitate relationships and to conceal the ego-self wearing it. It hides the Shadow – the mark of Cain!

The Shadow is the dark, denied part of ourselves, containing the rejected, unrealised, unresolved and repressed aspects of the psyche. Shadow aspects are projected onto others enabling us to hold them responsible for our 'badness' and scapegoat them. The Shadow is a cornucopia of riches that must be expressed and integrated as the soul progresses towards individuation; a process that is facilitated by *depth homeopathy* and is in keeping with Hering's Law of Cure: from within outwards.

The Id is the vital force of the Cosmos; it works always towards expression and contains the basic instincts of sex (procreation) and aggression (self-preservation).

The Superego is the internal critic, developed from norms and values derived from the father figure and society; it sets up the image of an 'ideal self' and punishes the ego with guilt feelings if the ego fails to meet its standards; it forces the ego to repress upsetting urges and needs originating from the Id; it contributes to the contents of the Shadow.

Archetype:
The word archetype derives from the Greek '*archétypon*', which is a compound of *arché* signifying: beginning, origin, cause, primal source or principle; and "*typon*", meaning: 'blow', but also the imprint of a blow: 'mould, type, pattern, image, form, model'. *The archetype* can, therefore, be defined as the primal or original pattern or model from which others of the same kind are copied or moulded. In its highest form, the archetype is a quintessential ideal or paragon, but it always

possesses its antithesis: a dark, perverted or shadow form. This ambivalence is characteristic of the relative sphere, which rests upon the co-existence and interaction of opposites. The spiritual culture hero, the Christ figure, will always be opposed by the Antichrist.

The archetypes constitute a dynamic template of fundamental role models and innate tendencies, capable through resonance of influencing, moulding and transforming the personal unconscious of the individual and thus shaping behaviour. This substratum may also be visualised as an underlying web of archetypal potential woven out of history, culture, tradition, myth and fantasy. By unconscious affinity, predisposition, miasmatic influence and destiny, all individuals are irresistibly drawn to one or other of the archetypal forms, which provide the foundation upon which they construct their reality and their experience of life, coloured by their culture, beliefs, circumstances, life events and personality.

The universal nature and scope of the archetype is evidenced in that the same archetypal pattern may be represented by a mythical god – Apollo; by a star – the sun; by a continent – Africa; by a metal – gold; by a feline carnivore – the lion; by an organ – the heart; and by certain humans: a corrupt, wealth-addicted Midas – an ambitious, achievement-driven business tycoon – a suicidal depressive – a magnanimous, noble-minded ruler – and a god-like spiritual master: five distinct archetypes all belonging to a single universal archetype: Aurum (Gold).

Collective unconscious:

Whereas the personal unconscious is the storehouse of experience unique to the individual, Jung proposed the existence of an inherited, universal or collective unconscious, innate and common to all: an eternal, psychic energy field archiving the archetypal images of every aspect of the creation, all forces, all forms and all life, and systematically chronicling the history of the universe, including all human experience, thought, imagination and memory. The structure of the collective unconscious is constituted by the archetypes: a matrix of potential possibilities, which find expression and representation in the human psyche, in the forces and fabric of the material world and are played out on the stage of life.

References

1 Shakespeare W. *Hamlet*. London: Oxford University Press, 1968. Act 1 Scene II, lines 70–71. p60.

2 Lilley D. *Healing the Soul. Volume 1. The lives of Samuel Hahnemann and William Lilley*. Glasgow: Saltire Books. 2014.

3 Campbell J. *The Hero with a Thousand Faces. The Collected Works of Joseph Campbell*. Novato CA: New World Library, 2008. Chapter One.

4 Shakespeare W. *Hamlet*. London: Oxford University Press, 1968. Act V Scene II, lines 211–216. p188.

Part one

THE ARCHETYPE

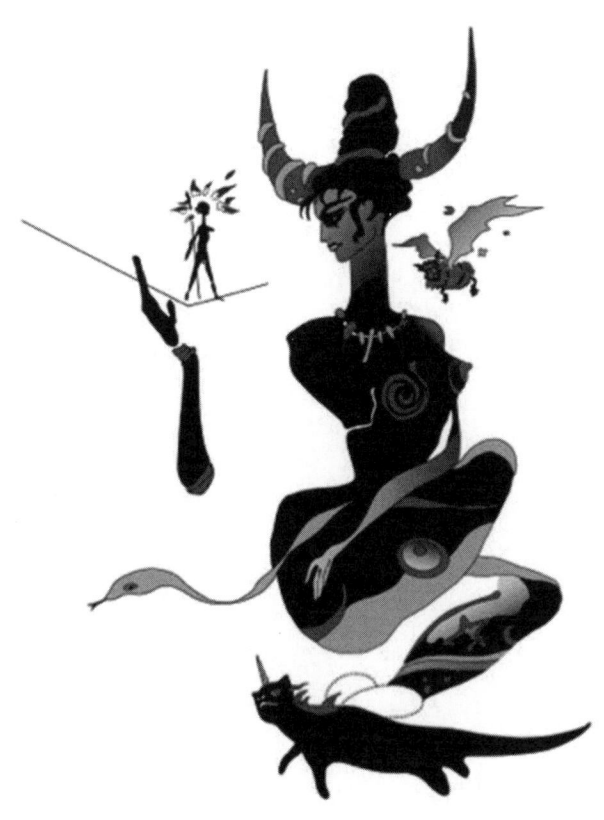

1

THE ARCHETYPE

The Collective Unconscious – Realm of the Archetype

Like an iceberg, the human being presents as a discrete consciousness, but beneath the guise of the ego-self/soul complex, lies a far more comprehensive and complex *personal unconscious*, filled with infinite potential. Unlike the iceberg, however, the personal unconscious, which archives experiences unique to the individual, is confluent with the vastness of the *collective unconscious*, the universal repository of Cosmic memory and wisdom.

Nothing is totally insentient, everything has memory, even the rocks hold impressions of the volcanic upheavals and mighty forces that weathered and fashioned them. Geologists, archaeologists and palaeoanthropologists can wrest and tease fragmented images of past ages from the strata and sediments of the earth and chronicle a collage of the planet's heroic past, but these are kaleidoscopic frames compared with the limitless, panoramic history of universal experience contained within the collective unconscious. If the hand, with fingers extended, is visualised as the *unconscious*, then each finger represents a separate personal unconscious holding the unique personal experience of an individual, while the palm embodies the unbounded, collective unconscious common to all. Just as the collective unconscious flows into the personal unconscious, the personal feeds into the collective, imparting its content to the common pool of experience.

It was Carl Gustav Jung (1875–1961), the Swiss psychologist and psychiatrist and founder of analytical psychology, who first postulated the concept of the collective unconscious. He defined it as follows.

> . . . in addition to our immediate consciousness, which is of a thoroughly personal nature and which we believe to be the only empirical psyche (even if we tack on the personal unconscious as an appendix), there exists a second psychic system of a collective, universal, and impersonal nature which is identical in all individuals. This collective unconscious does not develop individually but is inherited.

It consists of pre-existent forms, the *archetypes*, which can only become conscious secondarily and which give definite form to certain psychic contents.[1]

The collective unconscious contains not only the assembled experiences of human beings but those of all species, living or extinct. We may speak of a collective canine or feline unconsciousness, which when compounded provides a symbolic personification of the qualities and characteristics of the specific animal archetype. This is not limited to those species, which obviously possess a nervous system; the mighty oak possesses an identity, significance and presence equal to that of any animal. Nor is it limited to the organic world; the mysterious essence of all the elements and substances that comprise the inorganic world is held within the universal unconscious in the form of archetypal images. The brilliance of a diamond, or the splendid beauty of an emerald, sapphire or ruby can evoke archetypal responses, interpretations and personifications within us, which are spontaneous and intuitive. Mental forms and associations that may surface in thought or dreams when appropriately stimulated and cannot be explained by any experience in the individual's present life, hearken back to previous-life events or to primordial, innate and inherited images projected from the collective unconscious.

Contemplation of the collective unconscious may elicit the archetypal image of the *wise old man*, the sage, or *the wizard*, who through the experience of age, or many lifetimes, has attained a wisdom, with which he can offer guidance to others, often by means of stories, legends, fables or parables. He is a classic, literary figure and mythological character, exemplified in the person of Odin in Norse mythology, Nestor in the Iliad, Merlin of Arthurian Legend, and, in modern times, Tolkien's Gandalf. Like all archetypes, he has a dark, or fallen form, as depicted by Saruman, the shadow counterpart and opponent of Gandalf. The universal unconscious may also be likened to a *wise old woman*, who has ministered to the suffering and bitter experiences of men and women down the ages; who emanates wisdom and authority, and tutors with sternness tempered by benevolence. In Greek mythology, she is embodied in *Metis* and *Athene*, the Greek Goddesses of Wisdom, but most of all she is personified in *Hekate*, Goddess of the Crossroads and the Underworld. In psychological terms, Hekate is Goddess of the Shadow, she who holds the key to the treasures and terrors of the benighted realm of the unconscious mind: a goddess the homeopath has much reason to invoke. Greatest of all is *Kali*, the black goddess of Hinduism, Divinity of the Dark Unconscious, Goddess of the Void, who in her love for humanity and indifference to the demands of the ego-self seeks its death through the disruptions and jars of life that she may dance her dance of perpetual becoming on the burial ground of material desire.

The patriarchy in closing its ears to her counsel, has typically emphasised the sinister, malevolent and destructive aspect of the wise woman archetype, portraying her as *the witch*, a malicious, seductive sorceress, like Morgan le Fay, intent on the downfall of the hero, King Arthur, or as remorseless Destiny, deaf to the cries of her mortal children.

Sri Ramakrishna, the enlightened Bengali saint, regarded the darkness of the unknown and the impenetrable to be the Ultimate Mother or Kali:

> The night sky between the stars is perfectly black. The waters of the ocean depths are the same; the infinite is always mysteriously black. The inebriating darkness is my beloved Kali . . . she is indivisible Reality, Awareness, and Bliss.[2]

The image of the collective unconscious as a deep source of wisdom and love is supported by our dream-life. Often during times of difficulty, anxiety, stress and perplexity, dreams are experienced that provide instruction and direction. They are usually significant, giving the dreamer the distinct awareness that that they are out of the ordinary and demand attention. Usually they are vivid, intense, and do not dissipate from the memory as quickly as the common or mundane dream. They possess an emotional after-effect, which remains for a considerable time after waking and may colour the emotions of the following day. The content is archetypal, in the form of a fable, parable or personal myth, and requires analysis and interpretation in the light of the history, current emotional state and circumstances of the dreamer. During sleep, the personal unconscious gains greater access to the collective unconscious, and in response to powerful images generated in the conscious and unconscious mind, archetypal wisdom is unlocked from this universal source through resonance. Intense or habitual repression of emotions induces a numbing, psychic inertia which blocks this natural flow and may induce a chronic, dreamless state, that must always be regarded with concern.

The homeopathic potency, which carries a specific, archetypal energy pattern derived from the substance from which it is prepared, is capable of acting upon both the personal and the collective unconscious. When administered to a sensitive prover in a pathogenetic trial or proving, the potency elicits an archetypal response within the deepest levels of the unconscious and projects this image onto the surface permitting the prover to experience the singular qualities and characteristics of the substance, be it a mineral, plant or animal. The most important symptoms are those that influence the temperament, the emotions and the feelings of the prover, particularly their perception of life, their self-image and their relationship to others; their anxieties and fears and their dreams. These are also the central characteristics that must be evaluated and matched remedially in every patient receiving homeopathic treatment, no matter the condition they are suffering from. Only in the most acute conditions may this precept be modified or bypassed, and, even then, an outstanding emotional symptom, particularly if arising during the acute episode, may be the deciding factor in remedy choice. In chronic cases receiving constitutional treatment directed to resolving health problems that originate at soul level, dreams are of great value in not only selecting the most similar remedy, but also for evaluating progress, particularly where a frequently experienced dream theme, although still occurring, becomes less intense, less frightening, less disturbing and less negative.

The well-selected remedy, possesses an energy pattern most similar to the archetypal presentation of the case and therefore has the capacity to pass beyond the interface between the conscious and the unconscious minds, past the restraints of the super-ego (the internal critic) and the obstructive ego-self, and into the farthest reaches of the personal unconscious where it merges with the collective unconscious, the immeasurable ocean of Cosmic and Spiritual Wisdom (the wise old man or woman within us all), whose tides constantly and insistently urge the psyche towards expression, resolution and sublimation. Here, the remedy, suited to the archetypal energy of the patient and working in harmony with the healing force of the collective unconscious, weakens the barriers of repression between the two and permits repressed and distorted energy to flow from within outwards. Healing extends from the soul to the mind and the emotions and from thence to the body. In the process, dreams will be experienced, which are often revelatory and directive.

The concept of the collective unconscious shows that nothing in the psyche is ever lost or erased, and that which would appear to be lost has been repressed and hidden and must find expression if it is to be resolved or to function at its highest level. There is widespread mistrust and fear of the deeper, instinctive layers of the psyche. They are regarded as dark, unpredictable, non-rational, chaotic and uncontrollable – qualities that have been designated as feminine and inferior. The same logic assumes that the only ordering principle in the psyche comes from the masculine exercise of the reason. It is not generally understood that there is in the personal as well as the collective unconscious an innate and inherent intelligence that is more comprehensive than the intellect. Through the application of what I would term *depth homeopathy* it is possible to access this source of wisdom whilst releasing repressed emotions and the rejected aspects of the psyche.

The collective unconscious is the domain of the archetype. The homeopath needs to be familiar with this realm and with the concept of the archetype. The homeopathic materia medica is an unmatched archive of archetypal knowledge. *Homeopathy is archetypal medicine!*

The lore of the archetype

It was in 1919 that Carl Gustav Jung first used the term 'archetypes' to describe what he had previously referred to as 'primordial images' and which he directly linked to Freud's 'archaic remnants': mental forms whose presence cannot be explained by anything in the individual's own life and which seem to be aboriginal, innate and inherited shapes of the human mind.[3]

The word archetype derives from the Greek *archétypon*, which is a compound of *arché* signifying: beginning, origin, cause, primal source or principle; and *typon*, meaning: 'blow', but also the imprint of a blow: 'mould, type, pattern, image, form, model'. *The archetype* can, therefore, be defined as the primal or original pattern or model from which others of the same kind are copied or moulded. In its highest form, the archetype is a quintessential ideal or paragon, but it always possesses its antithesis: a dark, perverted or shadow form. This ambivalence is characteristic of the relative sphere, which rests upon the co-existence and interaction of opposites. The spiritual culture hero, the Christ figure, will always be opposed by the Antichrist.

Collectively, the archetypes constitute a timeless, universal, dynamic field of fundamental role models or innate tendencies, capable through resonance of influencing, moulding and transforming the personal unconscious of the individual and thus shaping behaviour. This substratum may also be visualised as a cosmic web of archetypal potential woven out of history, culture, tradition, myth and fantasy. By unconscious affinity, predisposition, miasmatic influence and destiny, all individuals are irresistibly drawn to one or other of the archetypal forms, which provide the foundation upon which they construct their reality and their experience of life, coloured by their culture, beliefs, circumstances, life events and personality.

The universal nature and scope of the archetype is evidenced in that the same archetypal pattern may be represented by a mythical god – Apollo; by a star – the sun; by a continent – Africa; by a metal – gold; by a feline carnivore – the lion; by an organ – the heart; and by certain humans: a corrupt, wealth-addicted Midas – an ambitious, achievement-driven business tycoon – a suicidal depressive – a magnanimous, noble-minded ruler – and a god-like spiritual master: five distinct archetypes all belonging to a single universal, masculine archetype: Aurum (Gold).

In like manner, a specific archetypal pattern may be epitomised by a mythical goddess – Artemis; by a celestial body – the moon; by a morphogenetic field – the East; by a metal – silver; by a feline carnivore – the cat; by an organ – the ovary and uterus; and by certain girls or women: excelling in sport and physical pursuits – lovers of nature and the wild – feminists, fighting for the welfare of animals, children, women and the planet – compulsive talkers, eloquent and gifted in debate – anxious, restless hypochondriacs: five distinct archetypal aspects all belonging to a single, universal, feminine archetype: Argentum (Silver).

The collective unconscious is the domain of the archetype. Whereas, the personal unconscious is the repository of experience unique to the individual, the collective unconscious is inherited, innate and common to all: an eternal, psychic energy field archiving the archetypal images of every aspect of the creation, all forces, all forms and all life, and systematically chronicling the history of the universe, including all human experience, thought, imagination and memory. The structure of the collective unconscious is constituted by the archetypes: a matrix of potential possibilities that find expression and representation in the human psyche, in the forces and fabric of the material world and are played out on the stage of life.

Plato: archetypal forms and ideas

By the 5th century B.C.E., Greek philosophers had developed the logic of the archetypal principle as a means of interpreting and clarifying the apparent chaos of life in this world. This logic was associated with the figure of Socrates and was expressed in its definitive form through the dialogues of Plato. Beneath the fickle and ever-changing façade of concrete reality, which is open to interpretation, opinion and conjecture, the universe was apprehended as being ordered by a multiplicity of timeless, primordial essences or transcendent, fundamental principles that give form, meaning and significance to the shifting confusion, imperfection and inequality of the material plane. Plato conceived these universal, changeless absolutes or paragons as archetypal *Forms* or *Ideas*.

Plato regarded these Forms or archetypal principles as primary, and the objects of conventional reality to be their direct derivatives, and therefore secondary. In this sense, *the Forms possess a superior degree of reality to that of the material world.*

Platonic archetypes form the world and also stand beyond it; they manifest themselves within time and yet are timeless. They constitute the veiled essence of things.[4]

Though transcendental, they are immanent.

Plato insisted that for the attainment of true knowledge, the philosopher's attention must be directed beyond appearances to the essence, beyond particulars to the universal, and beyond the finite and relative to the infinite and absolute. These absolutes exist in immutable, true and perfect form unsullied by the empirical world. They are in a permanent state of *Being*, whereas, all manifest phenomena exist in a constant state of *becoming*: transforming from one state to another as they germinate, attain their zenith and decay. Behind this world of change and *becoming* lies a higher Reality, the world of Forms and Ideas, which while giving rise to transformation is changeless and in a constant state of *Being* that is dynamic, yet static. Every aspect of existence is permeated and patterned by these specific, definite, enduring, immutable fundamentals, structures or essences, which remain distinguishable and stable regardless of the ceaseless flux of our inner and outer worlds.

Because of their eternal, immutable nature, the Forms and Ideas can be regarded as immortal and likened to divinities. In the pre-philosophical Greek mind, the archetypal principles took the form of mythical personages, whose persuasive and not always subtle presence was recognised in human nature and in the phenomena of the physical world. While physical beauty will wane and wither, the archetypal Beauty that gives beauty existence remains untouched by this transience. The Beauty of Aphrodite is transcendental and eternal; it belongs to a superior Reality. That which is deemed beautiful can be said to 'participate' in the absolute Form or Idea of Beauty, personified by the Goddess of Beauty.

In their ultimate, immutable form, the archetypal Ideas are immaculate, perfect and numinous; they express absolute moral and aesthetic values. The Ideas of the Good, the Beautiful and the Just, like the qualities of Truth, Perfection and Love, exist as independent, yet interdependent and overlapping, unchanging aspects of Reality; they are unconditional, pure, eternal and Divine. Only the virtues are absolute; their opposites, the vices or 'sins', are relative. Absolute, unadulterated, 'pure' evil does not exist; it is only the shadow aspect or degradation of Good; it is always comparative. Behind that which manifests as good lies the virtue of the Idea informing it: Goodness itself, the absolute Form from which all good derives. Behind that which is beautiful exists absolute Beauty: Beauty itself, supreme, pure, eternal and Real, not relative to a specific person or thing. Behind evil there is no absolute evil, no Devil, no satanic force, only a comparative lack of virtue and goodness in an individual or group of individuals, acting out the archetypal shadow of Good, in the service of synchronicity, which always seeks the awakening of the sleeping soul.

Similarly, giving common form and character to all cats that pass through the material world is an archetypal or Divine Cat: the eternal, collective, feline paragon, which embodies and patterns classic cat characteristics. This archetypal patterning does not produce a stereotype, for, when reduced to the relative world, the collective becomes individualised and each cat manifests distinct peculiarities that denote its uniqueness. Likewise, when humans emotionally and physically 'participate' in the Form or Idea of the Divine Cat, through resonance with its archetypal frequency, they do so in their own peculiar way; the human-cat characteristics being uniquely coloured by the ego-personality of the individual. To be able to discern the presence of the Cat in the mannerisms and behaviour of a human, the archetype's timeless profile must be intuitively perceived, anthropomorphically accessed and held in consciousness. This faculty requires archetypal awareness: an artistic ability critical to the homeopath, whose alert and sensitive apprehension needs to extend well beyond the range of the average, conventional physician. To understand a patient's reality and the singular affinity that draws certain characters and events into their orbit, the homeopath must define the presiding archetype that motivates and modifies the patient's behaviour. To detect the Gold, the Oak, the Scorpion, the Serpent or the Wolf in man or woman and to interpret the cryptic symbolism of myths and dreams is a fine and subtle art that needs cultivating.

References

1 Jung CG. *The Archetypes and the Collective Unconscious*. London: Routledge, 1996. p43.
2 Hati K and Pramanik PK. *Sri Ramakrishna – The Spiritual Glow*. Bhatwan India: Orient Book Co, 1984. pp17–18.
3 Jung CG. *Man and his Symbols*. Reading: Cox and Wyman Ltd, 1964. p57.
4 Tarnas R. *The Passion of the Western Mind*. London: Random House, 2000. p6.

ARCHETYPAL SYSTEMS

Two distinct, but interrelated and overlapping, archetypal systems are of central importance to homeopathic practice: the *atavistic* and the *mythological*.

The essence of each atavistic or mythological archetype resides in the collective unconscious: a field of interactive images, forms and patterns of behaviour innate within all life and symbolically evidenced in all aspects of the material universe. When activated, these archetypal energies arise from the collective mosaic and exert a powerful functional and formative influence upon the constitution, personality and unconscious mind of the individual whose peculiar sensitivity and destiny resonate with the attributes of the archetype. The dynamic of the archetype pervades the psyche and is pivotal to the psychosomatic profile of the patient and their personal reality.

The atavistic or ancestral archetype

Atavism may be defined as a resemblance to remote ancestors – a tendency to reproduce or revert to an ancestral type in plants and animals – a strange and mysterious recurrence to a primitive past and a more primitive form.

This strange mystery is re-enacted at the conception of every human being. In accord with the diverse influences that synergistically contribute to the development of a unique individual (e.g. karmic, inherited, constitutional, miasmatic), the formative energy of an ancestral archetype, derived from the archives of the collective unconscious, pervades the economy of the newly-conceived and models its emotional, intellectual and physical development along lines determined by the archetype's ineffable presence.

Though subordinate to destiny and karmic influence, chronic miasmatic inheritance is the most decisive factor in evoking the specific, controlling archetypal force. Miasmatic disease is ubiquitous in humanity and constitutes a dysfunctional change in the frequency of the vital force: the animating, harmonising energy that maintains the homeostasis of the mind/body complex. This dissonance, reaching into the archives of the collective unconscious, causes an ancestral form or *atavistic archetype*, possessing the same vibratory pattern as the patient's disease-state, to rise out of the mosaic of archetypes laid down in the deep unconscious since time beyond memory. Being archetypal, the energised ancestral form – mineral, plant or animal – will present anthropomorphically – in human guise – and impose its image upon the psychosomatic state of the patient with a degree of intensity dependent on the amplitude of the dissonance.

In the book, *Homeopathic Practice* (2008), edited by Steven Kayne, I wrote as follows about the atavistic archetype:

> All elements, their salts and their compounds, are our inorganic forebears, archived in the collective unconscious and energetically latent within us. From the pre-biotic, inorganic world, arose the biological world and the first organisms, which, once established, rapidly diversified into a myriad of evolving life forms, our organic forbears: a continuum of life, culminating in the emergence of: *the beauty of the world; the paragon of animals*: Homo sapiens.
>
> Standing at the peak of sentient life, we possess within the matrix of our being, a mosaic of atavistic or ancestral archetypes: a field of dynamic images, which in health are maintained in homeostatic balance by the integrating action of the animating vital force. This balance is represented by an ordered and harmonious frequency. In illness, a dissonance develops, disrupting the harmony of homeostasis. In response, the vital force in league with the collective unconscious and the power of the Id, causes an atavistic archetype, which resonates most closely with this disordered frequency, to rise into relief out of the mosaic of ancestral forms.
>
> In the illness of Aurum, the metallic element gold responding to the summons of its specific frequency, emerges as a powerful metaphor, or symbol, capable of profoundly influencing the entire constitution, moulding or warping the form, features, functions, faculties and feelings of the patient. The patient sees life through the eyes or filters of gold, moves with the body of gold, thinks with the mind of gold and reacts to life with the passions, fears, and prejudices of gold. To all intents and purposes, the patient becomes one with the archetype of gold, their illness is gold, and their remedy is gold.[1]

And, so it is with hydrogen, the first atavistic archetype.

Hydrogen: the first atavistic archetype

In esoteric and archetypal terms, nothing in the Creation is inanimate – all is inseparable from, and pervaded by, the Universal Intelligence – the entire Cosmos is alive and sentient! Hence, humanity's ancestral, archetypal lineage extends back 15 billion years to the creation of the first atom, hydrogen, amid the expanding field of energy of the new universe. With hydrogen's birth, the primal atavistic archetype of the homeopathic materia medica materialised – the first, lightest and most abundant of the elements that construct the physical universe.

Hydrogen is an insubstantial, weightless gas, which, filling a balloon, floats up into the clouds and out of sight. This provides us with a clear human image of someone flighty, ungrounded – 'spaced-out' – not in touch with reality; a vacuous being, lacking common sense, full of fancy, irresponsible, impractical and accident prone. Being the youngest archetype, it will tend to be immature, hesitant and apprehensive, distractible, floating of into dreamland, unable to concentrate and plagued with learning problems; and, being a highly inflammable gas, the hydrogen child or adult will be hypersensitive and prone to explosive fits of anger if irritated.

Being derived from the first element to materialise from the vastness of space, the archetypal characteristics of Hydrogen noted by trialists are understandable. The incarnation of Hydrogen is a descent of highly individualised energy from a boundless force-field into the discreteness of a material form – a birth that parallels our own descent from the limitless freedom of the spirit realm into the dense confines of the material plane; it must be attended by fear, confusion, and disorientation, followed by wonder, curiosity and endeavour and finally revelation. A sequence of responses common to all who incarnate and common to the provers of hydrogen.

Their fears are highly focussed, specific and significant: *poverty, insanity and dogs.* Concern about money and *fear of poverty* reflect fear of scarcity, deficiency and destitution: all characteristic fears of *Psora*, the fundamental chronic miasm upon which all other miasms are based; fears that relate to physical security and survival. *Fear of insanity* is the same fear translated into the intellectual sphere: fear for the security and survival of the rational mind. Deeper still, *fear of dogs* is the same fear raised to the level of the psyche: fear for the survival or salvation of the immortal soul: a fear expressed in the rubrics: *doubtful of soul's welfare* – and – *religious affections: despairs of salvation.*

The presence of *fear of dogs* in the very first archetype to materialise out of the expanding field of energy after the 'big bang' creation of the universe has to be significant. Just as it has to be when found present to the highest degree in the very first archetype to enter the homeopathic materia medica, China officinalis: the first remedy to be proved by Hahnemann in the pioneer experiment that confirmed conclusively that *like cures like.*

But, how does *fear of dogs* relate to salvation of the soul?

Esoterically, archetypally and pathologically, the Dog, like the Wolf before it, is caught-up in the symbolism of rabies, the dread viral disease that simulates in its destructiveness the deception, rage, hatred and savage violence of the *beast principle* that lurks in the darkest and deepest region of the psychic abyss: the Shadow. It is this *Lucifer principle*, resident in all of us, that stalks 21st century society and perpetrates acts of indiscriminate savagery without concern for the grief and suffering that result. Hydrogen, first of elements and first of our ancestral archetypes, an atom with but a single proton and a single electron, already fears the presence of the Beast!

Even as I write these words on October 2, 2017, I hear the television in our lounge recounting a tragic event that has just taken place in Las Vegas: the merciless machine-gunning of a large audience at a music festival in Las Vegas by a 64-year-old man that has cost at least 59 lives, left over 500 injured and so many others permanently traumatised.

Since, Hydrogen is the fundamental building-block upon which all atavistic archetypes are elaborated, the primal fears held in its blueprint are fundamental and prophetic: they evidence that the potential for *Psora* and the *beast principle* was laid down from the very moment the material Universe came into being.

Separation

In addition to fear of dogs, poverty and insanity, the Hydrogen archetype experiences the *anguish of separation*, isolation and solitude – emotions congruous with being the first atom in the Universe and finding oneself seemingly disconnected and alone in an alien world. Hydrogen's perception of severance, which is common to all incarnated souls deceived by the limited, materialistic vision of the ego-self, is responsible for much of the fear and anguish that contributes to miasmatic disease; and, it is twofold: a separation from one's origin or source – the Universal Intelligence or God – which constitutes vertical severance; and separation from all else that is – humanity, Nature and the Cosmos – which constitutes horizontal sever-ance. Combined: the world becomes a lonely, scary place!

They have a sense of unreality; of being detached or removed from reality; of separation from the world and of being alone. They feel a division between themselves and others and feel estranged from family and friends. Despite their sense of being one apart, they have no urge to bridge the gap and get close: indeed, quite the reverse: *aversion to being touched* and *aversion to company*. They avoid the sight of people and feel relief at being alone. They are not fully integrated into life, their environment, their family or society. A feeling of *indifference* encroaches: everything seems dead, nothing makes a vivid impression on the mind. Distant and *detached* (Granitum); indifferent to loved ones; *emotionally numb*. Indifference to relations; feels rejected by relatives. A spaced-out, ungrounded feeling. Everything seems strange, unreal and ludicrous and they find themselves laughing at serious things. Related possibly to the 'ludicrous' nature of their own earthbound state, or the relief and release from gravity that balloons symbolise, they are moved to laughter on seeing or thinking of balloons.

Some, try to ground themselves and to immerse themselves more completely in life by being intensely *busy* or by *hurrying, driving fast* and being *adventurous*. Others, needing to escape society, *desire to get away into the countryside* (Sulphur, Lac lupinum, Mag-carb). Some, disengage from life's gravity by adopting an irreverent, flippant stance, minimising its impact by disparaging it as ludicrous and unreal.

Imaginings

Commensurate with their descent into a dimension of greater density and lower frequency, they become subject to odd impressions and sensations. For some, it is like passing through a 'near-death experience'. Others, have an impression of being drawn downwards; or of time becoming exaggerated and urgent – a paradoxical, frenetic speeding-up, quite 'out-of-synch' with the slower vibration of the earth plane. Some, feel diminished, smaller than normal; fancy their body is too small for their soul or is separated from their soul. Imagine themselves dirty, despised and persecuted; subject to all kinds of pranks or torments. They are mistrustful of people and have paranoid feelings. The sense of being 'badly done by' or victimised is clearly portrayed by the delusion: they have *insects on the back of their head*. Their underlying paranoia produces the dream: *wrongful accusations of crimes.*

Full moon

They are *sensitive to the full moon*, which impacts detrimentally upon their emotional life and nervous system. Like many lunar-sensitive archetypes, their sensitivity is attended by nostalgic, tubercular longing for an ideal love. Being idealistic, romantic, sentimental and foolishly fanciful, they are easily infatuated (moon-struck), easily seduced and often end-up discarded. Unable to disengage their emotions, they suffer the painful *effects of unrequited, disappointed or rejected love*. They may feel despised by the lover who has jilted them and resentful against life (providence, God) for their shattered dreams and ideals.

Id-related dysfunction

Given the drastic alteration in consciousness of this reluctant, hovering, imperfectly-incarnated archetype, confusion and disorientation are inevitable, and both were amply evidenced by Hydrogen trialists. Connection with the power of the Id is imperfectly established, the steady influx of universal energy is disturbed and the basic instincts of survival and procreation – the aggression and libido aspects of the Id – are perturbed. Certain Hydrogen symptoms clearly demonstrate this.

- *Universal energy – vital force:*
  Exhaustion; depletion. Excessive weakness, fainting-weakness, with nausea. Tremulous weakness. Terribly tired. Desire and inclination to lie down. Chronic fatigue syndrome, better lying down (Psorinum); must lie down. Lassitude after eating. Extremities feel heavy (Gelsemium).
- *Aggression:*
  Causeless anger. Indisposed to talk when angry. Throws things away when angry. Anger felt in the stomach (third chakra: centre of ego-power). Ailments from anger and from quarrels. Censorious, disposed to find fault or is silent. Irritability after the menses. Irritability from the smell of vinegar (which like smelling-salts penetrates their indifference and numbness). Irritability is at its worst when they are tired and 'stretched-out'.
- *Survival:*
  Difficulty coping with stress. Tendency to panic, nervous apprehension. Anxiety when lying on back and 'looking' at the ceiling (contemplating life). Irresolution about what to do with life. Desire to remain in bed in the morning. Unjustifiably blames self for problems. Reproach themselves in the morning. Aversion to being touched. Bites fingers. Picking at fingertips. Sighing.
- *Libido:*
  Confusion about identity; especially confusion about their sexual identity.

Disorientation

Disorientation impinges not only on their general and sexual identity, it affects their appreciation of time and their sense of location: *forgetful of well-known streets*. Their time-sense is warped: they have stepped out of timeless eternity into a material plane chased by time that seems to be flying by: a dimension in which a life-time seems a mere blink. They have difficulty grasping the chronological sequence of past events and their locality: confused about what happened when and where. The limitations of time and space are foreign to them: crude notions difficult to apprehend and assimilate, having no significance in the causative realm from which they have come. The pressures and constraints of time are an unbearable imposition that stretch them out and cause stress and tension – *they feel stuck in time*.

Cognitive functions impaired

- *Concentration difficult: vacant feeling on attempting to concentrate; during examinations; while calculating, driving, reading, working or writing.*
- *Averse to studying.*
- *Mistakes in speaking, spelling, writing.*
- *Mistakes in space and time.*
- *Mistakes the left and right sides.*
- *Absentminded morning – evening.*
- *Disjointed and jumbled thoughts.*
- *Trouble explaining the mental state.*
- *Tendency to lose things.*
- *Clumsy, inadvertent and accident prone.*

Depression

They feel overwhelmed by the stressful dynamics of the material world and the common sequence of fear-unresolved leading to anger – and – anger-unresolved leading to depression, may materialise. Negative thoughts and depression 'dog' them.

- *Depression, especially at the full moon.*
- *Despair, hopelessness.*
- *Silent, morose, introverted.*
- *Taciturn during headache.*
- *Self-pity.*
- *Apathetic, bored, ennui.*
- *Joyless, regardless of circumstances.*

- *Indifference, disinterest and emotional numbness.*
- *Indifference to loved ones.*
- *Resignation.*
- *Thoughts of dead bodies.*
- *Thoughts of death.*
- *Desires death – morning, on waking.*
- *Suicidal tendency.*
- *Dreams: wrongfully accused of crimes; of escape; animal suffering; dead people; death; murder, suicide – all indicative of fear of humanity, society and life.*
  - ○ Erotic dreams also occur – *dreams amorous.*

Esoteric speculation

However, there are those, who, like Belladonna, are fascinated by esoteric subjects and those whose minds, like Sulphur, are constantly theorising and speculating, dwelling on abstruse philosophies and seeking answers to questions about the mysterious and the arcane.

- *Interested in esoteric subjects.*
- *Search for unification.*
- *New age religions.*
- *Existential questions about existence and about God.*

Caught between dimensions, they ponder the significance of life, suffering, death and destiny. The state of dichotomy may be resolved, may bring conflict or may misguide them. Hence, the consequence of their speculations can prove uplifting, sobering, inflating, conflicting, dysfunctional or delusional.

- *Things look beautiful.*
- *Positiveness – especially on waking in the morning; constant, beatific smile.*
- *Sensation of heavenly peace.*
- *Overflowing love for humanity.*
- *Desire to sing in the morning: cheerfully, joyfully.*
- *Lightness and freedom: no boundaries or painful experience of earthly restrictions.*
- *Simplicity and sobriety: desire to go on a long retreat; sail by themselves; desire to lead a simple Amish-like lifestyle: averse to technology and computers.*

- *Egotism – pious self-righteousness.*

- *Conflict between higher consciousness and worldly existence.*

- *Problems of having to live in this world because of a sensation of universal consciousness and enlightenment.*
- *Brilliant, inquiring, innovative mind unable to function efficiently in the practical, material world (absentminded professor [Sulphur]).*

- *Delusion is in heaven; in the presence of God; or in Hell (Stramonium, Hyoscyamus).*
- *Delusion they are possessed (Stramonium, Hyoscyamus).*

These disquieting religious delusions indicate that Hydrogen's, Belladonna-like, compulsion for esoteric and metaphysical speculation may unhinge them. With further deterioration, the psychopathology of Hydrogen may approximate the deeper *Solanaceae* state of Stramonium or of Hyoscyamus.

Just as Aconite is the acute counterpart of Sulphur, so Belladonna is the acute counterpart of Calc-carb and true to this affinity, Calc-carb, like Belladonna and Hydrogen, may have an obsessive interest in religion. In all three, the religious or esoteric pre-occupation may develop precociously, in the very young, and assume unhealthy proportions. Calc-carb *wants to read the bible all day* (Aurum, Stramonium, Veratrum – add Hydrogen). Interestingly, Sulphur, the false-philosopher among this associated group of philosophising archetypes, *takes passages of scripture literally and acts accordingly* (Anacardium, Lachesis – add Hydrogen). Hydrogen shares with Sulphur a sense of superiority and eliteness stemming from their 'enlightenment' and 'higher consciousness', which places them above the worldly and the uninformed. Hydrogen can also 'lord it' over others and boast about their accomplishments – usually their psychic, esoteric or religious advancement. In contrast, China, also a primal, dog-fearing archetype and one of the most psychic, remains modest, humble and reserved about their often-considerable esoteric knowledge and personal experience of higher dimensions.

Averse to the material plane of existence

Intrinsic to both the distorted perceptions (delusions) and philosophy of Hydrogen, and its suffering, is the theme of *separation*. Despite their spiritual aspiration and 'higher consciousness' of rarefied spirit-dimensions and life-eternal, their elevated vision, or 'enlightenment', fails to give them basic trust or unwavering conviction of the Oneness of the Creation. 'God' and 'Heaven' remain abstract and elsewhere, not to be found on the material plane that is dirty, sordid and debasing. Consciously, life is distasteful and incompatible with their heightened sensibilities. People, including those closest to them, seem callow, crude and alien. Their sympathies lie with suffering animals, which, being like themselves, innocent and pure, unlike the rest of humanity, they can identify with – both they and animals being fated to live lives of torment inflicted by humans. Unconsciously, they cannot accept incarnation. They cannot surrender to life or participate in what it unfolds with active, enthusiastic positivity (*dreams of high places* – above life).

Chakra response

Fourth chakra – Anahata – the heart chakra

They are separated from their Source, separated from their fellow humans and separated from the world, hence, they are separated from Love. This separation, in an 'air' remedy, is a grave loss for their very essence is love. Air is the basic element of the fourth primary chakra, Anahata, which is seated at the centre of the chakra energy system; its colour is green, the central colour of the visible spectrum: the green of Mother Nature: the embodiment of love! Separation or disconnection from Universal Love impairs the function of the fourth chakra, which like a heart valve becomes stuck – either incompetent or stenotic – too open or too closed – or unable to open and close appropriately in response to external or internal stimuli. This is the plight of Hydrogen. If Anahata is too open, the Hydrogen archetype becomes a love-addict: at the mercy of infatuation, idealisation and dependency – love-sick – prone to *ailments from disappointed, unrequited love*. If Anahata is too closed, Hydrogen becomes cold, aloof, withdrawn: *indifferent to loved ones and friends* and *numb to the beauty of life*.

The fourth chakra is the most feminine chakra (*yin*). Defensive closing-off of Anahata to ward-off threat from the patriarchal world (*yang*), rifts the masculine and feminine principles: a divergence contrary to individuation, which demands union. The closing-off disturbs the function of the second chakra, Svadhisthana, which is the seat of *Yin-Yang* balance. In Hydrogen, this causes *confusion of gender identity*. Impacting on adrenal function it may promote *masculinisation*: a psycho-physical phenomenon, which begins with Hydrogen, develops further in Causticum, Ignatia and Nat-mur and attains its most outspoken form in Sepia and Lac lupinum. Hydrogen, like Sepia, has: *growth of hair on the upper lip in women*.

The full moon stands at the centre of the moon's phases, midway between the waxing and waning of lunar energy. It equates with Anahata, the chakra standing at the centre of the chakra energy system and the colour green, the colour standing at the centre of the visible spectrum. In disturbing the function of the fourth chakra, Hydrogen's ego-based perception of life not only distances the archetype from the concept of unconditional love, but also disturbs its relationship with the full moon.

Hydrogen's emotional sensitivity and exhaustion are markedly worse at the full moon.

Green is the combination of two primary colours: blue and yellow. Blue is the colour of the fifth chakra, Vishuddha, whose basic element is 'ether': an element more imponderable (ethereal) than 'air' and clearly analogous to the lightest of all atomic elements, Hydrogen. Yellow is the colour of the third chakra, Manipura, whose basic element is 'fire': an element also analogous to Hydrogen, which is violently inflammable in air and burns with a blue flame. Like Magnesium and the major tubercular remedies China, Coffea-crud, Phosphorus, Phos-ac, Stannum and Silicea, Hydrogen stands astride the fifth, fourth and third chakras: the chakras of ether, air and fire: the chakras of *Carcinosis, Tuberculosis* and *Syphilis*.

Fifth chakra – Vishuddha – the throat chakra
Ether carries sound waves, hence, when considering the fundamental element of the fifth, or throat, chakra, Vishuddha, 'sound' can be coupled to 'ether'. Sound and symbol are intrinsic to communication on the material plane. The throat chakra governs communication and creativity, hence, communication through creativity and communication through the arts – abilities that are embodied in the colour blue. Consonant with the function of the fifth chakra, Hydrogen is *hypersensitive to sounds and noises*.

The fifth chakra is the level of consciousness aligned with the cancer miasm, *Carcinosis*: the chronic miasm characterised by inability to communicate and express emotions and feelings, which are controlled, repressed and kept under lock and key.

Communication is the art of transmitting and receiving information through symbolic patterns – sounds, words and images. These patterns, made-up of information and ideas, surround us like an invisible force field from which we draw – receive – and to which we contribute – transmit. Communication is an act of connection, an act of union and expansion – expansion through union and union through expansion. Hence, the fifth chakra, constitutes a critical point of contention for the Hydrogen archetype, which by its very nature needs to expand, but due to its horror of incarnation, its paranoia and its aversion to life, people and the world, eschews union and seeks escape (*aversion to company; aversion to touch; desire to go into the country; dreams of escape*). Inability to surrender to the symbiosis of expansion and union generates a conflict between the two that impedes fifth chakra function: communication is disrupted, symbolic patterns are jumbled, artistic expression falters and the Hydrogen trialists report: *mistakes in speaking, spelling, writing; disjointed and jumbled thoughts; mistakes left and right sides; trouble explaining mental state.*

Third chakra – Manipura – the solar plexus chakra

This is the fire chakra that governs the metabolism and the radiation of energy to every part of the body. It is the seat of the will and the intellect and represents consciousness at the level of rational, logical thought, which is embodied in the colour yellow. The ego-power is centred in Manipura, radiating vitality, drive, motivation, ambition, confidence, courage and willpower to the psyche. If in excess: the individual becomes arrogant, over-bearing and boastful and if deficient: timid, hesitant, and procrastinating. The fire chakra is also the energy level of the syphilitic miasm whose prime psychological features are pride and paranoia.

Just as the acorn contains all the potential and information necessary to give existence to the mighty oak, so Hydrogen, the first and lightest atom, with its single proton and its single electron, contains the blueprint of all the miasms and holds the fundamental characteristics of each: the survival issues of *Psora*; the gender issues of *Sycosis*; the pride and paranoia of *Syphilis*; the romantic idealism and longing for love of *Tuberculosis*; and the repressed emotions and inability to communicate of *Carcinosis*.

The hubris of the Hydrogen archetype is elitist, centred round philo-sophical and religious superiority: a self-righteous sense of being elevated above others (*delusion: body enlarged*); they can be as boastful and egotistical as Sulphur. Their paranoia is pervasive, they are highly suspicious: others are not to be trusted, they are bent on tormenting, accusing, belittling and ridiculing them (*delusions: they are persecuted – the subject of all kinds of pranks – they are despised; dreams: wrongful accusations of crime; ailments: from embarrassment, from anger and from quarrels*).

More common, however, is weakened ego-fire, consequent to feeling diminished by their descent onto a lower plane (*delusion: all is diminished; they are dirty; they are despised*). This was born out by several trialists, who reported emotional improvement while testing hydrogen; a sure sign of a curative response based on resonance between substance and subject and indicative of mental and emotional characteristics that Hydrogen can disrupt or cure.

- *Relaxed attitude to work.*
- *More efficient than usual.*
- *Puts time to better use.*
- *Less driven to plan, make lists, constantly organise.*
- *Confidence improved.*
- *Less procrastination.*
- *Less nervous with strangers.*
- *Less tendency to bite and tear thumbs.*

- *Concentration and memory improved.*
- *More cheerful and positive in the evening.*
- *Alert and mentally active in the evening and night.*
- *Less irritable when tired or under daily duress.*

All these observations can be reversed and expressed negatively and recognised as indications for Hydrogen and characteristics of the ailing Hydrogen archetype.

Imbalance of the fire chakra manifests physically as either excess of fire: intolerance to heat and sensations of heat or burning; or deficiency of fire: intolerance to cold and sensations of cold or chill. Hydrogen evidences both extremes in its mix of physical sensations.

Excess of fire
- *Face: heat with weakness.*
- *Sensation of heat on waking.*
- *Headache with sensation of heat.*
- *Burning pain as from pepper in the nose.*
- *Sensation of hot vapour rising in throat.*
- *Pains: burning; cutting; stinging; stitching.*
- *Face discolouration red: worse for anger and emotional excitement.*
- *Aversion to hot or warm drinks; warm food; spices and highly seasoned food; coffee; tea; tobacco.*
- *Desire for cold drinks; carbonated drinks.*
- *Open air better.*

Deficiency of fire
- *Cold air blowing on ears, legs, feet.*
- *Coldness right leg.*
- *Sensation of coldness above mouth.*
- *Sore throat from cold air.*
- *Perspiration: cold sweat from anxiety.*
- *Perspiration: increased during coldness.*
- *Worse becoming cold; and tendency to take cold.*
- *Desire alcohol; tobacco.*
- *Better warm drinks.*

Similarities between Hydrogen and the acute fever remedies Aconitum and Belladonna extend into the physical sphere and are apparent in acute conditions. All three are noted for *suddenness of onset*, the rapidity with which their acute conditions develop, and all have paradoxical temperature reactions. Though very sensitive to cold exposure, the feverish Aconitum needs the open air and wants to be uncovered. Though Belladonna is vulnerable to exposure of the head to cold or wet, it is even more susceptible to sun-exposure and overheating. When feverish, Belladonna is intensely hot with a bright red face, yet wants to be covered and does not want the windows open. The pains of Aconite, like Hydrogen, are burning, cutting, stitching. Hydrogen mimics the action of atropine (Belladonna) on the mucous membranes of the mouth and throat.

- *Tongue adheres to the roof of the mouth.*
- *Sensation of dryness even with a moist mouth; food tastes dry.*
- *Drinking does not relieve the dryness of the throat.*

Hydrogen is most active at the full moon and at the key transition points of life when the psyche needs to enter a deeper stage of incarnation and does so with reluctance or trepidation. These psychic challenges, demanding the next level of commitment to life, arise at approximately seven-year intervals: at seven when departing infancy; at fourteen when puberty concludes childhood, at twenty-one when the young adult must take the stage – and so they march on into the summer of maturity, the autumn of mid-life and the winter of later years. To these common punctuation points, marking life's journey, must be added circumstances that call for greater groundedness and greater involvement in the responsibilities and events of life; all of which task the weaknesses of the Hydrogen archetype.

It is thanks to the proving of Jeremy Sherr[2] conducted in 1991 that we have these insights into the nebulous nature of the Hydrogen archetype, and to the work of Frans Vermeulen[3] that we have a compilation of its salient features, including clinical observations from Louis Klein FSHom and material from Dr Filip Degroote's *Dream Repertory*.[4]

Reflection on the effects of the primary atom on the human psyche, under double-blind trial conditions and during therapy, is an essential exercise, preparing the way for the study of the more complex ancestral archetypes that follow. Despite its atomic simplicity, the first element of the Universe highlights the potential for suffering and spiritual growth that descent into the arena of life holds for the incarnated soul; it also identifies key markers that define each of the chronic miasms.

Being insubstantial, ungrounded archetypal forces, the role of the gasses in homeopathic therapy is circumscribed, but, nevertheless, when indicated, vital. Like all archetypes, they represent a very definite clinical picture or emotional profile, but in the face of the deepest strata of miasmatic disease, their action is relatively superficial and transient. They gain access to the labyrinth of the psyche and commence the process of cure, unlocking the constitution and bringing subtle cues to the surface in the form of dreams, imaginings or changes in disposition, lighting the way into the obscure regions of the unconscious and offering guidelines to remedy selection. After acting, and fulfilling their role, they need to be followed by remedies with more weight and penetration. Through coupling with other more substantial elements, Hydrogen and Oxygen contribute their special qualities to a wide spectrum of deeper and longer-acting remedies.

* * * * *

Helium

The first-generation stars of the new Universe started life as massive spheres of hydrogen and helium atoms; hydrogen being predominant. In these stars, the action of gravitational pressure caused the temperature within the star to rise to the point where nuclear fusion took place. In this way, the star 'burned' hydrogen nuclei to form helium, releasing stellar heat and light in the process. When all hydrogen was exhausted, the next fuel to sustain the star against the force of gravity was Helium, aptly named after the Greek God of the Sun, Helios.

The second lightest and most abundant element of the observable Universe, Helium was the second atavistic archetype to evolve from the creative sequence. Another gaseous, ethereal archetype hovering reluctantly on the fringes of incarnation: alive, yet not fully alive; in the world, yet remote from the world. *Some, refuse to fully incarnate*, only partially participating in the life-experience; some become *autistic recluses*. They desire to be utterly alone; have no need for another soul; would prefer living on a remote island or to spend life sequestered in a monastery (*averse to company*). Being a stranger to the material world, the Helium archetype dreams of being alone in an unknown city.

An outstanding property of helium gas is its pressing need to defy gravity and levitate – to leave the earth-plane. True to this propensity, the archetype desires to walk alone in the high mountains; has an affinity for the rarefied air, snow and ice of high altitudes; and dreams of mountains, of snow, of being barefoot in the snow, and of hail beating down. *They are ungrounded* and describe a feeling of lightness in the whole body, as if floating; as if the body had disappeared; as if floating out into the universe; and of waves going through the body – their inner core, as if floating, not solid.

A parallel levity of spirit and humour translates into *light-heartedness and jocularity* with a sense of inner joy and laughter. Easy bursting into loud laughter, sometimes for no reason. Laughter is an expression of their very being – their inner self: they are the levity; they are the laughter, they are the mirth! Wanting to laugh and to make others laugh, even while sometimes in a bad mood. Taken further, their levity makes them feel like doing something exciting or crazy. They want to sing and dance. Giggling and silly laughing. Laughing and joking. With this, a desire for distraction and escapism: wanting to watch action movies.

At the other extreme, in vivid contrast to the ungrounded or autism-like state, but consistent with sudden arrival on the earth plane in mortal form, comes a startling *awareness of being*, accompanied by the revelation: "I exist!" This intense consciousness galvanises them. Their energy is boosted and an 'explosive' desire to affirm themselves, to refuse compromise and to realise their aspirations ignites them. If their endeavours are compromised or frustrated, they are moved to explosive anger.

Positive levitation of the psyche promotes a desire to meditate and fills them with a longing to be with God – a yearning to return to their source. This devotional urge is attended by a desire to listen to sacred music (church or organ music), particularly Bach; or a need to play the piano.

Matching either Helium's shying away from immersion in life, or its over-energetic plunging-in, the sensory nerves of the skin are either refractory and insensitive to stimuli or acutely hypersensitive.

- Hypoesthesia, even anaesthesia: insensitivity to cold, heat and touch, even when pinching or scratching oneself on the face or body.
- Unpleasant hyperaesthesia: worse for touch; skin hyperaesthesia with burning sensations.

The vision shares in this contradiction, evidencing either blurred vision and poor accommodation, or visual hyper-acuity: very clear vision, vision in every angle – or a mix of the two; distorted vision: own body or others' bodies deformed; everything in the centre of the vision very clear, foggy on the sides.

Similarly, Helium's reluctance or eager impetuosity are mirrored in their awareness of temperature – intense, inner cold or waves of hot flushes.

- *Icy cold in the bones, as if ice was freezing inside the body, a need for warm covering.*
- *Ice cold air in nose.*
- *Sensation of body warming up, waves of hot flushes, desire to undress.*
- *Hot fluid as if streaming inside the skull.*

Encasement in a physical body is unbearable for such an expansive archetype.

- *Locked up in a cage; locked up in self, as if something would burst.*
- *Strangulated feeling from throat to chest.*
- *Everything feels too tight: necklace, earring, spectacles, clothes.*
- *Want to take off everything.*
- *Pressure at the top of the head, like a cover or cap, better eating.*
- *Shoes as if too small in the morning.*

Helium dreams

Theme of being held captive – caught in past family dynamics, past relationships or past friendships.

- *Family arguments.*
- *Dead family members.*
- *Family secrets never revealed before.*
- *Ex-lovers.*
- *Meeting old friends.*

Common themes of incarnated life:

- *Embarrassment and failure.*
- *Pregnancy, birth, babies.*
- *Dirt – Sex – Violence – Death.*

Yet, in the background, the presence of the sacred feminine:

- *Helpful woman; kind people.*

This sketch of Helium, extracted and annotated from Frans Vermeulen's compilation in *Synoptic Reference 2*[5], when compared with that of Hydrogen, shows the significant archetypal shift induced by the acquisition of a single electron.

* * * * *

References

1   Lilley DJ. *The homeopathic materia medica*, In: Kayne SB. ed., *Homeopathic Practice*. London: Pharmaceutical Press, 2008. Chapter 5, pp80–81.
2   Sherr J. *Dynamic Provings* Volume One. Worcester: Dynamis Books, 1997.
3   Vermeulen F. *Synoptic Reference 1* (second edition). Glasgow: Saltire Books, 2015. pp972–974.
4   Degroote F. *Repertory of Dreams*. RadarOpus.
5   Vermeulen F. *Synoptic Reference 2*. Glasgow: Saltire Books, 2015. pp839–840.

3

THE BIRTH OF THE UNIVERSE

Cosmic purpose and design

Before proceeding with stellar alchemy – the sequence in which great stars forge the axial elements required as fuel for their survival – we should ponder how order arose out of primordial chaos at the birth of the Universe. The march of ancestral archetypes across the stage of life is not random; it is disciplined by order and design. Is there evidence that, from its inception, the Universe unfolded with intelligence and the express purpose of producing sentient life?

The second law of thermodynamics states that all change in a closed system – the Universe – is a change towards greater *entropy* or chaos. Chaos is overwhelmingly more liable to increase than to resolve. Chaos systematically leads to greater chaos. All about us, we witness the law of ever-increasing entropy in action: the death of stars, the erosion of mountains, the corrosion of metals, the diseases that afflict us, the aging process and not least of all: the destructive behaviour of the human ego. However, the second law of thermodynamics also states that if any subsystem in a closed system shows a tendency to greater complexity and order, it will be balanced by a greater loss of complexity or disorder in an interlocking subsystem. Hence, the chaos that surrounds us, even in its most dire aspect, is, paradoxically, essential reparation for something sacred and sublime that is ever-germinating from the chrysalis of disorder. Its effect is clearly discerned in the immaculate order of life's evolution towards higher forms. Although concealed within the psyche, the same order is operative in the inexorable ascent of the soul towards Divinity. Paradoxically, it is in league with what seems the most pernicious chaos of all: human disease. In the light of the second law of thermodynamics, however, disease exemplifies positive, compensatory entropy: it brings order and sublimation by facilitating the individuation of the soul, which is the very objective of the Creation. The realisation of this entropic law is defined in a vital concept: *the healing power of illness.*

Scientific atheists assure us that the Universe is insentient, governed by mechanistic forces; that evolution has no purpose or direction; and that human beings are the consequence of random mutations in genetic material, screened by natural selection and survival of the fittest. Notwithstanding all these empirical convictions, the unprejudiced, intuitive mind is persuaded that the glory and grandeur of the Creation must be the work of a supreme artist. Science, itself, has revealed the presence of such a Supreme Consciousness.

Creation

In 1992, the American astronomer, Edwin Powell Hubble (1889–1953), established beyond any doubt that our universe is in a state of continual expansion: every part of the expanding universe receding from every other part. The further a galaxy is situated from us, the faster it is receding; the most remote objects are moving away from us at immense speed: over 90% the speed of light (275,00-kilometres per second). An inescapable corollary of this is that in the past, all parts of the universe must have been much closer together and in fact, going back to the beginning of space and time, all mass and energy must have been compressed to infinite density – infinitely dense, infinitely small and infinitely powerful. Here, the laws of physics and mathematics fail us: the finite cannot analyse or comprehend the infinite. This point of absolute values of energy and mass is aptly called a 'Singularity' – it is the domain of the philosopher, not the scientist. Beyond and within the Singularity lies the Ultimate, Un-manifest Cause, the Universal Intelligence: omnipotent, omniscient and omnipresent – known to Hindu philosophy as Brahman. This Omniscience is indivisible from the Divinity resident at the heart of the soul – the Atman: the human Spirit. The Universal Intelligence, poised in the infinite potential of the Singularity, conceives and carries the design and destiny of the Creation, from the atom to the galaxy; from the monad to the God-woman or God-man.

At the beginning of the present cycle of our Universe, some 15–20 billion-years-ago, the infinite potential of the Universal Intelligence, symbolised in the Singularity, moved and became manifest in a cataclysmic event – the 'big-bang' of creation: an inconceivable cosmic convulsion – an ultra-hot expansion that brought into being time, space, causation – the vital force, the four fundamental forces of the universe, energy – and matter; the entire phenomenon pervaded by the Universal Intelligence from which it emanated. From the moment of creation, the Universal Energy, of which the *Id* and the 'instinctively perceiving' *vital force* conceived by Hahnemann are part, is intelligently at work, presiding over the critical values and balance of the four fundamental forces: the gravitational and electromagnetic interactions and the strong and weak nuclear interactions.

In 1964, this scenario was confirmed when radio telescopes detected, from every direction of space, a tell-tale *microwave radiation* at 3 degrees above absolute zero on the Kelvin scale (3K): the fading glow of the prodigious heat, trillions upon trillions of degrees, generated at the very instant of creation!

It would seem logical that the explosive expansion of a Universe in space and time from an infinitely powerful, infinitely small, infinitely dense epicentre must result in a perfectly even or 'smooth' distribution of energy and mass in all directions. Yet, we find ourselves in a Universe manifestly populated by 'lumpy' aggregations of matter: planets, stars, galaxies, clusters of galaxies and even super-clusters. 'Embryonic' galaxies must have been present in the early Universe before matter formed as minute fluctuations of energy density, which later formed gravitational nuclei for the concentration and cohesion of matter.

In 1992, microwave radiometers, on board the Cosmic Background Explorer (COBE) satellite, detected minute 'ripples' or structure in the microwave background radiation indicating the existence at the birth of the Universe of the very fluctuations of energy needed to bring about the formation of galaxies. It would have done Hahnemann's heart good to have shared in the excitement generated by this discovery, confirming his conviction that a universal, governing, harmonising and unifying force exists: an 'instinctively perceiving' energy acting with purpose upon the universal substrate. The microwave 'ripples' evidence the finger of the Creator: moving with artistry and design, foretelling the evolution of *Homo sapiens* and the sublimation of the human soul.

The earliest evidence of the regulatory action of a unifying (vital) force upon the expanding universe is to be seen in the remarkable patterns linking the four fundamental forces and the quantities associated with them. Simply stated, these fundamental ratios are so critically selected from a vast range of possible values that one cannot but conclude an exquisitely precise fine-tuning of the Universe, setting-up conditions for the emergence of galaxies, stars, solar systems, planets and life. A simple, but critical example, is the expansion rate of the Universe; a rate that must have been set at the 'big bang' – the crucial value being the strength of gravity.

- If gravity had been *a little stronger*, it would soon have become dominant and caused the new Universe to collapse prematurely.

- If it had been *weaker*, the expansion would have become uncontrolled, not permitting time for stars and galaxies to form.

In another way, the strength of gravity is crucial to the existence of life in the universe.

- If it were *weaker*, it would be unable to compress the material in a star the size of the Sun strongly enough to ignite thermo-nuclear reactions – then – only very massive stars would be able to radiate energy in this way but would exhaust their energy too rapidly for evolution of life to occur.

From the very birth of the Universe, we recognise that it possesses very special, not arbitrary or random, properties, governed by a cosmic, unifying influence: the universal Vital Force.

These signs have persuaded some scientists to deduce that the Universe has been 'finely-tuned' to favour the appearance and survival of intelligent life. The postulate that human consciousness was inevitable and intended because of purposeful design has become known as the '*strong anthropic principle*'. Looking back in time from this vantage point: our very existence defines the necessary structure of the Universe. Nevertheless, most mainstream scientists discount the strong anthropic principle as a metaphysical concept. Fortunately, as homeopathy has revealed, conventional science is neither the yardstick nor the arbiter of truth.

The predetermined properties of the Universe predict that *the sequence* in which the ancestral archetypes enter the Creation, *the stage* on which they act and *the script* that informs them are 'fine-tuned' and meticulously orchestrated and that individuals markedly aligned, through disposition and constitution, with a respective archetype will tend to experience events in their lives that match its archetypal profile. This phenomenon is a well-recognised theme in homeopathic practice. When archetypal similarity is clearly defined in an individual, it can be confidently anticipated that the young are destined to face challenges characteristic of the archetype's myth and the older have already faced them, are currently doing so, or will certainly do so in the future.

These reflections on the living nature of the Creation beg a question: what is the likely fate of the Universe? Science presents three possible scenarios, all dependent on the amount of matter contained in the universe. Firstly, *a static universe* in which the force of gravity and the force of expansion equalise and establish a *cosmological constant*, resulting in a non-expanding, non-contracting universe: a postulate that Einstein first espoused, but later, hearing of Hubble's evidence for an expanding universe, discounted as "the greatest blunder of my life".[1] Secondly, *an open universe*, which most astronomers believe in, proposing an ever-expanding universe that must ultimately peter-out in exhausted nothingness; its galaxies irretrievably scattered, their star-fires spent and cold. Or, thirdly, *a closed universe* in which gravity finally overpowers expansion, causing the universe to involute, ever-contracting until all matter collapses to a point of infinite density and power: the very Singularity that gave it birth.

A closed universe is the model that accords with the philosophy and destiny of the soul and the postulate: 'as above, so below' – the macro- and the micro-cosmos imaging each other. The entire Creation is characterised by rhythm and cycles: ever-repeated spiralling sequences of birth – life – death – rebirth. What is true for the soul: emergence from Divinity and return to Divinity, must hold true for the Universe: expansion from a Singularity and retraction into a Singularity. A vast cycle – in absolute terms: transient – a wave in the immensity of time – known to Hindu philosophy as a *kalpa*: a pulse-beat in Eternity.

A Universe is not infinite; it is a closed system; it is measurable. Infinity demands an infinity of Universes, all ceaselessly expanding or contracting – every contraction followed by an expansion – a vast, boundless expanse of rhythmically pulsating universes, each passing through majestic cycles of creation, preservation and dissolution, ever-repeated into the timeless-reaches of Eternity. Endless cycles that on a cosmic scale parallel the spiral sequence of *Psora* (creation) – *Sycosis* (preservation) – *Syphilis* (dissolution)

All things return to their origin. Nothing is created from nothing or returns to nothing. Change is the germination of potential – dissolution is a return to that potential; nothing is lost or gained; for everything 'Is', always was and always will be. The human Spirit arises from the Universal Spirit, as a wave on the ocean of Divinity, and individualises as the human soul. At the point of individuation, soul and Spirit become one and the Spirit subsides into the loving embrace of the Universal Spirit. We come from 'God' and we return to 'God'.

Standing between the soul and the Holy Grail of individuation is the ego-self, the perennial adversary, a mythical being, that never was, nor ever will 'Be': an illusory artifice created by the soul to compensate for the loss to consciousness of its divine qualities and consequent to its failure to live with basic trust. The highest calling of the homeopath is to *heal the soul* of its ego-based disease by facilitating the dissolution of this pseudo-being through *depth homeopathy*. The elemental tools needed to achieve this are fashioned in the laboratory of the Cosmos through *stellar alchemy*.

* * * * *

Stellar alchemy

In the evolutionary epic of the atavistic archetype, it is the history of stars with a mass of about twenty-five suns that provide the early narrative, for they can complete the full cycle of stellar alchemy that culminates in a supernova and the fabrication of the heaviest elements and their expulsion into space.

As we have seen, all stars start life by fusing or 'burning' *hydrogen* nuclei, converting them into *helium*. When all the hydrogen has been consumed, helium provides the next fuel, and in turn produces *carbon*. Eventually, after millions of years all the helium is exhausted. While burning helium, the centre of the star remains hot enough to support the weight (gravitational force) of its outer layers. When helium burning ends, the compression of the inner core by the weight of the outer layers of the star forces temperatures up beyond 60 million degrees Kelvin, to the point where carbon burning begins. Carbon burning produces *neon, magnesium and oxygen*. When all the carbon is exhausted, the gravitational collapse of the star sets in again and the temperature rises above one billion degrees, and neon burning begins with the production of more magnesium and oxygen. At 1.5 billion degrees, oxygen burning begins and when two oxygen 16 nuclei collide, they produce a variety of elements, including *silicon, sulphur, phosphorus* and more magnesium. At this point of stellar alchemy, silicon is the key ingredient, because at the following stage of nuclear burning, at a core temperature of 3 billion degrees Kelvin, silicon becomes involved in a sequence of hundreds of nuclear reactions, yielding as their end-product the 'ultimate stellar ash': *iron 56*.

While the burning of hydrogen and helium takes millions of years, carbon burning takes only about 600 years, neon burning lasts only a year, oxygen burning six months and silicon burning is over in less than twenty-four hours. Each stage is attended by further inward collapse of the star; the core becomes hotter and hotter and the nuclear reactions more violent. The nuclear fuels are becoming less and less efficient, and, at the high temperatures generated, neutrinos are created, which in escaping freely from the stellar inferno remove energy faster than the star's surface can radiate. The star runs out of energy and the stage is set for a cataclysmic event!

All the energy the star derives from thermonuclear reactions comes from compressing protons and neutrons more tightly together in atomic nuclei. In iron 56, this compression has reached its limit; no more energy can be provided by nuclear fusion. However, the destiny of such a great star demands that it shall give birth to the more massive nuclei – such as gold, silver, lead, uranium – all of which are less tightly packed than iron 56. To forge these heavier elements, more energy is needed. What happens next provides that energy!

Reduced to a sphere of iron about as massive as our sun, with no energy being produced by nuclear fusion at its core, the star has no means of support. The result is dramatic, instantaneous and violent. The inner regions of the star are crushed inwards and the pressure on the iron nuclei at its core becomes so massive that electrons and protons fuse to form neutrons. In an instant, the core shrinks dramatically while retaining the same mass. The surrounding stellar material plummets inwards upon the neutron core at immense speed; the star implodes and immediately explodes, bouncing back from the colossal compression. Neutrinos escaping from the neutron core and generated by its compression, fire and boost the expanding shock wave and blow apart the outer layers of the star in a titanic explosion: *the supernova!*

The supernova shines for a few weeks as brightly as an entire galaxy of stars and the remnant core persists as a rapidly-spinning, neutron star emitting radio and other waves. This hyperactive, stellar relic is known as a *pulsar.*

In the violence of the explosion, the materials of the star's outer layers are superheated; multiple, complex, nuclear reactions elaborate the elements heavier than iron, which are expelled into space to form the interstellar gas and dust that over aeons concentrate, coalesce and collapse to form the next generation of stars, such as our Sun.

Surveying this immense Cosmic landscape, we are informed of the sequence of archetypes that form the axis from which, stellar alchemy forges the elements that form the substance of the Universe. The sequence is always:

Hydrogen ‡ Helium ‡ Carbon ‡ Neon ‡ Oxygen 12 ‡ Silicon . . . ‡ Ferrum 56 (Iron).

Significantly, at each stage of stellar evolution, from carbon through to silicon, magnesium is elaborated, and the fusion of oxygen 16 atoms produces not only the key element silicon, but also sulphur and phosphorus and more magnesium.

Knowing that the 'Mind of God', or Universal Intelligence, is purposefully at work and that nothing is by chance, it is reasonable to cast an archetypal eye on this alchemical progression to see what can be divined from it. Focusing on the substantial rather than the gaseous archetypes, a design takes shape: a declaration of intent discernible billions of years before its enactment. Hydrogen and Helium, the lightest elements of all, representing reluctant, fearful archetypes hovering hesitantly on the fringe of reality, are immediately followed by carbon, the element destined to become the keystone of organic life.

Reference

1   O'Raifeartaigh C. Einstein's Greatest Blunder? *Scientific American* Guest Blog. February 21, 2017. Available online at: https://blogs.scientificamerican.com/ guest-blog/einsteins-greatest-blunder/ (Retrieved 11.03.2018.)

4

GRAPHITES – 1

Fundamental Psoric Archetype

Building block of life

Appearing as the first substantial element in the axial sequence of stellar alchemy, carbon confirms its fundamental importance. Carbon is the building block from which the first living molecule and subsequently all life came into being; it is the pillar of the organic world and through its giant molecules and complex combinations evidences nature's supreme artistry. The purest form of naturally-occurring crystalline carbon is *graphite,* which always contains a trace of iron (4%). Historically, Graphite was called black lead or plumbago because of its confusion with similar-looking lead ores, particularly galena. Although generally considered black, graphite is a grey metallic-sheened mineral. Most graphite is produced

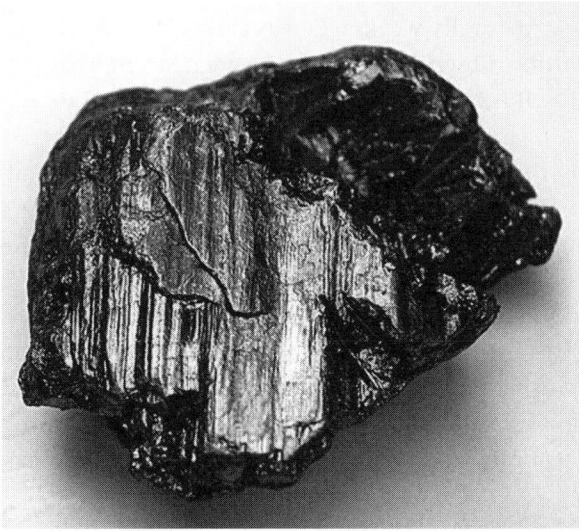

Figure 4.1 Graphites

through the metamorphosis of organic material in rocks; even coal is occasionally transformed in this way. The natural affinity that exists between graphite and iron is born-out by the nodules of graphite that are frequently found within iron meteorites that have hurtled to Earth from space.

Science reveals the existence of cosmic graphite, which is considered an important constituent of carbonaceous dust detected in the interstellar medium. Some graphite is to be found in igneous rock that is formed through the cooling and solidification of volcanic magma or lava, showing an archetypal relationship between Sulphur (volcanism), Silicea (magma) and Graphites (carbon). In the theatre of life, Silicea provides the platform, Graphites supplies the actors and Sulphur invents the plot.

Transmutation

When graphite is exposed to exceptionally high temperature – high pressure conditions, such as exists at depths of 150 kilometres in the Earth mantle, it is slowly transformed over billions of years to another allotrope of carbon: *diamond*. This metamorphosis of carbon, one of the most sombre of substances, into a peerless, brilliantly-reflective crystal may be likened to the transformation of the human soul, through the tests and trials of life-times, from ego-based ignorance to spiritual enlightenment. The aptness of this analogy is supported by the radical change in atomic configuration that converts graphite to diamond. The carbon atoms of graphite are tightly-bonded in two dimensions, forming sheets that can slide easily over each other and are structurally weak, whereas carbon bonds in a diamond, form an inflexible three-dimensional lattice of great strength and hardness. The cardboard ego-self is contrasted with the adamantine might of the deathless soul!

Graphite is the stable form of carbon; even diamonds at or near the surface of the earth are undergoing an extremely slow process of transform-ation into graphite. Their difference in structure results in a profound differ-ence in the properties of graphite and diamond. Graphite is one of the softest materials; diamond is the hardest. Graphite is a good lubricant; diamond is the ultimate abrasive. Graphite is opaque and grey-black; diamond is translucent and adamantine. Graphite is a conductor; diamond is an insulator or semi-conductor. These disparate qualities mirror the contrasting attributes of the Graphites and Diamond (Adamas) archetypes.

Key properties

Graphite has three special properties:

- *It has good electrical conductivity* – the only non-metal to have this quality, hence a property of major archetypal significance: anthropomorphically indicative of unusual psychic, aesthetic, emotional and physical sensitivity.
- *It is an excellent lubricant*, evidencing a nature that is soft, gentle, yielding, impressionable, vulnerable and compliant; a protecting, caring, loving disposition; but also, a person, who can be slippery, manipulative and flatter for favour.
- *It is an inert substance* – it is not chemically reactive – in human terms, an archetype that lacks drive and is indolent, slow to react and slow to decide, but, once committed, stubbornly resists change and persistently adheres to a predetermined course (habit, belief, tradition, creed – *ideas fixed*).

The lubricating ability of this carbon allotrope stems from its unique structure. Graphite is made up of extremely thin layers of multiple carbon hexagons, which can glide easily over one another. This ability is responsible for the remarkable lubricating qualities of the substance, but also for its intrinsic *weakness*, which is notable when compared with Diamond, another carbon allotrope. This fragility pervades the nature of the archetype and colours its vision of itself, which is typified by a sense of inferiority and inadequacy, lack of self-esteem, self-consciousness, great anxiety and many fears. It also evidences vulnerability to impinging emotions – which can dislocate the inner, dynamic balance of the psyche without visible evidence – particularly grief from the loss of a love source or love focus.

- *Industriousness.*

A further property, stemming from the carbon atom itself is *industriousness*. Gaia's teeming life forms are testimony to the *industry* and *artistry* of the carbon atom, all achieved through its capacity to fashion giant molecules into a diverse array of incomparable living masterpieces. *Creative, artistic, loving, caring activity* must be an essential prerequisite for the health and happiness of the fundamental carbon archetype.

Archetypal pointers – Doctrine of Signatures[i]

Lead pencil

Hahnemann obtained his preparation of Graphites from the purest black-lead taken from 'an English lead pencil of the best quality'. The ability to mark paper and other surfaces gave *graphite* its name, chosen in 1799 by the German mineralogist, Abraham Werner. He derived this from the Ancient Greek: *graphein*, which means *to write* or *draw*. Although, modern pencil-lead is commonly a mixture of powdered graphite and clay, in Hahnemann's time all pencils were made with leads of English natural graphite.

Experience reveals that the mystery of the archetype clings to everything related to it, even the seemingly mundane. Once this is appreciated, nothing is overlooked or discounted, and gems of insight are uncovered where least expected. This is true of the humble *lead pencil*. It presents several elements for archetypal analysis: its creative uses – its anomalous name – its idiomatic meaning – and its tell-tale colour. We shall consider each of these as we proceed.

Colours – black and grey

Since colour is Nature's most expressive symbolic code, defining in a single statement much of the salient nature of the subject displaying it, the colours *black* and *slate-grey* must be added to Graphites' special properties when constructing its archetypal profile, which represents – far more than Sulphur – the fundamental nature of the psoric mind.

The Void: dominant feminine archetype

In the process of stellar alchemy, *lithium, beryllium* and *boron* are formed before Graphites (*carbon*), but unlike Graphites, these lighter elements are not integral to the alchemical process. The sequence of axial elements, essential to the life of a great star is: *hydrogen, helium, carbon, neon, oxygen, silicon*, and *ferrum*. Of these, Graphites is the first substantial axial element and the source of all life; a dark-grey substance bearing the blackness of night, paled with the grey of dawn, imaging the emergence of the Creation from the blackness of the Void – the womb of the Great Mother – the Cosmic, or Sacred, Feminine. Within her vastness, the Great Goddess encompasses the Cosmic Masculine represented by the 4% Ferrum (*iron*)

---

[i] See also Chapter 5.

that even the purest graphite contains. At the instant of creation, the Feminine releases the Masculine, which gives motion, force, form and direction to the creative force. At the end of a *kalpa* (cosmic cycle) the Masculine is withdrawn and subsumed once more into the Void of the Great Mother Goddess. Graphites symbolises this Sacred Relationship. It is an archetype that embodies the feminine, generative energy of the Great Mother; her presence evidenced in its grey-blackness, high conductivity and protective, lubricating softness. But, it also embodies the critical presence of the Masculine, evidenced in its iron content, which grounds Graphites and imparts practical efficiency and common sense to the predominately feminine archetype.

Iron content: recessive masculine archetype

Ferrum, the archetype of iron, is synonymous with Ares and Mars: respectively, the Greek and Roman Gods of War. Esoterically, every archetype bestows its myth and mystery upon all in its domain and so it is with Ferrum and Graphites. In the 16th Century, a huge deposit of graphite was discovered in Borrowdale, Cumbria, England, and, during the reign of Queen Elizabeth 1, this graphite was used as a refractory material to line moulds for cannonballs, resulting in rounder, smoother balls that could be fired further, contributing to the strength of the English navy. The Borrowdale deposit of graphite was extremely pure and soft.[1] This, seemingly inconsequential, anecdote, metaphorically portrays a profound event: the 'launching' of the Cosmic Masculine from the pure enveloping softness of the Cosmic Feminine at the instant the Singularity manifested the expanding Universe.

Returning to Mother Earth from the far reaches of space in the form of solid-iron meteorites, this most masculine of all elements, embodying the Warrior Archetype, bears within its structure, nodules of pure graphite, token of the Cosmic Feminine that sent it forth to 'do battle' in the Universe – just as knights of old bore a protective talisman from their beloved and warriors of today carry photos of their dear ones.

Such observations must not be disregarded as transports of the romantic mind, they acknowledge a higher Reality that informs the world about us; revealed also in dreams that require interpretation in the light of similar vision.

The Ferrum presence within the Graphites psyche can be persuasive or ineffectual. When assertive, it empowers and imparts level-headedness, common-sense, practical ability and drive, but when muted, Graphites lacks drive, decisiveness, confidence, courage and perseverance.

The diamond: Self-realisation

These deliberations support a fundamental relationship between Graphites and Calc-carb (organic calcium carbonate derived from the middle layer of the oyster shell). Whereas, Calc-carb, the oyster, gives birth to the pearl, Graphites, carbon, gives birth to the diamond, both processes metaphorically representing the individuation process that gives 'birth' to the Spirit: the Pearl or Diamond that symbolise the goal of Self-realisation: the Atman!

Archetypal characteristics:
Conductivity – Lubrication – Inertia

Conductivity – Sensitivity

Good electrical conductivity points to an archetype that is sensitive on every level – psychically, aesthetically, emotionally and nervously – as well as an unusually impressionable archetype (Aurum, gold; Argentum, silver; Cuprum, copper – and – Carcinosin, Lac humanum and Lac lupinum: apex archetypes of the materia medica). Graphites is hypersensitive to mental and sensual impressions – *to odours, especially the fragrance of flowers, to pain and, above all, to music.* All impressions create reaction quite out of proportion to the stimulus.

Flowers
Sensitivity to the odour of flowers aligns Graphites with Phosphorus – certainly, the most ethereal of substances and the most psychic and artistic of archetypes – and with China, another highly sensitive, psychic, artistic archetype. These relationships, suggest hidden qualities in the Graphites psyche, not immediately apprehended in such a basic, down-to-earth individual: refined qualities of feminine softness, sensitivity and aesthetic appreciation deep to their sturdy, stolid, appearance, and an unexpectedly keen intellect. The same sensitivity relates Graphites physically to the atopic, allergic, remedies: Allium cepa, Nux-vom, Sabadilla and Sanguinaria – all of which suffer allergic rhinitis (hay-fever) from inhalation of pollen.

Music
Music moves them to tears and may induce sadness and even the deepest melancholy. It is significant that the archetype personifying the first non-gaseous element to fuel a star in the expanding Universe and the key

element upon which all life is founded should be sensitive, not only to music, but especially to church music – sacred music – organ music!

Being the stable and purest form of carbon, Graphites is the signature archetype of *Psora,* the miasm that typifies the anguish of the soul separated from its source and origin – seemingly abandoned, forsaken and utterly alone; left to its own deserts in a vast, intimidating Universe. Like Hydrogen and Helium, fresh 'cast-out of paradise', Graphites unconsciously longs to return to that sacred dimension. The rich, enveloping, sonic power of the organ in the vaulted majesty of a great cathedral touches the aching nostalgia in the depths of their being and moves them to tears. The shedding of such tears temporarily relieves their emotional state (Pulsatilla). These tears are not only due to tender sensibility and what may be considered a species of 'homesickness', they spring from a primal psoric fear, or unconscious conviction, that their 'expulsion' from paradise was due to spiritual unworthiness: the blight of 'original' sin (*anxiety about salvation*)

This susceptibility to sacred music is mirrored in two exemplary archetypes: Lac lupinum, 'man's noble, unsullied sibling and Aurum, gold, the archetype that in its highest form epitomises the realised soul. Both, are entranced and uplifted by sacred music and moved to tears. In ominous contrast, two base archetypes, Lyssin and Thuja are averse to sacred music. Lyssin, the nosode of rabies and thus the very incarnation of the Lucifer archetype is accordingly disquieted by the sound of a church choir singing and inexplicably overcome by anxiety on hearing church bells ringing. Thuja, the signature archetype of *Sycosis,* the miasm of profligacy and deceit, shares these negative responses. Known as the *Arbor vitae,* Thuja is the living embodiment of the Tree of Knowledge of Good and Evil, the mythical tree that harbours the satanic serpent that conspired the fall of 'man'. Myth and materia medica tell the same story!

Pain

Graphites subjects have a low pain threshold and are extremely sensitive to and intolerant of pain (Mag-carb). This sensitivity is exaggerated by their anxiety about their health, their fears of disease, of dying and of death. They may dream about disease and obsess about death. Every chest pain convinces them that they have heart disease. They are oversensitive to the least bodily discomfort. Like Goldilocks, everything is either too hot or too cold, too big or too small, too hard or too soft. This preoccupation can delay or override any task or activity that needs to be done. Graphites is not the type to stoically disregard discomfort and press on regardless.

- *Sensitive to pain.*
- *Delusions:*
  - *Has heart disease.*
  - *Is sick.*
  - *Is about to die.*
- *Dreams: of disease.*
- *Death:*
  - *Presentiment of death* (2).
  - *Sensation of death.*
  - *Thoughts of death* (4) *with sadness* (4).

Trivia

Being emotionally sensitive, Graphites easily takes offence and the offence is usually trivial and not worth the emotion. They take umbrage from the least misconstrued word, expression or action.

- *Offended easily; takes everything in bad part.*

They are easily moved to anger, which is typically out of all proportion to the provocation. Once riled, they can be harsh and abrupt in manner and display a rudeness, even insolence, which seems quite out of character. Though easily offended and vexed, the passion soon passes and unlike Sepia, Nat-mur, Staphysagria, Nit-ac and Petroleum, the majority soon dismiss it from their minds. With some, however, it lingers.

- *Dwells on past disagreeable occurrences; at night.*

Small things excite them excessively; when speaking their hands become unduly hot. They take fright from anything unexpected and the effect of the fright lingers (*ailments from fear, fright*). Everyone impinges on their peace of mind and every disturbance, or interruption, vexes them, therefore, they prefer to be alone and seek solitude.

A typical aspect of Graphites sensitivity, which proves a millstone round their necks, is their *over-reaction to trivialities* and their *unhealthy preoccupation with minutiae and inconsequential detail*. They are unable to prioritise, unable to distinguish the important from the unimportant and fail to show resolution and decisiveness even in the smallest matters.

- *Trifles seem important.*
- *Conscientious about trifles: occupied with trifles.*
- *Irresolution, indecision – about trifles.*
- *Depression about trifles.*
- *Anxiety about trifles.*

- *Grief, even to despair, about the most trifling matter.*
- *Extreme scrupulousness; cannot take anything lightly.*
- *Extremely fretful and impatient; irritable about trifles and very critical.*

Like Silicea, Graphites has a penchant for great attention to detail and superfluous elaboration that amounts to fussy and obsessive perfectionism. This fastidiousness proves their downfall. Even the clever and gifted are hindered and worn down by it: they can never complete their work; it is never finished, something must always be added or changed; it is never good enough; and besides, such meticulous perfectionism can never be gratified: it leads to anxiety, fretfulness, discouragement and finally exhaustion and despair. Like other related carbons, Carbo-veg (charcoal) and Kali-carb (pot-ash), they may suffer from 'brain-fag' and 'burn-out'. Their incapacitating worry over detail and preoccupation with petty things exasperate those who live or work with them. This is exacerbated by their constant 'nit-picking' and fault-finding that will not overlook or condone the least discrepancy or inaccuracy (Kali-bich; Nit-ac).

Apart from these obsessive traits, another notable cause for getting bogged-down in trivia is their indecisiveness, procrastination and equivocation, which lead to the neglect of priorities, even urgent matters. They busy themselves with whatever catches their eye, rather than with what really needs to be done. Their *lack of confidence, indecisiveness* and *inertia* (lack of motivation, lack of drive, indolence) compound and conspire against them.

- *Aggravation from trivialities.*

Trivialities provoke anxiety, fear, apprehension, indecisiveness, frustration, discouragement, depression and weeping.

Eventually the same emotions are experienced without cause!

- *Causeless emotions – emotions without cause.*

These inexplicable emotions are an exaggeration of the same mental state. They experience causeless foreboding, causeless apprehension and anxiety, causeless anger, causeless depression and weep without cause.

Clairsentience

At a deeper level, the singular capacity of graphite to conduct electricity, denotes that the Graphites archetype, like the Gold, Silver and Copper archetypes, possesses a heightened ability to intuit and sense the qualities, emotions, feelings and motives of other people. They can tune in so intimately that they experience the other person's moods and emotions. If the bond is psychically intensified because of protracted proximity or intimacy, Graphites may find themselves becoming one with the other person: as if they were losing their identity and being taken over or subsumed within the being of another. Like the Mercurius archetype, they may easily pick up mannerisms, accents, vocabulary, stance and energy patterns of those who attract their attention. Intellectually, this rapport may enable them to pick up on the thinking of another person and to describe their point of view better than they can their own. Empathetically, they can sense emotional distress or physical illness in others (Lyssin). Such is their clairsentience, they may find their thoughts and feelings being invaded by those of others; so much so, that they can be in doubt as to whether the feelings they entertain are truly their own or picked up from someone else. These marked sensibilities resemble the psychic vulnerability of Phosphorus and the hypersensitivity of Nat-carb to certain people, places and things. These similarities are flagged by shared symptoms: in the case of Phosphorus: sensitivity to the odour of flowers; and in Nat-carb: sensitivity to music. Nat-carb is particularly sensitive to the sound of the piano; and Graphites to that of the organ. All three archetypes are *hypersensitive to mental and sensual impressions* (Carcinosin).

Their acute sensitivity to ambience, mood and emotion, although taxing, can prove a great boon, particularly as it facilitates their natural Mother Goddess urge to care for and tend to others. Empathetically, they are deeply affected by other people's lives. Reciprocally, other people pick up on this receptivity and are naturally drawn to confide in them (Nat-mur). Graphites is an excellent listener and able, better than most other archetypes, to set aside personal feelings and to understand and evaluate the other person's problems objectively and pragmatically. They are gifted in their ability to identify what will be best for the other person's welfare. Graphites, like Nat-mur, is *the archetypal wounded-healer*, unable to act efficiently, decisively and dispassionately on their own behalf, but singularly able to impersonally and objectively advise and direct others.

Lubricant

Soft, impressionable, vulnerable, lack of confidence, feminine, caring, embracing

Duality – hard yet soft
Crystalline graphite is made-up of tightly-bonded carbon atoms arranged in two-dimensional sheets that yield to pressure by sliding over each other.

This quality makes graphite an ideal dry-lubricant, used to protect the surface of moving-parts. The mineral appears hard and resistant, but is soft and has a greasy, slippery feel. It appears black but is dark-grey with a metallic sheen. Graphite's apparent hardness is impressed upon the mind because it is frequently found in massive pieces and looks dark, rugged and tough.

This soft, yielding quality, in a substance that looks hard and metallic, is archetypal and miasmatic, revealing in its duality, the presence of *Psora*: the split between the soul and the ego-self, and the promise of *Sycosis*: the split between virtue and vice.

Several personality traits and tendencies can be deduced from these distinct and opposing features. They signify a tender vulnerability masked by a compensatory façade of imperviousness (Lycopodium); a reserved, faint-hearted, beta disposition concealed by alpha posturing and bravado; or, at a positive level, an unsuspected feminine sensitivity and empathy in a dour, silent, undemonstrative individual that only comes to the fore when others are in distress and in need of help.

Impressionable

The softness of graphite, suggests an archetype with an impressionable psyche, over-susceptible to the influence of circumstances, events and the major role players in their life. Like Pulsatilla, Graphites is too easily impressed, persuaded and led by others. Although their innate nature and miasmatic constitution are primary influences, the conditioning, imprinting and nurturing they receive in early life have a disproportionate influence on their life perspective and prove too long-lasting and too resistant to change. This exaggerated effect is often due more to the archetype's exceptional sensitivity than any severe neglect or trauma in their upbringing.

Fundamental to their self-image is the 'delusion' that others have what they lack. Whereas, others are well-rounded, inherently valuable and loveable, by comparison they are not as good, worthy or deserving of love.

Certain family scenarios are inclined to foster these feelings.

- An exceptional role model in the immediate family: often a parent or grandparent, who appears to the young Graphites to be extraordinarily gifted or capable.
- A parent who takes up a lot of psychic space, being highly emotional, unstable, histrionic, dramatic and extrovert or who is influential, powerful and lauded by others – leaving the young Graphites feeling in comparison insignificant and of no consequence.

- A parent with a strong masculine energy that comes across as autocratic, dictatorial, critical, derogatory, belittling and intolerant; most often the father, but, not infrequently, a cold, aloof, intimidating mother.
- An influential sibling:
  - More central to the family dynamics – favoured, indulged, praised.
  - More assertive, winning or manipulative.
  - More outstanding: extrovert, attractive, talented.
  - Disadvantaged: with special problems demanding the attention and focus of the family.
- A large family: an environment in which Graphites felt unnoticed, unimportant and neglected.

These are children who felt overlooked and neglected when they were young. It seemed that other's needs were more important than their own. They had no voice and were seldom heard (a perception that impinges on the function of the fifth chakra). Knowing that their needs (priorities) would not be heeded, they learned to 'numb' and forget themselves (fall asleep). They turn their attention away from their real wishes and needs and became preoccupied with small comforts and substitutes for love (trivia). In the development of this defence strategy, Graphites' problem of recognising and responding appropriately to even urgent priorities and their tendency to divert their focus to minor, inconsequential trivia can be discerned and understood.

They grow up with *a sense of invisibility* – of being *a 'grey', inconspicuous being* – and a *resignation* that they will never amount to anything, never become significant, valued or truly loved – either by others or themselves. Having no sense of value or worth, they assume that they will never get love from any source; nor do they believe they deserve it.

They sacrifice their wishes for the wishes of others and compliantly go along with other people's priorities and enthusiasms, adopting them as their own. They expect that their viewpoint, needs and plight will be discounted or ignored. They often get dragged along by the preferences and wishes of others (Alumina). From this, comes their tendency to comply and conform and their *inability to say "No"*, which they fear will cause rejection, separation and alienation. This negation or 'forgetting of self', makes others the active agents in their lives; a submission that accounts for their *indecisiveness*, their inability to take a personal stance, their *stubbornness* and their *reactive anger*.

Their indecisiveness becomes a major characteristic that hinders their efficiency, impedes their progress and causes them endless frustration. They are often pulled in different directions and unable to choose which to follow, they sit on the fence in a state of uncommitted limbo or inertia. Their stubbornness, which is as marked as that of Calc-carb, is of the same order: a stubborn reluctance to decide and to get moving and an equally stubborn resistance to change direction once committed. *Behind the obstinacy lies a deep anger* – at not being heard – at being neglected and disparaged – often self-inflicted through warped ego-perspective and lack of self-love. From this, comes anger at having to comply with the wishes of others – due to their dread of being discounted and alienated – and anger at being over-looked or reprimanded if they do not comply. Their decision is to make no decision – to be angry and hide it – to seemingly go along with what is decided by others, while inwardly remaining divided, angry and resentful.

The resigned demeaning of themselves manifests in various ways. They are apologetic, self-effacing and uncomfortable with:

• Attention being focussed upon them.
• Taking up their own space.
• Taking up others' time.
• Asking to be seen or heard.
• Calling attention to themselves.
• Expressing themselves in a group.

It is apparent that the descent into life has 'disconnected' the Graphites psyche from Universal Unconditional Love. Their subjective, ego-filtered vision tells them that *love is localised and conditional* rather than boundless and unconditional. This is their personal 'delusion'. From this unconscious misconception comes *the fixation that who they are is not inherently loveable*, valuable, significant or worthwhile. They experience themselves as discon-nected from the unconditional, loving, goodness of life. The core of this fixation is an *'inferiority complex'*: a self-image based on insufficiency, inad-equacy and inferiority (Psorinum, Carcinosin, Lac lupinum, Lac caninum, Lac humanum). Their delusion of separation from Love, and the resultant inability to respect and love themselves, influences the life they experience and their responses to it.

Lack of confidence
Behind an affectation of composure, joviality or truculence, Graphites is timid, hesitant and lacking in self-confidence. This diffidence particularly relates to their *competence, social skills and ability to make a correct decision*. Several rubrics highlight their social fears, their desire for solitude, their standoffishness and their prickly sensitivity.

- *Confidence – want of self-confidence.*
- *Timidity – bashful – timidity about appearing in public.*
- *Fond of solitude.*
- *Aversion to company.*
- *Company aggravates.*
- *Disturbed – averse to being disturbed.*
- *Conversation aggravates.*
- *Irritability when spoken to.*
- *Averse to being spoken to (2).*
- *Reserved.*
- *Seriousness, earnestness.*
- *Inclination to sit (3).*
- *Indisposed to talk; desire to be silent – a person of few words.*
- *Temperament phlegmatic.*
- *Aversion to being touched – ticklishness.*
- *Offended easily.*

Social phobia
Social intercourse does not come easily to Graphites: they are self-conscious and shy and not good at small-talk; striking-up a conversation with someone they don't know and making new friends is difficult for them. They are socially awkward. Their natural tendency is to shy-away from others, especially strangers, and to avoid unfamiliar situations. In company, they have little to say and feel tongue-tied. Even when a topic is of interest to them and they have a definite viewpoint, they lack the courage to express their opinion (Ignatia; Lycopodium; Petroleum; Silicea). They remain silent and later reproach themselves for being cowardly (*cowardice: afraid to express his opinion; will: weakness of will*). Their social fears, reticence and lack of rapport with people, leave them one apart, on the outside looking-in – the proverbial wall-flower (Ambra-gris, Nat-mur, Kali-carb, Calc-carb, Nat-carb). They are never so lonely, miserable and bored as when in company. They cannot wait for the social engagement to come to an end and release them from their ordeal. In the company of friends and family, they come into their own and often have a ready wit and a jovial disposition.

- *Fear of people – fear of a crowd.*
- *Fear the approach of others.*

Feminine energy
The intrinsic softness of graphite, though belied by its hard, shiny, metallic-guise, signals the presence of a pervasive feminine energy within the archetype. This aligns the archetype with feminine values and feminine

sensitivity. This bias, when manifest in the fundamental, psoric archetype, engenders a mistrust and fear of the masculine.

- *Aversion to men.*
- *Fear of men.*

The aversion and fear of men, found in both male and female Graphites subjects, is not so much a fear of their predatory sexuality, but rather of their masculine aggression, competitiveness, assertiveness and autocratic egoism, which is daunting to the timid, Graphites ego-self. They much prefer the company of women, which they find less challenging and intimidating. *The fear of men* embodies also a fear of the bureaucracy, fear of the patriarchy and *fear of authority figures.*

The oversensitive Graphites archetype is distressed by the sordid side of life – injustice, the abuse of animals, women and children and the exploitation of nature – and unable to come to terms with these harsh realities (China). In the face of human savagery, the suffering of its victims and the relentless and unconscionable despoiling of the planet, they doubt there can be a loving God in heaven or the least divinity in man. Unlike the militant Causticum activist, who fearlessly tilts against injustice and the establishment, Graphites succumbs to despair and resigned inertia. They evidence a marked carbon trait: *the inability to process and digest life.* Physically, this is often born out in gastro-duodenal inflammation and ulceration.

The *gentle, yielding, sensitive, feminine* nature of the Graphites archetype requires comparison with Pulsatilla (meadow anemone): the archetype that personifies more than any other the fundamental, immature, feminine, beta-type personality (Chamomilla [chamomile] represents the immature, masculine, alpha-type personality). The younger Graphites often comes across as being simple, not world-wise, innocent and emotionally immature: characteristics we might anticipate in such a fundamental archetype. These qualities often bely their natural intelligence and the intricacies of their inner world.

PULSATILLA-LIKE

Graphites and Pulsatilla are similar in many ways. They are both *shy, mild, gentle, timid and impressionable* in disposition, but the emotions of Graphites are more deeply-rooted and complex. Pulsatilla is generally shallow, changeable and often flighty. With familiarity, the initial shyness and timidity of Pulsatilla are soon set aside and replaced by a self-assured, extroverted vivaciousness, which can be flirtatious, provocative and manipulative. Graphites remains reserved and introverted, keeping quietly to the periphery, even in familiar company. The admixture of iron keeps them grounded, level-headed and serious. While Pulsatilla loves comfort, luxury, opulence and the good things of life, Graphites, like other carbons, is less sophisticated, more 'down-to-earth', has simpler interests, needs and tastes and is not afraid of work or getting their hands dirty and calloused. They are often men and women of the earth with a love of nature, gardening, growing their own vegetables, cooking, the arts and crafts and raising their children to be productive members of society. Pulsatilla is far too spoilt, precious and indulged to seriously tax themselves in such ways. Whereas, the eccentricity of Graphites lies in their preoccupation with trivia, Pulsatilla entertains strange notions about diet, exercise, sex and religion, which can become dysfunctional and fanatical. Both are easily moved to tears, but while Pulsatilla laps-up sympathy and consolation, Graphites does not wish to be consoled and would rather be left alone. Both Graphites and Pulsatilla are inclined to become overweight (Calc-carb; Ferrum), but, whereas, Pulsatilla loves sweets, doughnuts and cream-cakes, Graphites is generally averse to sweets. Their temperature reactions may distinguish between them, but even here there is a similarity. Pulsatilla is warm-blooded and averse to heat; Graphites is chilly and averse to cold, but, like Pulsatilla, Graphites cannot bear stuffiness, needs windows open, needs fresh, open air and wants to keep the head cool (Ars-alb), dislikes becoming overheated and is intolerant of the warmth of the bed.

EARTH MOTHER

The dominance of the feminine principle in the psyche of Graphites is fundamental to the archetype, producing a woman, or man, who personifies the warmth and caring qualities of the Great Mother Goddess – She who gave birth to the Creation and with whom Graphites is so archetypally bonded. Graphites can be an 'Earth Mother', possessing a gentle, caring, mothering nature, that feels deep compassion for humans and animals and is always prompted to take them under her wing. Often a plump, jovial, uncomplicated, charitable person, practical and efficient, helping others for the joy of it; fully dedicated to being of help, yet able to remain objective, not permitting her generosity of spirit to interfere with family and home.[2] They are often to be found in one of the caring professions. These mothering characteristics are also true of Calc-carb and Mag-carb. All three, create homes that are warm, welcoming havens: good places to be!

Both Graphites and Calc-carb are homely women, of cheerful disposition, who take great joy in creating a happy, welcoming home and bustling over those who cross its threshold. Their kitchen, sewing or crafts room are their sanctuary from which they produce all manner of edible and useful commodities for friends, family and sometimes the local market.

Like, Mag-carb, Ficus religiosa (Bodhi tree) and Lac lupinum (the Wolf), friendships mean a great deal to Graphites. Apart from family, they usually have an intimate circle of very close friends on whom they are dependent. Any rift or discord in such a relationship causes them great distress, which they cannot just shrug off.

- *Ailments from discord between relatives and friends.*

The feminine bias of the Graphites psyche reduces intellectual pride and swings the dynamic of the psyche towards the integrity of the soul rather than the intrigues of the ego-self. Graphites is more inclined to respond from the heart than from the head and from kindness than from ego-preference. At the same time, however, they keep their feet on the ground and remain practical and level-headed.

Foreboding

Not only does Graphites lack confidence in themselves, they lack confidence in others – their affections, their motives and their integrity – and, more profoundly, they lack confidence in life itself and what it holds in store for them. *Forebodings of misfortune* hang over them, like a sword of Damocles, robbing them of peace of mind and intruding into their dreams that are fraught with difficulties, mishaps and danger. In every way, they epitomise the lack of basic trust that so characterises the *grey*, psoric perspective of life – a sure sign that the structures of the ego-self are firmly in place.

Hesitancy

Their timidity and lack of confidence make them hesitant and indecisive; their worry about making the right decision robs them of confidence. It is a vicious circle that makes Graphites one of the most irresolute of archetypes; an indecisiveness that is exacerbated by several factors.

- *Lack of confidence.*
- *Fear of making the wrong decision.*
- *Fear of making a critical and irremediable mistake.*
- *Mistrust of the future.*
- *Conviction that misfortune is ever waiting to pounce; that bad-luck is their inevitable lot.*
- *Cautious to a fault, scrupulously meticulous and terrible conscientious.*
- *Preoccupation with unnecessary detail.*

- *Inability to discount anything or take anything lightly.*
- *Every possibility and eventuality must be weighed and measured.*
- *An overdeveloped conscience evokes guilt even before a decision is made: for it might prove wrong!*
- *An excessive sense of responsibility and accountability renders decision-making painfully onerous.*

Defensive strategies

Because of their standoffishness and want of social graces, Graphites may come across as rude and lacking in good manners. They do not go out of their way to endear themselves to others. Their behaviour is calculated to keep people at a distance. Other, less than attractive, characteristics behind which they may hide and which are not thought of as typical of Graphites are:

- *Rudeness.*
- *Insolence, impertinence (2).*
- *Harshness, roughness (2).*

- *Mocking sarcasm.*

An unpleasant trait they share with closely related Carbo-veg (vegetable carbon): an equally unsociable individual, who suffers from social fears.

- *Quarrelsomeness without waiting for answers (2).*

This characteristic is only noted in Graphites and Ambra-gris: both timid archetypes, shy of social interchange, easily embarrassed and self-conscious. The quarrelsomeness is protective of a sensitive ego. They lack the confidence required for temperate debate and discussion and attempt to carry the day by adopting an uncompromising, quarrelsome manner, which does not give the other party opportunity to make their point or disagree – or scares them off.

- *Affectation.*

They are not devious or dishonest by nature, but they may hide their shyness and awkwardness behind a veneer of affected self-assurance, composure and indifference, which makes them appear aloof and snobbish. It is an attempt to project a confidence and nonchalance they do not feel [Lycopodium]. Their authentic self is hidden by a false persona.

- *Humour.*

Graphites hides timidity, self-consciousness and embarrassment not only behind rudeness and sarcasm, but also a light-hearted, jocular front of teasing, laughter, humour, wit and flippancy. For those whose psoric vision sees life as grim and tragic, a superficial, comic response diffuses tension and permits them to dissociate from their anxiety and despair.

- *Teasing* (1). *Teasing in children.*
- *Teasing, laugh at reprimands* (unique) – to hide their discomfiture.
- *Reproaches, laughing at reproaches* (unique).
- *Laughing at reprimands* (2).

This kind of behaviour proves infuriating to parents, but as in the comic response of the stressed adult, inappropriate and ill-timed laughing, joking and teasing in a Graphites child is often an unconscious, protective strategy to deflect admonishment and chastisement or to shield a vulnerable ego from the embarrassment of rebuke and scolding.

Despite these defensive responses, which can give one a poor impression of them, under this dour, rough, rude, quarrelsome, sarcastic, irritable, impatient, unsociable demeanour there is often a heart of gold that becomes evident on deeper acquaintance or when someone needs help. Like graphite they appear hard but are in fact soft.

- *Sympathetic, compassionate.*
- *Affectionate.*
- *Sentimental.*

Inertia

The third cardinal property of graphite, every bit as important as electrical conductivity and lubrication, is *inertia*. It is a characteristic that pervades the Graphites archetype psychically, emotionally and physiologically. At the subtlest level, the inertia of Graphites mantles the soul, inducing a state of somnolence and indolence in which the soul 'goes to sleep', abdicating sovereignty over the psyche and deferring to the opinions, preferences and prejudices of the ego-self that informs it. At the physical level, the inertia of Graphites permeates the organism inducing a slowness of function and performance that touches every aspect of the economy. The tendency to sluggishness, stasis and torpor is characteristic of all the carbon remedies, but especially Graphites, Carbo vegetabilis and Carbo animalis. Sepia, a closely-related carbonaceous remedy, is characterised by endocrine imbalance, venous stasis, muscular hypo-tonicity and prolapse and on the emotional level by sadness, depression, apathy and indifference.

The psychic cause and consequences of inertia are detailed under the heading Grey.

Obesity

The basic metabolic rate is slow, evidenced early in life in a tendency to put on unhealthy weight. Like many of the carbon archetypes, the Graphites constitution is inclined to obesity. This obesity is not the healthy, solid flesh, that belongs to a strong, hearty individual, but the soft, flabby kind found in Calc-carb, indicating impaired function. These two remedies run parallel in the treatment of such 'morbidly' fat, unhealthy individuals. Both Graphites children and adults tend to be overweight with poor muscular tone and enlarged abdomens; they lack stamina and energy and are easily tired. Anaemia may contribute to their tiredness. They look pale and puffy but may flush bright-red when emotionally stressed and this can precipitate a nosebleed – all signs that confirm the close relationship between Graphites and Ferrum, another archetype inclined to corpulence. As noted, Graphites always contains an appreciable amount of iron in its structure.

Graphites must always be remembered for fat children with unhealthy skins: the younger with eczema and the older with teenage pimples and acne; yet, strangely enough, youngsters and adolescents with no interest in sweets or decidedly averse to them.

Graphites subjects usually have big appetites and are very hungry, suffering hunger pains plus-minus two hours after a meal, which are relieved by eating. They eat too quickly and with too much relish.

However, it must not be forgotten that Graphites can be indicated for emaciated states brought on through illness, e.g. a child, greatly emaciated, little or no appetite, very restless, passing acrid, highly-offensive stools of brown fluid mixed with undigested particles. The remedy also has a notable keynote contradicting its general tendency: *emaciation of the suffering parts.* Diarrhoea, in Graphites cases, may be caused by the suppression of a skin eruption, such as eczema.

Slow function

The Graphites slowness of function is summed up in a keynote from the materia medica:

Suited to women, inclined to obesity, who suffer from habitual constipation; with a history of delayed menstruation.

- Hypothyroidism – nodular goitre.
- Adrenal fatigue.
- Insulin resistance.
- Sleep:
  - *Excessively tired, weary and sleepy.*
  - *Sleepy during the day.*
  - *Does not feel fresh in the morning.*
  - *Dullness in the morning.*
  - *Dullness after siesta.*
- Eyes:
  - *Light aggravates: extreme photophobia.*
- Inner ear:
  - *Sensitive to motion; worse motion and travelling.*
- Digestion:
  - *Fatty food aggravates (Carbo-veg, Pulsatilla).*
  - *Gastric stasis or paresis.*
- Intestines:
  - *Constipation: large difficult stools united by mucus threads.*
  - *Fermentation rather than digestion: abdominal distension and excessive flatulence.*
  - *Rectal prolapse.*
- Menses:
  - *Delayed menarche (late onset of puberty).*
  - *Getting the feet wet delays menses (Pulsatilla); causes painful swelling of the ovaries.*
  - *Menses scanty, pale, irregular, painful.*
  - *Menses too late with constipation; obstinate constipation and delayed menses occur together.*
  - *Leucorrhoea instead of menses (acrid and excoriating; in gushes, day and night) or leucorrhoea before and after the menses.*
  - *Retroverted uterus; uterine prolapse; weakness of pelvic floor.*
- Sexual female:
  - *Libido low or lacking; decided aversion to sex.*
  - *Anorgasmia.*
  - *Lack of lubrication: vaginal dryness.*
- Sexual male:
  - *Tardy orgasm or failure to achieve orgasm despite every effort (both sexes).*
  - *Averse to sex, lack of sexual enjoyment.*
  - *Erectile dysfunction.*
  - *Premature ejaculation.*
  - *Sexual debility from sexual excesses.*

- *Sexual debility with increased desire.*
- Nervous system:
  - *Cataleptic condition: conscious, but without power to move or speak.*
  - *Numbness is more common than pain.*
- Body temperature regulation:
  - *Easily chilled and just as easily overheated.*
  - *Chilly person who is sensitive to a warm room and craves the open air.*
  - *Chilly – lack of body heat, must wrap up; sensitive to the least draught of air.*
  - *Easily overheated, makes them ill; cannot withstand the heat of summer.*
  - *Exertion rapidly overheats; aggravates all symptoms.*
  - *Warmth of bed aggravates, e.g. itching of skin.*
  - *Worse hot drinks – a general (stomach: better warm drinks, especially milk – a particular).*
- Circulation:
  - *Venous stagnation.*
- Blood:
  - *Anaemia, especially young girls with menstrual difficulties: delayed puberty; amenorrhoea; menses late, scanty, painful.*
  - *Anaemia with easy flushing and redness of the face.*
- Lymphatics:
  - *Lymphoedema.*
- Skin:
  - *Slow to heal: unhealthy skin; every little injury suppurates.*
  - *Skin heals with keloid formation.*
  - *Old scars break down and ulcerate.*
  - *Dryness of the skin without eruption.*

Mental slowness

The constitutional sluggishness, slowness and incapacity of the archetype can impede the mental functions and impair emotional responses. Mental inefficiency is often accompanied by aversion to work, especially mental work, indolence and *lack of drive*.

Graphites covers the entire spectrum of intellectual ability from the dullard to the scientist. At the lower end of the scale, Graphites is a slow thinker – slow of wit and comprehension; his hands quicker and surer than his mind. He is often physically industrious and efficient but shies away from mental work and at school is mentally lazy, easily distracted, lacks concentration and has no urge for scholastic endeavour. He may be over-weight but can put this to good use in a rugby scrum or in martial arts – i.e. putting his iron content to good use. These non-academic Graphites youngsters are slow, inefficient thinkers and lack motivation, but they are not mentally backward or handicapped as many Baryta-carb, Borax, Calc-phos, Nat-mur, Bufo and Mercurius children may be.

- *Mathematics, calculating; inept for.*
  - ○ *Inept for algebra.*
- *Slowness and sluggishness from mental overwork, fatigue and burn-out.*

Though Graphites does wonderful work in such dull, slow-thinking children and adults, it is far more often called for when, as in Carbo veg, this slowness and inefficiency of the mind has come on from overwork, mental or physical, or dates from some illness – a state of 'burn out' in those who have overextended themselves in prolonged, sedentary, mental work – the scholar, the student, the author, the artist, the scientist. They are played-out and their mental powers fail them.

- *Prostration of the mind, mental exhaustion, brain-fag, after mental exertion; from scientific labour* [unique].

Laziness – indolence
The laziness may be either mental, or physical, or both. Indolence with an inclination to just sit and do nothing. *They have a severe lack of drive.* There is utter lack of zest for any form of activity – in extreme cases almost taking the form of a catalepsy.

- *Laziness (indolence) although very intelligent.*

Two carbons, Graphites and Petroleum, appear in italics in this rubric. Other remedies are Alumina, Ammonium carbonate (another carbon) and Conium, an archetype close to Graphites in the treatment of menopausal women and cancer.

In their indolence, like Sulphur, they can become neglectful of their appearance and hygiene, and unaffected by untidiness.

Graphites is a remedy to be thought of when a person has lost their drive and when an aversion to work, especially mental work supervenes. *Dreads and avoids mental work.* Averse to business. In a state of mental exhaustion and incapacity. *Mental dullness is increased by sleep. Dullness of the mind, worse in the morning on waking.* Work impossible after an afternoon sleep.

- *Unfit for mental work after the noon siesta; for four hours.*

Dullness, stupefaction in the head

The dullness and difficulty in thinking of Graphites is felt as a physical symptom in the head, or is associated with headaches or vertigo, both of which are worse in the morning after waking – especially after a sound sleep.

Stupid feeling in the head; intoxicated in the head; gloominess in the forehead; weakness in the head, can hardly think – *all worse in the morning on waking.*

Slowness must be regarded as an important general in Graphites.

Everything is too late: puberty, menstruation, stool, orgasm, skin healing, mental processes, decisions and emotional responses.

Inefficient mind

The following rubrics reflect the inefficiency of the Graphites mind.

- *Slowness of the mind [2].*
- *Slowness of purpose [unique].*
- *Aggravation from mental exertion [2].*
- *Absent-mindedness [2].*
- *Concentration difficulty [3] – in children – concentration impossible.*
- *Abstraction of the mind [2].*
- *Aversion to mental work – dreads and avoids mental effort.*
- *Mental work impossible.*
- *Aversion to thinking.*
- *Thoughts wandering.*
- *Obscurity of thought.*
- *Vanishing of thought – afternoon.*
- *Deficiency of ideas – ideas fixed.*
- *Confusion of the mind [2]:*
  - *Morning – on and after rising – on waking.*
  - *As if intoxicated.*
  - *During menses – after menses.*
  - *After sleep.*
  - *Ameliorated by walking in the open air.*
- *Mistakes – makes mistakes.*
  - *Talking:*
    - § *Misplacing words.*
    - § *With vertigo.*
    - § *Using wrong words.*
  - *Writing:*
    - § *With vertigo.*
- *Stupefaction – as if intoxicated – morning – during vertigo.*

- *Forgetfulness.*
- *Memory – weakness of the memory.*
  - *For what he has just done.*
  - *Recent facts.*
  - *What has happened.*
  - *Mental labour.*
  - *With vertigo.*
- *Prostration of the mind – after slight mental exertion.*
- *Mental work fatigues.*

Graphites is for older people who forget what they or others have just said or done yet, retain good recollection of the past.

The forgetfulness of Graphites can be due to age; a sign of constitution-ally-slow mental processes; or stem from deep psychological issues. Being the fundamental carbon archetype, Graphites represents the young, incarnated soul that in descending from a higher dimension *forgets* its true nature and finds itself in a holding environment that seems unloving, threatening and unpredictable. In defence of its 'naked vulnerability' and sense of being unlovable, insignificant and without worth, the untrusting soul retires behind a compensatory pseudo-self that studiously avoids pondering life's significance and purpose and unconsciously attempts to dull what seems an intolerable experience by distracting itself with irrelevant things. This skimming over the surface of life and preoccupation with trivia leads to *absentmindedness and forgetfulness* – the superficial equivalent of the soul forgetting its own inherent preciousness.

Self-forgetting is also built into the seemingly-praiseworthy, Graphites trait of always considering the others person's needs and problems rather than their own. They forget and neglect their inner nature while directing their attention to the needs of the environment and of others. Their own needs are considered less important and are, therefore, neglected. They listen and respond to the needs and plight of others, but this altruism is yet another Graphites way of neglecting a priority in favour of a more superficial activity. In imitation of how they perceived their early caregivers to be – not caring, nurturing, attentive or loving – Graphites turns a deaf ear to the cry for attention issuing from their own inner voice. Conditioned to feel fundamentally unimportant, insignificant and inferior, they tune themselves out of consideration and busy themselves attending to others. Hidden by a generous, caring, loving nature lies an undermining lack of self-respect and an inability to love, protect and cherish themselves – deficiencies that must be overcome to attain Cosmic Love. Reconnection with this Divine Aspect dispels the pervasive sense of inferiority, and, despite adversity, imbues all experience with spiritual significance and purpose, dissipating the greyness, indolence and inertia that so beset Graphites.

References

1 Norgate, M, Norgate J. *Old Cumbria Gazetteer, black lead mine, Seathwaite*. Geography Department, Portsmouth University, 2008. (Wikipedia.)
2 Bailey PM. *Homeopathic Psychology – Personality Profiles of the Major Constitutional Remedies*. Berkeley CA: North Atlantic Books, 1995. p71.

5

GRAPHITES – 2

The Doctrine of Signatures

Lead pencil analogies

Creativity

Archetypal analogies can also be drawn from the source of Hahnemann's Graphites. The lead pencil is the symbol of the author, the poet, the musician, the artist, the draughtsman, the architect, the builder, the engineer, the mathematician and the scientist. All these abilities and occupations may be inherent in the multifarious Graphites archetype.

Sex

At a ribald level, not out of place considering the jocular, earthy, sometimes coarse, twinkle-in-the-eye nature of Graphites: 'putting lead in one's pencil' is a colloquial expression for achieving an erection. This is one of Graphites' notable areas of influence and it covers the extremes of satyriasis and impotence and the unfortunate in-between situation where tormenting sexual desire and fantasies are attended by flaccid inability to perform, or where the promise of prolonged, passionate pleasure is thwarted by premature ejaculation.

- *Immoderate sexual excitement – persistent erections – priapism.*
- *Tormenting and persistent sexual thoughts and fantasies; intruding even against the will (also occurs in women); whilst lying in bed, unable to sleep.*
- *Sexual 'wet' dreams that mirror his conscious state.*
- *Sexual debility (erectile dysfunction) with increased desire.*
- *Sexual debility due to excessive indulgence or excessive masturbation.*
- *Impotence.*
- *Loss of erection during intercourse; worse from anxiety.*

- *Lack of enjoyment; want of sensation during intercourse; a remarkable indifference to sex and little excitement during it.*
- *Premature ejaculation.*
- *Failure to ejaculate despite all efforts.*
- *Cramps in calves during intercourse.*
- *Intercourse is followed by severe prostration.*
- *Intercourse followed by irritability.*
- *Thoughts; persistent; sexual – tormenting.*

Aqua marina; Asterias rubens; Cantharis; Conium: Graphites; Lycosa tarantula; Ozone; *Staphysagria*.

Here, the presence of four key remedies for cancer of the breast must be noted: Asterias, Conium, Graphites and Lycosa.

Graphites also covers:

- *Itching, moist eruption of the scrotum.*
- *Oedema of the prepuce and scrotum.*
- *Herpes genitalis.*

The Graphites woman suffers the female equivalent of impotence: low libido or complete aversion to sex and aptly, considering the properties of graphite: vaginal dryness and inability to lubricate adequately during intercourse. Graphites is a remedy for peri-menopausal, atrophic changes in the vaginal mucous membrane and for senile vaginitis. The menopausal woman may also parallel the male by experiencing persistent and tormenting sexual thoughts.

Menopause: art and creativity

In the lead pencil simile, two elements of the libido aspect of the Id are metaphorically aligned: the creative (artistic) and the sexual – thereby, signalling an important relationship, especially critical to the health of the mature Graphites woman: the need to find artistic, creative fulfilment, particularly when the sexual and reproductive life is undergoing involution. It is said that *what Pulsatilla is to puberty, Graphites is to the menopause* – and this is very true!

Midlife can be a time of crisis for the Graphites woman. Previously, she found meaning, identity and fulfilment in the challenges of family responsibilities and an outlet for her mothering nature in caring and worrying about others (Mag-carb). She is now faced with an empty nest as the children leave home; many will be on their own, without a partner, through death, divorce or desertion. Graphites, like Pulsatilla, is dependent on family, but, unlike Pulsatilla, she is also dependent on nurturing others; which, in this archetype, is often a substitute, or compensation, for *unfulfilled creativity*. As Coulter tells us: always consider Graphites for a middle-aged woman, who is clearly gifted, yet, is unfulfilled, unhappy in her life, dejected and filled with self-pity.

Two dreams provide commentary on this:

- *Dreams of admirable buildings.*
- *Dreams of excelling in mental work.*

These dreams, in such a frustrated woman, are not wishful thinking or merely dream fantasy, they clearly indicate unconscious awareness of very real potential and talent. She is being prompted by her higher-self to achieve fulfilment in some intellectual, artistic or creative work. She needs some focus, some stimulus and some challenge to ignite passion and joy and light up the drab 'greyness' of her menopausal sky. *The stereotyped, domestic role of the middle-aged wife and mother does not fulfil Graphites.*

Energy repressed is energy distorted and this is of significant concern in the major carbon remedies: Graphites, Petroleum, Kreosotum, Carbo-veg and Carbo animalis, because of carbon's carcinogenic potential. To comprehend the immense, creative energy latent in Graphites, we have only to contemplate the reaction of carbon to the great mass extinctions of the past: e.g. the 'Great Dying' of the Permian-Triassic extinction event, some 252 million-years-ago in which over 90% of all species were wiped out. Carbon 'dusts-itself-down', and *'pencil-in-hand'* addresses the almost empty canvas and sets about the task of restoring bio-diversity; each time doing so with added finesse and refinement. A sobering thought in this respect is the fact that due to human activity since 1900, the present rate of extinction has exceeded the normal, standard or 'background extinction rate' of earth's biological history by over 1000 times. Given that it is carbon that is dying and carbon that must restore, and knowing of the sentience innate in all aspects of the Creation, we cannot doubt that these events touch the 'unconscious of carbon' and are held in the psyche of the Graphites archetype. Like Causticum, Graphites cares deeply about human transgression against the planet, but needs to free herself from her psoric *resignation, self-doubt and lethargy* to follow Causticum's banner. In doing so, she will align herself with the drive of her carbon essence and find emotional fulfilment and physical health.

Encouraging the peri-menopausal Graphites to find an artistic or altruistic outlet is an essential part of therapy. This is not always easy to achieve, because of Graphites' *poor self-esteem, sense of mediocrity, timidity, indecisiveness and lack of drive*, and a constitutional tendency towards *inertia*. In

Coulter's words: 'she is afraid to stretch her wings and fly.' Without the beneficial effect of achievement or artistic fulfilment, Graphites is inclined to lapse into self-pity with feelings of being unappreciated, taken for granted, badly done by, and *singled out for misfortune* and misery. Their unfulfilled creative urge may be translated into heightened libido with the intrusion of tormenting sexual thoughts and fantasies, or the libido may sink into inertia: reduced to a mere glimmer, or totally extinguished, with *aversion to sex*.

To the actively creative and artistic Graphites, their talent is a precious gift, vital to their emotional and physical wellbeing, giving them self-worth, identity, meaning, joy and, most salutary of all, fulfilment. Once engaged, Graphites, like Silicea, breaks free from self-doubt, procrastination and indolence; they become focused, determined and enthusiastic; but always with the danger of overextending themselves and declining into brain-fag or burn-out.

Lead – saturnine temperament – Lycopodium

A further analogy pertinent to the *lead* pencil relates to its anomalous name, a designation that has become traditional despite the pencil never having contained any lead. Historically, graphite was called black lead or plumbago, the latter name being commonly used for massive pieces of the mineral. Both names arose from confusion with the very similar-appearing lead ore: galena, also called lead glance: one of the most abundant and widely distributed sulphide minerals. Galena is lead-grey in colour and has a silver sheen. Deposits of galena often contain appreciable amounts of silver, e.g. 1–2%, which, by no coincidence, is an effective remedy for chronic lead poisoning. Just as nature places *Arnica montana* on mountain slopes where it can prove most useful, so silver is found in lead deposits. The Lead archetype personifies much that is reprehensible and toxic in human nature and in accord with the traditional belief that evil creatures of the night, such as vampires and werewolves, can only be killed by silver weapons, experience reveals that silver combats the toxic effects of lead! At every corner, we find myth and materia medica shadowing one another.

Resemblances invariably have archetypal significance. The ease with which large chunks of graphite and galena can be confused – soon dispelled by comparing their weight – signals that the Graphites and Plumbum (metallic lead) archetypes will share certain characteristics and it is to the heavy metal we must look. Only on lead's terrain can the two approximate, for the masculine in lead is so dominant, cold and self-absorbed, it has no means to mirror the gentle, mothering image of Graphites. Knowing its toxicity, we can be sure Plumbum provides a window to a dark side of Graphites.

From medieval times, the *saturnine* temperament was attributed to the influence of the planet Saturn: it was also identified as symptomatic of lead poisoning. The alchemists perceived a mysterious association between the planet and the metal: just as gold was recognised as the metal of the sun and silver the metal of the moon, so lead was believed to possess an affinity for the planet Saturn. The god Saturn, after whom the planet was named, was the Roman counterpart of the ancient Greek god, Kronos, a self-serving, cruel and cowardly deity, who emasculated and overthrew his father, Ouranos, the primal sky-god, and devoured his own children by the Earth Goddess Rhea, that he, in turn, might not be overthrown. The need to gain ascendency over parents, to 'emasculate' them, whether father or mother, and to lord it over one's own children, to 'devour' them, due to an innate sense of inadequacy, is an unpleasant trait typical of the Lycopodium archetype, which has much of Graphites and Plumbum in its emotional make-up.

Lycopodium clavatum, club-moss, is the diminutive cousin of the huge *Lepidodendron* (30 metres high and up to 1.5 metres in diameter), the largest of the Lepidodendrales: the primitive trees that some 300-million-years-ago dominated the Carboniferous coal swamps and provided the bulk of the organic material for the coal beds that covered most of Earth's tropical land areas. Climate change caused the collapse of the vast rainforest system and colder, dryer conditions, resulted in the great forbears of the club-mosses dwindling drastically in size to the point where the tiny, Lycopodium club-moss evolved. What a falling-off was there, from the towering Lepidodendron, monarch of the swamps, to the humble ground-creeper of today. The Lycopodium archetype still feels this reduced status: a sense of inferiority that accounts for their compensatory arrogance and chauvinism. Similarly, Graphites compensates for low self-esteem by adopting a standoffish, truculent or over-jovial, flippant persona.

The archetypal relationship between Lycopodium and coal is fundamental and formative; it links Lycopodium to the industrial revolution, the world of technology and the left-cerebral intellectualism of the modern world. Coal and graphite are comparable in appearance and colour; both are carbon minerals produced by the transformation of organic material by exposure to high temperature and high pressure. Consequently, Graphites and Lycopodium share many points of similarity, not least of all their *diffidence, procrastination and sexual difficulties*. When detected, the often subtle, feminine bias of Graphites is a good distinguishing point.

Lycopodium is prepared from the small, yellow spores of the plant. These have a hard, resistant, outer capsule that protects a soft centre containing finely-divided oil. The impervious capsule masking a soft centre faithfully portrays the tender vulnerability of the archetype concealed beneath a veneer of egotistic hardness. This metaphor of emotional duality is matched by the outer cragginess of a lump of graphite when compared to its intrinsic softness. Another parallel relates to lubrication. Lycopodium spores were used as a dusting powder before the days of talcum powder, protecting the skin from chaffing and often proving of benefit in cases of eczema in the bends of the joints and folds of the skin (intertrigo), for which it is frequently of value when given in potency. As noted, Graphites is an excellent dry lubricant; protecting mechanical surfaces exposed to constant friction; used medicinally, it is an outstanding remedy for weeping eczema. When matching the patient's constitution and given systemically, both remedies can cure vaginal dryness and lack of sexual lubrication that makes intercourse difficult or painful.

The similarity between Lycopodium and Graphites extends to their ability to present the *saturnine temperament* of Plumbum. To best 'plumb' the nature of this unpleasant temperament, it is well to contemplate and feel a piece of lead. It is a dull, grey, heavy, ponderous substance and, for a metal, rather soft. Dropped from a height it has no timbre; it hits a hard surface with a dull, muffled thud. Translated into mood and behaviour, this conjures a sluggish, sombre, gloomy, melancholic demeanour – a brooding, morose, sullen, taciturn and unsociable disposition, which, if at all forthcoming, is sour, cynical and sardonic with a penchant for surliness, insolence and cruelty. Emily Bronte aptly describes Heathcliff, the anti-hero of her novel, *Wuthering Heights*, as saturnine. Though charged with the potential for rage, malice and violent doings, this baleful temperament denotes a prevailing state of *passive aggression* – the dark side of Graphites – part of its emotional inertia.

Colours – black lead – grey plumbago

Black

Although graphite is dark-grey in colour, the first impression on seeing a large piece of the material is of a metallic-black, coal-like substance; only closer scrutiny apprises the eye that its blackness is yielding to a lighter shade. It depicts grey emerging from black, a transition that images the stirring of the Singularity and parallels the opening paragraphs of Genesis.

In the beginning, God created the heaven and the earth.

And the earth was without form and void; and the darkness was upon the face of the deep.

And the Spirit of God moved upon the face of the waters.

And God said, Let there be light: and there was light.

And God saw the light, that it was good: and God divided the light from the darkness.

And God called the light Day, and the darkness he called Night.

And the evening and the morning were the first day.

Graphites denotes the first evening and morning of the psyche, seemingly lost to the warm embrace of the Infinite and precipitated from the blackness of the Void into the chill, grey dawn of incarnation's day. It images the deceptive, half-light of the human intellect kindling the coming of *Psora* out of the serene blackness of the primitive animal will – the very moment, captured by the ancient text, when first man and woman, at the instigation of the serpent, 'more subtle than the beast of any field', partook of the fruit of the tree of Knowledge of Good and Evil and the duplicitous ego-self usurped the dominion of the soul. In Graphites, we hold the blueprint for the evolution of *Psora* and a chronicle of psoric thinking; its archetypal picture documents the onset of miasmatic disease and reveals the ego-delusions that cause and maintain it.

Black embodies the Void and the qualities of the Great Mother Goddess – she, who is the life force in matter; the sacred energy of creation – hence, the attributes that are innate and potential in her three personifications: the Virgin, the Mother and the Crone. These feminine archetypes are intrinsic to the feminine-orientated Graphites archetype.

Carbon, as graphite, is 'black', the primal colour from which all others emerge; carbon, as diamond, is 'white', the transcendent colour to which all others return. The greatest paradoxes are the Light within black and the Divinity within the soul. These are innate and potential in Graphites; they are its mystery and its magic.

Black is infinite potential and presents the greatest polarity and the greatest paradoxes of any colour. It symbolises both the potential for enlightened spirituality and perfidious evil.

Out of the darkness all things emerge and into the darkness all things return. Black is the beginning and the end, just as the day begins and ends in darkness and just as we are born from the darkness of the womb and slip away into the darkness of death. Our life begins in the unknown and ends in the unknown. Graphites represents the beginning: it stands at the beginning of the soul's journey – at the crossroads of choice; but it also ushers in the final chapter: it holds the mystery of light and dark, expressed in the proverb: *'light at the end of the tunnel'*. It conducts us into the personal Shadow that we may discover the Universal Light. This is what it means to face ones' own Shadow. When the Shadow impinges on awareness it brings feelings of *guilt, shame, unworthiness and fear of rejection*, all of which fall within the ambit of Graphites. Within the personal Shadow is the *leading and kindly light* that can guide the soul towards spiritual unfoldment and individuation.

Black is silent, but if we listen intently to that silence, we hear a sacred sound – *"Om"* – the music of the Divine. In the retreat of silence, Black brings us face to face with the personal death that brings liberation: the death of the ego-self! That Black is the confrontation with the Shadow: *'the dark night of the soul'* – where all that the ego-self represents and cherishes is swept away – the cataclysmic psychic catharsis known to Nordic tradition as *Ragnarök – The Twilight of the Gods* or *War of the Wolf* (see *The Wolf*).[1]

There are aspects of Black that must be swept away to achieve emotional and psychic health. Graphites, the fundamental substance emerging from black, addresses these negative aspects.

Black is a person, who needs to *control, hold on and repress*: characteristics that begin with Graphites and *Psora* and peak in Carcinosin and *Carcinosis,* the cancer miasm. Control prevents the archetype from feeling their emotions. Any emotion that is not felt, be it love or hatred, or any other emotion, acts as a barrier to perceiving Cosmic Love as the fundamental force of the Creation.

Behind the need to control lie *anxiety, fear and lack of trust*. Fear of the future and its unpredictability; fear of a merciless world: random, purposeless and chaotic. Black symbolises control, and, the desire to control, for Black holds onto every colour within itself and lets no colour escape. Black represents those who *maintain control by hiding and repressing their feelings, by not confiding in others and by withholding what they know* – keeping things to themselves, keeping their own counsel. This silent, stubborn stoicism is represented by the hard, external appearance of graphite; the concealed sense of martyrdom is part of its softness. When someone habitually wears black, it shows they have something bottled up inside, something they cannot face and are repressing, or something they have not resolved. They are stuck; unable to move on; caught in circumstances. Black is like the womb, a safe and hidden place to be in a threatening world.

After the death of her beloved Prince Albert, Queen Victoria habitually wore black: the 'trappings and the suits of woe' – tokens of grief, of mourning and of tradition. Graphites is a major remedy for *relentless grief, wearing black* to honour it, and steadfastly *observing tradition*. In addition, Graphites matches the stout, dowdy, matronly appearance and fecundity of the British matriarch – 'the grandmother of Europe' – *her obstinacy, her blunt honesty, her benevolence and her self-imposed seclusion.*

Black desires silence and solitude, but when negative, fears to be alone, or, falls between the two, preferring solitude, but needing someone within call (Lycopodium). Black is restricted, limited and formal: it is reserved, conventional, conservative, orthodox, regimented, punctilious, fastidious, proper, correct, straight-laced, prejudiced, judgemental and traditional. Black is caught in the trivia of protocol, precedence, rules, ritual and dogma; their immense potential tethered by the inconsequential; their minds conformed by consensus creed. This Black sees only black or white and admits no grey. Here, the closeness of Graphites, the carbon of life, and Kali-carb, the carbon pot-ash of plants, is revealed through the medium of Black.

Negative Black magnifies and warps these values and seeks to impose them on others: desire to control 'self' (repression) becomes desire to control and dominate 'the other' (expression corrupted). Judgement and prejudice directed against 'self' (rejection) become judgement and prejudice directed against 'the other' (bigotry and fanaticism). That which is dis-owned about 'self' is repressed into the black of the psyche, the Shadow, and the corrupted energy, inflamed with contempt, hatred and malice, is projected upon 'the other', who is demonised, scapegoated, victimised and destroyed. The Inquisitors wore black; the Gestapo wore black; and the 'baddy' in the movies wears black! In this negative Black, the archetypal profile has shifted by natural progression from fastidious, unsociable, gentle Graphites, where its basic structures are laid down, into either of two poten-tially destructive archetypes: Arsenicum, the fanatical perfectionist or Anacardium, the sociopath. In Ennea-type terms: Graphites, Ennea-type Nine, the carer and mediator, has inclined to either of its wing personality archetypes: Arsenicum, Ennea-type One, the arch-perfectionist, or Ana-cardium, Ennea-type Eight, the arch-bully and anti-social personality type. The anger of Graphites may be intense and can be violent, but it is short-lived and never malicious; it is mostly a controlled, repressed anger that finds expression indirectly through *passive aggression.*

These archetypal dynamics are predictable. They follow a psychically determined pattern, in which Graphites is fundamental and central. Arche-types are not fixed and static, they are dynamic and always in a state of ascent, descent or fluctuation, as one or other of the adversaries in the conflict between the soul and the ego-self gains the upper hand, or as their respective fortunes wax and wane. In the configuration of Graphites, Arsenicum and Anacardium, a close relationship is demarcated showing how the fears, anxieties and controlling perfectionism of Graphites can over time cause the archetype to transmute into a fanatical Arsenicum and how fear, anxiety and controlling repression can over time precipitate it into a destructive Anacardium state. Conversely, it is apparent that the healing of an Arsenicum or Anacardium state can archetypally lift the constitution towards Graphites. Familiarity with the Enneagram, and the nine fundamental personality types it outlines, is of inestimable value. It patterns the ego-based delusions that torment the psyche when, through lack of basic trust, the soul loses contact with its Essential or Spiritual Perspectives and views life through the warped, subjective filters of ego-based vision. These delusions fuelled by fear lie at the root of disease. According to our attunement to one or other of our lost spiritual perspectives these delusions, imaginings or misconceptions are potential and common to us all. We play out our lives on a stage set by our Ennea-type, an archetypal persuasion that constitutes our unconscious perception of reality (see *The Wolf*[1]).

Black encompasses another emotional spectrum, which belongs fully to Graphites: *sadness, depression and despair.* Mistrust of life and anxious foreboding create an archetype with a *doom and gloom* perspective. A pessimistic anticipation of misfortune, troubles and failure. The depression and despondency are often extreme: a profound melancholia – *feels miserable and unhappy.* Characteristic of the archetype, a mere triviality may plunge them into disproportionate gloom. Their anticipation of failure pertains also to their spiritual wellbeing causing religious depression: the belief that they have *sinned away their day of grace* and are beyond salvation.

- *Dejection with great heaviness of the body or of the feet.*
- *Feels unfortunate.*
- *Dwells on past disagreeable occurrences – at night; lying in bed.*
- *Despair and discouragement over trifles, worse on waking in the morning (2).*
- *Discouragement with much weeping (2).*
- *Sad and melancholic – feels he must weep – with sighing.*
- *Causeless weeping – without provocation (2).*
- *Weeping – pities himself.*
- *Weeping relieves (2).*
- *Music makes him weep (2).*
- *Indifference – no pleasure in anything (2).*
- *Suicidal disposition.*

Sadness and weeping tend to be worse during the menses; at puberty; and at the menopause.

At night, while lying in bed sleepless, their minds are haunted by tormenting and unpleasant thoughts (compare Carbo-veg; Carbo-an; Kali-carb).

Their despondency tends to be worse in the evening and their apprehension and anxiety are worse in the morning on waking – i.e. when they have to face the day.

Sadness, despondency, dejection, depression, gloom and melancholy have these modalities:

- *Evening or night in bed.*
- *At puberty (2).*
- *During menses (2).*
- *At the menopause (2).*
- *With sighing and weeping (2).*
- *About trifles (2).*
- *From music (2).*
- *With suicidal disposition.*
- *With heaviness of the body.*
- *From pressure about the heart and chest.*
- *During chill and fever – during perspiration.*
- *Ameliorated after eating.*

There is much sighing and a wretched feeling of having been singled out for misfortune. *They are filled with self-pity.*

Unfortunate: feels unfortunate; that he has been ill-used by fate, life, destiny, God; singled out for misfortune (other archetypes with the same italic grading are: *Chelidonium; China; Lycopodium; Sepia* [cuttlefish ink: another black carbon remedy]; *Staphysagria; Tabacum*).

This important rubric highlights the *disconnection from love* (Ennea-type Nine) that shapes the archetype's character and persuades them that they are unworthy and unlovable and singled out for misfortune (punishment); it also sums up their conscious or unconscious relationship with their Creator: a relationship built on fear, mistrust and being badly done by. At its root, separation from unconditional, universal love is separation and estrangement from 'God'. Held unconsciously in the Shadow, such a sense of abandonment and isolation is crippling and erosive and can culminate in malignancy, especially of the organs of creation: ovaries, uterus and breasts (Carbo animalis, Kreosotum – both carbons).

Grey

In the archetypal transition from black to dark-grey, the Graphites archetype is born. The birth is primordial, graphite being a considerable constituent of the carbonaceous dust in interstellar space: a dust that contributes, with hydrogen and helium and other supernova material, to the formation of new stars.

Grey is the colour that provides a window into the psyche of this fundamental substance.

Reflecting on Grey with the mind of a shaman reveals a wealth of analogy that elaborates and confirms our understanding of the closely-related Graphites archetype. This is a useful exercise that can be applied to all colours of the spectrum, e.g. Green and Mag-carb; Red and Ferrum; Orange and Cuprum; Yellow and Sulphur; Blue and Nat-mur. Apart from encouraging lateral thinking, communing with colour brings intuitive insight into the subtleties of chakra energy, which can be applied in practice and when analysing dreams.

Grey is first light: dawn; and last light: dusk – times of transition or change: hence, grey is also birth, puberty, menopause, death – times of Graphites power. At birth a baby's eyes are grey; it enters a grey Graphites world. Grey is also half-light or *twilight* – a time of imagination, inspiration, exaggeration and distortion, when shadows loom large and fancy is rife – the time of the poet, the author and the creative mind; time of *Pulsatilla* fear: a plump, immature, timid archetype that weeps for trivia or without cause; time of *Phosphorus* terror: an artistic, psychic archetype that fears the dark, ghosts and thunderstorms and is averse to the scent of flowers; and time of *Calc-carb* dread: an earthy, stout archetype that bustles and mothers and is enraptured by sacred music. All Graphites connections that fall into place like pieces of a mosaic – the mosaic of the materia medica – a work of art conceived in the collective unconscious.

Grey also pertains to the eerie shadows cast by the haunting half-light of the full moon, a time when imagination dwells on the fantastical, the frightening and the fiendish: time of Graphites, but also time of Arg-nit: an apprehensive archetype that suffers performance anxiety and panic attacks; time of Ars-alb: an archetype that fears death and is restlessly anxious, fastidious and controlling; time of Calc-carb: an archetype that values solitude, is beset with a legion of fears, especially of disease and is offended by the least ridicule; time of Lycopodium: an archetype that feels inferior and inadequate, fears men, flatters for favour and projects an image of strength to mask a lack of self-confidence; time of Phosphorus: an archetype that is feminine and creative and undertakes many things but perseveres with none and is easily distracted away from priorities; time of Pulsatilla: an archetype that is gentle, timid, indecisive, impressionable, feminine and feels self-pity, whose menarche is late and menses are delayed from getting the feet wet; time of Silicea: an archetype that lacks confidence, is slow to get started, but once committed stubbornly persists, cannot be stopped, and burns out; and time for the Wolf and the Raven: archetypes that guide the analyst into the darkest recesses of the psyche.

More pieces of a mystic mosaic, here, pointing to the similarities between the major 'full-moon-remedies' and Graphites, but also, in as much as they all refer to different key aspects of Graphites, highlighting the archetype's central position: its primal influence radiating outwards, like the rays of the moon, illuminating related archetypes. Graphites is essentially a feminine archetype, hence, intimately related to the full moon, Luna, and the prime archetype of the moon Argentum (silver) and its leading salt, Argentum nitricum (silver nitrate), with which it shares many social and performance fears. The moon exerts a powerful influence over the emotions and hormonal functions, hence, the Graphites modalities: worse at the full moon and worse during and after the menses and its singular affinity for the initiation of the menstrual life at puberty and its termination at menopause; all indicative of this lunar relationship. The menstrual symptoms of Graphites are violent colicky dysmenorrhoea, morning nausea and vomiting, and exhaustion. Luna has menstrual cramps with bearing down pains and, like Graphites, is better in open air and cool air.

Grey signals birth from the Void – the emergence from paradise into the first grey-light of life on Earth – an illusion that warps Reality and deludes and disconnects Graphites from unconditional, universal Love! Grey is the misty, undefined boundary or divide between dimensions: between spirit life and birth . . . between death and spirit life; between the conscious and the unconscious; between the personal and the collective unconscious. Potent junctions of transition and flux, hence, of anxiety, indecision and foreboding – the territory of Graphites. Crossroads that call for the guidance of the Divine Crone, Hekate, and the Messenger of the Gods, Hermes: deities that conduct the soul across divides and dimensions, which are embodied in the atavistic archetypes the Wolf, the Dog, the Horse, Mercurius, the sun wolf, and Lycosa, the wolf spider. All allies of Graphites, the archetype that faces the anxiety and fear of deciding and initiating change. Given appropriately, Graphites can overcome *procrastination, equivocation and indecision* and enable forward movement.

As noted, Graphites is a feminine archetype. The 4% iron that the purest graphite contains reflects the recessive or subordinate role the masculine plays in this key archetype. In mythological terms, the sacred feminine is embodied in three distinct archetypes: the Maiden or Virgin – the Woman or Mother – the Crone or Wise Woman. All three are inherent in Graphites. The archetype's influence is frequently called for at the 'grey' points of transition from one feminine form to another, especially puberty and menopause. Here, it helps emotionally and hormonally, facilitating maturation and assisting the young girl or woman move into the next stage of life confidently and creatively. At each point, it interfaces with other associated archetypes: the Maiden: Pulsatilla, Staphysagria, Cimicifuga – the Mother: Mag-carb, Calc-carb – the Crone: Calc-carb, Sepia.

Grey is a bridge between Black and White – between origin (the Void) and destination (Illumination); it encompasses the entire individuation path of the soul: confirmation of the wide compass and cardinal importance of Graphites. But, Graphites is often missed! It is a 'grey' archetype, a retiring, reticent and reclusive archetype, frequently overlooked unless it draws attention because of an exuberantly, oozing eczema, for which it is renowned. Here lies a pitfall into which many fall: no tears – cannot be Pulsatilla; no talkativeness – cannot be Lachesis; no depression – cannot be Aurum; no nastiness – cannot be Nit-ac; and no eczema or history of eczema – cannot be Graphites. All untruths on a plane where paradox persistently plays out her perversity!

Grey is the mist that clouds vision; it diffuses light and blurs focus. Descending upon the mind, 'grey' clouds the intellect, causing it to wander, grope, falter, stumble and slow to a snail's pace; feeling its way hesitantly, *at a loss for words, thoughts, ideas, recall, purpose and direction*, and exhausting itself in the process. In accord with the natural rhythm of Graphites and its affinity for transition: the mental confusion and inefficiency of the archetype are worse after sleep, on waking, after rising and in the morning, and *during and after the menses*: times peculiarly affected by Graphites. The confusion of the mind is *ameliorated by walking in the open air*, which dissipates the grey, mental haze. In the morning, the mind feels stupefied, as if intoxicated, and there may be an associated mild vertigo. Black is asleep, white is awake, grey is a state of semi-somnolence: the mind half-awake, half-asleep – sluggish, indolent, unmotivated. While black sleeps and white acts, grey sits around and does nothing. Grey and Graphites can be lazy, indolent and unmotivated!

Garnering negative connotations of Grey from tradition, provides a remarkable inventory of Graphites feelings, perceptions and behaviour, all tainted by the grey mind-set of *Psora*.

Grey is Psora: the dawn of disease: a colour and a state that embody the *lack of confidence* and *pessimistic fear of life* that typify Graphites.

Reference

1 Lilley DJ. *The Wolf – A Mythological and Comparative Study*. Glasgow: Saltire Books. 2017. pp27–31.

6

GRAPHITES – 3

Fear, Grief and Guilt

Fear

If fear has a colour, that colour is grey – as grey as the stones! Dread haunts the features and imparts an ashen hue. Being timid, anxious and sensitive by nature, Graphites invariably lives with fear. The fear that haunts them is often conjured by a negative imagination. *Grey is lack of faith,* therefore, they have a *fear of failure* and *fear of losing,* and often, like Lycopodium, would rather not try than fail or lose. They approach all aspects of their life with hesitancy, circumspection and uncertainty. Their excessive wariness, caution and indecisiveness leads to inhibition, delayed response, lack of initiative, procrastination and eventually having to face and deal with crises.

- *Fear causes weeping and weeping brings relief.*
- *Fear in the morning on waking and in bed: of death, misfortune, suffocation, insanity, business, and thunderstorm.*

We have noted their social fears, their fear of people and their specific and innate fear of men. Their severance from Cosmic Love, leaves them in a frightening world, at the mercy of an unfeeling, merciless fate. *Grey is ominous and threatening.* Their belief that they are unworthy, unlovable and singled out for misfortune, convinces them that only troubles, trials and adversity lie ahead. Hence, they *fear the future* and live with a persistent *sense of foreboding* that some mishap, calamity, or tragedy will befall them, or their loved ones.

- *Fear of the future.*
- *Fear something will happen.*
- *Fear of misfortune.*

A typical psoric fear haunts them: *fear of poverty*: the fear that they will be unable to provide for their family and themselves. This is a fundamental survival fear (Hydrogen), found also in Arsenicum, Calc-carb *Psorinum* and *Sepia* – all archetypes extremely close to Graphites. This fear may result in avarice and miserliness: an uncharacteristic thriftiness and pinch-penny attitude in an otherwise generous, caring person.

Their emotional timidity extends into the physical sphere; they are not very brave. Their pain threshold is low; hence, they *fear pain and suffering*. This makes them very cautious and careful in what they do; they avoid activities that could expose them to injury. They are especially *afraid of falling*. Always anticipating and dreading mishaps, they have a great *fear of accidents* and are very nervous drivers. Their anxious pessimism causes them to worry constantly about the welfare of their family: that they will be involved in an accident or come to some harm – *fear of losing loved ones*.

Grey is the colour of illness – the colour of mental cloudiness – the colour of Psora. Not surprisingly, Graphites *fears illness*, they are *hypochondriacs* (3). This often centres around their abdominal symptoms, which they interpret in the worst light, and their mental health: *fear of getting some dread, incurable disease* and *fear of losing their reason* – of developing senile dementia or Alzheimer's disease – of lapsing into the grey, ghastly, twilight world of insanity. Connected with these fears are *fear of old age, infirmity and dependency*. The thought of death fills them with trepidation; they fear the act of dying and the suffering it may entail, and they fear the mysterious unknown that looms beyond death. Some have doubt about their soul's welfare and *fear damnation*. Despite their fear of death and dying, Graphites is an archetype that can commit suicide rather than go through the pain and suffering of a dread disease.

Their nervous system is overwrought: *they take fright easily and are easily startled*. This is worse at night, lying in bed, when the least noise makes them fear that intruders are trying to break in. The effects of a severe fright or shock may stay with them for a lifetime (Opium). Like Phosphorus, they are *afraid of the dark, of ghosts and thunderstorms*.

Caught in a grey dimension between light and dark, they are emotionally susceptible to both and may seek sanctuary in one or the other. When stressed by the frenetic pace of life and the importunities of others, they find solace in the solitude and silence of darkness, but when they are down and prey to depression, the dark feeds their gloom and despair and the long nights of winter become intolerable. Like Stramonium and Lac-can, they may fear what the dark conceals and what the light reveals.

Having lost God, evil steps into the vacancy and becomes a predatory force which they give credence to and fear; either as an independent, autonomous force, or as a destructive influence acting through humans and especially through men – which, given history, is a just contention! *Fear of evil* is a primal psoric fear, symptomatic of loss of basic trust; induced by the superstition of the ego-self and magnified by the puritanical, psoric superego, which rules the ego by fear, forcing it to repress all that the superego deems reprehensible into the Shadow. Small wonder that when bigoted religion straight-laces the Graphites' mind, sexual fantasies rise insidiously out of the shadows to tease and torment them.

Because of its primal nature, *fear of evil* is a huge rubric, but the black letter archetypes, though few, are significant: Calc-carb; China-sulph; Kali-iod and Psorinum. Calc-carb and Psorinum are the psoric archetypes standing closest to Graphites. China-sulph and Kali-iod need to be understood in the light of the rubric. We are inclined to consult a rubric for the express purpose of selecting from the remedies listed, the one most likely to match the patient presenting with the symptom described by the rubric. If the symptom is very pronounced, we are more likely to favour and compare remedies that appear in highest grade: i.e. 'black-letter' in patient = 'black-letter' in rubric. But, we do not always ask why the archetype is there, how its essence compares with others in the rubric, or investigate the special significance of its high grading. China-sulph has two components: China and Sulphur. China is, along with Phosphorus, the most psychic, imaginative and artistically creative of archetypes. Marry this visionary psyche to Sulphur, the most unsophisticated, fundamental and super-stitious of archetypes and a rich blend of psychic awareness, credulous fantasy and superstitious fundamentalism assures that Satan is out and about, and *fear of evil* can reach obsessive levels. Kali-iod also has two components, Kali (potassium) and Iodum (iodine), and the same high grading as China-sulph, but the dynamics of the archetype are totally different. The Kali archetype rigidly observes the ideology, tradition, customs and culture of its forbears; the Iodum archetype is often scapegoated and perse-cuted for belonging to a certain nation, race or religion. Married in a molecule, these influences produce an archetype that carries in its cellular memory, in the very fibre of its being, *the knowledge that evil truly exists*, not as a superstitious fantasy or disembodied dark force, but in the form of brutal, bigoted, racist stereotypes that perpetrate acts of religious and ethnic persecution. Being a fundamental archetype, Graphites has both the fantasy-laden *psoro-tubercular fear* of China-sulph and the hard-core, prag-matic *syphilitic fear* of Kali-iod.

Fears of Graphites

- *Fears are experienced especially in the morning; or in the evening, or night, while lying in bed* (2).
- *Dark.*
- *Death* (2).
- *Dying.*
- *Suffocation – better eating* (2).
- *Disease – being incurable.*
- *Insanity – losing their reason* (2).
- *Something unfortunate will happen.*
- *Misfortune* (2).
- *Accidents* (2).
- *Confrontation.*
- *Evil – in the evening.*
- *Falling.*
- *Approach of others.*
- *People – anthropophobia.*
- *Men.*
- *Authority figures.*
- *In a crowd – socialising* (2).
- *Public speaking.*
- *Failure.*
- *Business* (2).
- *Poverty.*
- *Thunderstorm* (2).

Anxiety

A component of fear is anxiety. Grey has been described as the colour of the tortured mind, forever trying to escape from some unknown anxiety and this is so true of Graphites and its acute counterpart, Arsenicum. The Graphites mental state is dominated by *anxiety and gloomy depression.* The two emotions come together in their *foreboding of some misfortune, failure or accident.*

- *Being beside oneself with anxiety.*
- *Extreme apprehensiveness; did not know how to overcome it.*

The level of anxiety in Graphites is high and intensified by the least challenge: e.g. the risk of confrontation; having to face authority figures; or having to discipline subordinates. Their anxiety is often, therefore, *anticipation anxiety* before something they must do, intensified by negative thinking. Graphites is not listed under *performance anxiety* and it should be. Like Carbo-veg and Lycopodium, both closely related remedies, Graphites is an extremely self-conscious person, with serious social fears and dread of the limelight. The thought of *public speaking* is terrifying, an ordeal to be avoided at all costs. If faced with the inevitability of having to perform in public, Graphites can be thought of in the same light as Argentum nitricum and Gelsemium. All three tremble from anxiety, but, unlike the other two, Graphites is not inclined to develop diarrhoea from anxiety.

Anxious overeating

Many Graphites subjects respond to anxiety by overeating. Consequently, chronic anxiety and obesity are a frequent archetypal combination. A characteristic of the greedy, overweight Graphites, often differentiating them from other corpulent archetypes, is their disinterest in, or aversion to, sweet things. When present, this is a strong indication, but it must be remembered that there are some who do desire sweets. They are averse to foods that many overeaters love and indulge, but a liking for beer can be their downfall. They prefer chicken and bland foods. Their aversions are numerous: meat, fish, cooked food, salt, sweets and even soup. Distaste for salt can be a major characteristic. Some complain that hot drinks disagree with them. However, most are relieved by warm drinks and warm milk is often the best solution for stomach pain (gastralgia). Graphites is a good remedy for unusual thirst and acute and chronic gastritis after the abuse of alcoholic drinks (Phosphorus). They are usually thirsty. At times, there may be a pressing need to drink, to cool themselves internally; without true thirst. *Both their anxiety and their gastralgia necessitate eating, which brings temporary relief.* Because their hunger and greed are spurred on by anxiety, they tend to eat too much and too fast, which further aggravates their digestive problems. Graphites eats with an urgency and relish that draws the attention (Lac lupinum; Raven).

- *Anxiety ameliorated by eating.*
- *Greed, cupidity; eating*
- *Hurry, haste, while eating.*
- *Fear of suffocation relieved by eating* can be considered a strange, rare and peculiar (SRP) symptom.

The anxiety of Graphites causes restlessness; it impels them to move – from place to place – they cannot keep still (Arsenicum). The anxiety is increased by attempting close, mental work; the more focused and intensely they concentrate, the more restless they become. Their agitation is transferred to their legs, which are constantly jigging up and down or swinging from side to side, towards and away from one another.

- *Fidgety feet whilst sitting studying* (Zinc met).
- *Restlessness during mental work* (Borax, Fagopyrum, Indigo, Kali-phos, Nat-carb).
- *Restlessness whilst sitting at work* – Graphites and Ars-alb.
- *The anxiety is relieved by walking about in the open air and by warmth.*

The restless nature of their anxiety confirms the close relationship between Graphites and Arsenicum, both fastidious, controlling archetypes consumed by trivia, conservative and narrow-minded and fearful of life and death. Arsenicum has three common allotropes, or structural forms: yellow, black and metallic grey; the last two confirming the strong connection between the two archetypes. Although often needed as a chronic, constitutional remedy, Ars-alb is the acute counterpart of the carbons and of both Thuja and Mercurius, hence, a remedy that can be called for in the treatment of acute and chronic conditions of psoric, sycotic or syphilitic origin.

The anxiety of Graphites is particularly liable to encroach when they are lying in bed. Anxiety worse in the morning, on waking. This is when they dwell on their business worries and the transactions of the day. Anxiety worse in the evening in bed, with insomnia and tormenting thoughts.

Anxiety rubrics:

- *A sense of inquietude, often worse in the morning, on waking* (3).
- *Restlessness and anxiety at night – on waking in the night – driving out of bed* (2).
- *Before midnight – after midnight – 2.00 a.m.* (Ars-alb).
- *During sleep; with disturbed sleep.*
- *On waking – on waking from frightful dreams.*
- *Full of cares and worries in the evening in bed.*
- *With weeping – ameliorated by weeping* (3).
- *Driving from place to place* (2).
- *About the future.*
- *About salvation* (2).
- *Anxiety of conscience – anxiety about past actions – guilt.*
- *About trifles* (2).
- *About business.*
- *Hypochondriacal – anxiety about health – fear of incurable disease – from pains in the stomach, abdomen or head.*

- *During manual work.*
- *From sedentary life.*

Their anxiety and fear can precipitate *panic attacks* with concomitant physical symptoms.

- *Agitation, compression of the heart and anguish, as if at the point of death, or under the fear of some calamity, often with headache, vertigo, nausea, and perspiration.*
- *Great anguish and oppression, with a very disagreeable sensation in the stomach.*
- *Great anguish in the evening, as if a misfortune had happened, with heat in the face and coldness of the hands and feet.*

A sense of compression behind the sternum induces a great fear that a heart attack is imminent. He often feels as if his end is near, or as if the greatest misfortune impended. Constant tormenting thoughts of death; a presentiment of death – often feels as if his end was near, or as if threatened with the greatest misfortune.

- *Thoughts of death* (3) as intense as Aconitum.
- *Thoughts of death with sadness.*
- *Sensation of death* (2).
- *Presentiment of death* (2).

Given the intense and ongoing level of anxiety that stresses Graphites it is apparent that they have an 'ulcer personality'. This is borne out by their digestive symptoms. Graphites has cured many cases of gastric and duodenal ulceration. Their anxiety is felt in the stomach with an incessant sense of hunger and a need to eat. They are driven to eat to relieve a feeling of suffocation and a burning, gnawing in the stomach.

- *Pain in the stomach relieved by eating.*
- *Gastric pains worse from cold drinks and better by warm milk.*
- *Heartburn and acid eructations.*
- *Severe flatulence and relief from belching is as marked as in Carbo-veg.*

The dreams of Graphites are indicative of the anxiety and fears that beset the archetype. Life is an alien dimension fraught with danger and difficulty. Their conscious fears are portrayed in dream form: *dreams of misfortune, accidents and difficulties* – of striving and struggling against unequal odds. And, the emotions engendered by their dreams continue into the day that follows (Psorinum). They experience dreams related to disturbed dynamics of the psyche – the distortion of reality brought on by an ego-based perspective – and the comatose state of the Graphites soul (*dream: fainting; comatose sleep; unconsciousness*). In sleep, the eagle eye of the Graphites superego is dimmed and the repressed and inhibited libido energy finds expression in sexual dreams and conservative sobriety gives way to abandoned pleasure – *dream: carousing.*

The fundamental all-embracing nature of the Graphites archetype is emphasised by *dreams of dogs*, which are solar, and *dreams of cats*, which are lunar. The special affinity for cats is highlighted by the dream of *cats without number*, highlighting the predominantly feminine nature of the archetype. Further indication of the archetype's fundamental position in the archetypal hierarchy is revealed in *dreams of fire and water* – which, together with earth and air, represent the fundamental elements of the Creation. Water is the symbol of the unconscious mind, hence, *dreams of danger from water* points to intuitive awareness of the intense bottled and corrupted energy held in the Graphites Shadow and the inherent danger of it being projected negatively upon others, or, of its controlled, unexpressed force impacting on the emotional and physical health. Depending on their context, dreams of fire may point to destructive syphilitic energy, but positively fire is a beacon or symbol of the passion of the creative mind. Intuitive awareness of their unrealised creative and artistic capacity is revealed in: *dreams of excelling in mental work; of admirable buildings; dreams: impressive; fantastic.*

Dreams of Graphites

- *Anxious* (3) – *with anxiety ameliorated on waking* (2).
- *Frightful* (3) – *hideous* (3) – *vexatious* – *vivid.*
- *Continued after waking.*
- *Misfortune* (2).
- *Accidents* – *of fatal accidents* (3).
- *Difficulties* (2).
- *Danger.*
- *Striving.*
- *Exhausting* – *of lethargy.*
- *Dead bodies* – *of dead people.*
- *Embarrassment.*
- *Morose.*
- *Mental exertion.*
- *Business of the day.*
- *Ghosts, spectres, distorted images* (2) [unique].
- *Distorting everything* (2).
- *Events distorted* – *of previous day.*

- *Animals:*
  - *Dogs.*
  - *Cats – of cats without number [unique].*
- *Amorous – with orgasm (2).*
- *Lewd, lascivious, voluptuous (2).*
- *Carousing.*
- *Water – of danger from water (2) (Mag-carb).*
- *Fire.*
- *Excelling in mental work.*
- *Admirable buildings [unique].*
- *Impressive.*
- *Fantastic.*
- *Historic.*
- *Visionary.*
- *Fainting – of comatose sleep – of unconsciousness [all unique].*
- *Things heard, read, thought or talked about.*
- *Persistent – recurrent (2).*
- *Pleasant (2).*

The delusions or imaginings of all archetypes, like their dreams, are coloured by their anxieties, fears and perceptions; and, conversely, their fancies and dreams reveal fears and perceptions-of-self that would not otherwise be obvious. Further insights into hidden layers of the psyche can be derived from encouraging the subject of analysis to court their fancies through deliberately setting aside time before sleep, to permit their thoughts and feelings to range freely without coercion or restraint. The process should be likened to taking one's dog for a walk and at a given point (sitting alone in the dark and in quiet, unreflecting self-observation) letting it off the leash (abrogating all intellect and logic) and permitting it to run free and unin-hibited (instigating a journey of self-discovery). Keeping with the same analogy, the dog (and dogs are peculiarly significant to Graphites) will run here and there, sniffing at this and that and inevitably honouring some tree or object with special attention by cocking its leg. So, it is with the mind; it must be permitted to run at will; the owner being an observer, passively noting its circumambulations, what attracts it and where it tarries. The mind must remain impersonal, unprejudiced and non-judgemental: the internal observations being faithfully gathered without omission, even that which seems unimportant, irrelevant, unpleasant, painful or reprehensible. Such an exercise, which should always be employed if participating in a pathogenetic trial of a substance (proving), is of great assistance during homeopathic therapy and can be likened to the *free association* technique of Freud. It often provides insight into repressed, disowned and unrealised aspects of the unconscious; clarifications that are invaluable because of being un-rationalised and unfiltered by the guarded ego-self and the puritanical watchdog, the superego.

The dog analogy comes naturally to mind, since, it images the technique of the exercise and assists in executing it. The metaphor is archetypal, for the Dog archetype, like the Wolf, is a guide and conductor of souls through boundaries and dimensions. Any doubt about this connotation is allayed by consulting the rubric: *dreams of black water*, a tiny rubric where Ars-alb (2) and Lac caninum (Dog) are found. While water, in general, pertains to the emotions and the unconscious, black water alludes to the darkest, deepest and most obscure regions of the psyche: a region the homeopath must gain access to, for it contains the demons that haunt the unconscious mind and provides the therapeutic means to exorcise them. The rubric confirms the singular ability of Dog and Wolf to access this dark dimension. The presence of Ars-alb in the rubric is relevant to Graphites for the Arsenicum archetype, as previously noted, is the acute counterpart of Graphites; both share, in highest grade, fussy perfectionism and restless anxiety and both can be puritanically straight-laced and bigoted while repressing a seething, sexual prurience. Lac caninum and Graphites are also closely associated, complementary archetypes. Graphites dreams of dogs and both Graphites and Lac-can archetypally represent the C-type personality – a psyche that suffers from the *disease to please* – that cannot say "No" and sacrificially defers to others – a personality often associated with the cancer diathesis and the cancer nosode, Carcinosin.

The delusions of Graphites are informative. Graphites is not a grandiose, inflated syphilitic archetype, quite the opposite, it is rather weighed down with psoric humility, yet it may sense itself to be *a great person*. Like the dreams of *excelling in mental work* and of *admirable buildings*, this incongruous perception points to unconscious awareness of soul qualities deep to the timid, ineffectual, introverted personality erected by the superego/ego-self alliance. The perception that *everything, even the familiar, is strange* is awareness at soul level of the warped reality ego-based vision produces. The sense that *someone is in bed with them* is not a sycotic-based duality; it is awareness of the psoric birth of the ego-self within the domain of the psyche due to loss of basic trust, and the division of soul and ego-self that results. This parallel alignment is central to the dynamics of the psoric miasm.

The imaginings of Graphites reveal other key features of the Graphites mind: the sense of being singled out for misfortune by a malicious fate: *they are unfortunate*; their ever-present hypochondriasis: *they are sick and about to die*; and their pervasive sense of guilt: *they are a criminal*; their psychic sensitivity: *sees dead persons*; their imaginative, hence creative ability: *sees frightful images on closing the eyes* – an act that takes them into the grey, twilight divide between the conscious and the unconscious, indicating, besides richness of fancy, vision of corrupted energy in the darkness of their unconscious. Finally, the ubiquitous *water* theme, which ties their imaginings to their dreams of *danger from water*: danger from the contents of the unconscious – a threat that can be adulterated and expunged by the action of Graphites in dynamic form.

Delusions (misconceptions, imaginings, misapprehensions) of Graphites

- *They are a great person (2).*
- *Everything is strange (2).*
- *Familiar things are strange.*
- *Evening in bed.*
- *Assembled things, swarms, crowds.*
- *Someone in bed with them.*
- *They are a criminal.*
- *Criminals – about criminals.*
- *They are unfortunate.*
- *They are about to die.*
- *They have heart disease.*
- *They are sick.*
- *Visions on closing the eyes.*
- *Sees images, phantoms – night – on closing eyes – frightful.*
- *Sees dead persons.*
- *Fanciful.*
- *Hearing.*
- *Water (2).*

Grief

Grief is grey! Grey is the colour of the shroud, of the wraith and of ash, which, coming from the funeral pyre and the cremation oven, is associated with death, mourning and the departing soul. The association of grief and ashes is ancient: 'the Children of Israel covered their heads with ashes to give expression to the poignancy of their grief'. 'Earth to earth, ashes to ashes, dust to dust' is the intonation of the priest as the bereaved cast earth upon the coffin of the newly deceased.

Grief is often a major causative influence in the history of the Graphites archetype and it tends to become persistent and long-lasting. Their grief is a potent cause of suffering; it is inconsolable and casts a shadow over their lives. Their tears bring relief, but not recovery.

A common response to intense, deep-seated grief or bereavement is to give Ignatia or Natrum muriaticum, and often they are of great assistance, but where they fail to bring a satisfactory conclusion, Graphites should be considered. In grief, Graphites must be compared with Ambra grisea; Aurum; Causticum; Cocculus; Helleborus; Ignatia; Lachesis; Nat-mur; Phos-ac; Staphysagria (all 3). Graphites, the 'little grey archetype' (1), having the lowest grading, is likely to be missed, unless eczema is a concomitant feature. But, grief must be regarded as a major indication for Graphites.

Relentless, helpless, self-pitying, determined grief points to Graphites. There is much *sighing and weeping*, which temporarily gives them a sense of relief, but unlike Pulsatilla, *their tears and sighs are not a solicitation*; they are not attention-seeking; they do not welcome consolation; they shun society and would rather be left alone in their misery. The sadness and weeping are affected by their hormonal cycle, being worse during the menstrual flow or if their menstruation is delayed. If the cause of the grief occurred in the years of puberty or menopause, this must be regarded as an added indication for Graphites. *The grief is personalised* (Nat-mur): the experience and heartache are peculiar and exclusive to them; no one else has ever been so singled out for such awful suffering. They feel most unfortunate, badly done by and deeply sorry for themselves. Words of comfort and encouragement are resisted, or resented, and wise counselling evokes a superficial response, which proves short-lived; once the supporting influence is removed, they visibly relax and sink back into the quicksand of their grief, giving the impression that they prefer this over the effort and change of perspective needed to extricate themselves from its grip. Their default mode is emotional inertia!

The 'death' that bereaves may be the death of a relationship or marriage rather than the passing of a loved one. Grey is the colour of the long-term partnership or marriage in which the fire in the conjugal hearth has burnt out and not even glowing embers remain, only ash; a situation that often coincides with menopause. Graphites is primarily a woman's remedy; the archetype, female or male, presents with a dominantly feminine energy. Starved of love, respect and empathy and partnered with a patriarchal, chauvinistic archetype (such as Lycopodium), Graphites has lost her joy, her self-esteem, her lubrication and her libido. Being Graphites, she hangs onto the grey, miserable status quo. Eventually, he moves on, possibly into the arms of someone else. Graphites is devastated and despite their history and her unhappiness, feels rejected, unwanted and unlovable, finds reason to blame herself for the rift and imagines herself heartbroken. She clings to whatever vestiges remain of the relationship without respect or care for herself. Graphites can free her from dependency, give her the resolve to start a new life, the confidence to reinvent herself and find a creative, healing outlet.

Graphites is a remedy for grief due to the loss of a beloved pet, be it a dog or a cat. As noted, they have a special affinity for cats and often dream of them.

- *Dreams of animals.*
  - ○ *Of dogs.*
  - ○ *Of cats.*
    - § *Of cats without number.*

And, remember: *All cats are grey in the dark!*

This is an adage that first appeared in a book of proverbs written by John Heywood in 1546, notated as: '*When all candles be out, all cats be grey.*'

The expression was used by Benjamin Franklin in 1745 in a letter of advice he wrote to a young man regarding his best choice of mistress. After counselling the young man to rather marry and settle down, Franklin goes on to recommend that if, however, he decides to remain fancy-free, he should, in all his amours, *prefer old women to young ones.* Supporting this advice, he cites several reasons: older women are world-wise, knowledge-able and converse agreeably; they are more caring and attentive, more prudent and discreet, more sexually practiced and 'there is no hazard of children'. He further justifies his contention by asserting that 'in all animals that walk upright', the ravages of time beset first the upper body – the face, the neck, the breast – 'the lower parts continuing to the last as plump as ever . . . *and as in the dark all cats are grey*' – the sexual pleasure to be derived from consorting with an older woman 'is at least equal, and frequently superior – every knack being by practice capable of improvement'.

Given the apposition of cats and grey in the saying, does this tongue-in-cheek, sexist missive, disclose an archetypal Graphites pattern? Certainly, the writer expresses Lycopodium sentiments; Lycopodium and Graphites are closely related archetypes; and cats and grey certainly belong to Graphites. But, is there a pattern, and if so, what is it?

Graphites is a feminine archetype, therefore, the archetypal pattern pertains not to the man, but to the woman in the anecdote. Turn the tale around and it is the mature, experienced peri-menopausal woman, who chooses to take a young man as lover and reignite her languishing libido with his youthful passion and potency. The paradox of certain Graphites women is their patent sexual inertia, loss of sexual desire and aversion to sex (Sepia) – born of miasmatic, constitutional inheritance, disenchantment with men, a bad marriage, hormonal changes after childbirth and the jading effect of domestic life (Sepia) – and yet, the concealed presence of a reservoir of latent, sexual energy that may stir and seek fulfilment in midlife when the children have left home (Sepia). Circumstances, opportunity and attraction will determine whether this happens or remains a wishful fantasy, for often, an imbedded Graphites conservatism and hesitancy must first be overridden. With apathy, indecision and reserve set aside and the primordial, propagating drive of carbon prompting her, Graphites can rediscover her youth and sensuality, surprising herself and her younger partner.

But, such scenarios carry a risk of ever-increasing attachment and dependency, which, given the circumstances of the woman and her lover, their age-difference and the selfish fickleness of young men, must lead to disappointment, heartache and *grief*!

A mature, attractive woman with grown-up children has a considerably older husband she both admires and respects, but their sexual relationship has long since petered-out and become platonic. Now, he has a disease that has rendered him infirm and dependent. She meets a young man and a strong attraction matures into a clandestine and intense love-affair. She benefits greatly from the liaison; it stimulates and vitalises her, releases a sexual ardour she has never known and compensates for the sacrifices she must make in caring for her handicapped husband; but, she is torn apart by it – torn between gratification and guilt! Her husband's health takes a turn for the worse and as his end approaches, so her own 'loss of grace' looms ever more reproachfully and incriminatingly over her. *Anxiety of conscience* besets her, giving her no peace. In despair, she abruptly breaks off the relationship and devotes herself exclusively and sacrificially to nursing her dying husband. He dies, and she adds the grief of his death to the grief of her lost love; a love she can never retrieve because of the cherished memory of her husband and her uncompromising guilt at having betrayed him. Thus, two inveterate emotions of Graphites – *grief and guilt* – become entwined, taking away all joy and hope.

This Graphites history is a collage taken from real lives and events; the details may differ, but the archetypal theme is the common denominator: a theme that presents, with variations, in homeopathic practice. Yet, unless the heroine is a lady of ample proportions and has a history of exuberant eczema, Graphites is unlikely to be thought of.

Conium (poison hemlock) is another archetype that in midlife benefits emotionally and physically from an active and fulfilling sex life; grieves the loss of a sexual partner; and may be prey to a combination of grief and guilt.

The theme also makes one think of Sepia, an archetype, which, being prepared from the carbon-rich, grey-black ink of the cuttlefish, shares many characteristics with Graphites. The affinity between the two is affirmed by Sepia's archetypal connection with *grey-eyed* Athene, the Greek Goddess of Wisdom, the Strategy of War and the Arts and Crafts. Athene wears an aegis, or shield, adorned with the severed head of Medusa, a hideous woman with a tangled mass of venomous snakes for hair, whose visage was so horrifying that any 'man' who gazed upon it was instantly turned to stone: its hatred of men analogous to the male antipathy of Sepia and Graphites, and its appearance very Sepia-like with its eight arms writhing around a parrot-beaked mouth. The cuttlefish has enormous eyes relative to its size. Large eyes are considered a sign of wisdom: the prime attribute of the goddess Athene and her totem bird, the Owl, whose large eyes are rendered more conspicuous by its feathered facial discs. The grey, wraith-like bird silently sweeping through the shadows in the eerie light of the moon is the owl. Grey is the colour of the owl, of Sepia and of Graphites – the colour associated with age and wisdom – and the colour sacred to grey-eyed Athene, Goddess of Wisdom.

Wisdom is silver-grey and possesses the following connotations, all of which relate to the higher Graphites.

- Secure, stable, reliable.
- Intelligent.
- Mature.
- Experienced.
- Wise.
- Staid, sober, serious, grave.
- Modest.
- Humble.
- Conservative.
- Prudent and judicious.
- Unprejudiced.
- Just.
- Impersonal.
- Transpersonal.
- Venerable.

Guilt

Guilt is grey, and guilt is *Psora*, just as shame is *Sycosis*. Graphites easily takes on guilt even when innocent and even when they are the one being exploited or wronged. It may start with Christian indoctrination that imprints the young Graphites mind with the warped concept of original sin. But, even without such brainwashing, the archetype has an innate tendency to find themselves wanting and guilty of error or omission (Psorinum; Carcinosin; Alumina; Ars-alb; Chelidonium; Digitalis; Nat-mur; Staphysagria; Sulphur). They are forever blaming themselves for anything that goes amiss. Guilt shadows them because of their painstaking scrupulousness and their hair-splitting analysis of every word and action, no matter how trifling the circumstances. They are extremely conscientious and constantly dissatisfied with their efforts and what they achieve. They always anticipate that their endeavours will end in mediocrity or failure and this may instil a sense of guilt even before they make a start. Being overcritical of themselves, they are also overcritical of others; they can never relax and accept things as they are; they must always fuss and fret. This engenders great anxiety and such a sense of guilt and failure that *they feel like a criminal*. Typical of Graphites, this is all without realistic cause.

• *Anguish and hurry chase them around like a criminal.*

As Hering states: "A desperate state of mind!"[1]

Eventually, their anxiety and guilt may take on a religious slant, with fear for their salvation and fear of evil, which becomes a tangible force in their lives, capable of doing them harm, conspiring their downfall and damnation. These are fears of an unsophisticated, gullible mind. They point to other traits of Graphites: their impressionability and defenceless *vulnerability*. Like grey, a hue which is often thought of as colourless, they can be easily persuaded towards either white or black; they lack a discriminating mind of their own. In this light, grey signifies qualities previously sought after by the Church and by Victorian society and particularly commended in the raising of refined young girls: *innocence with ignorance* – ingredients for manipulation, seduction and disaster! At another level, grey represents *intelligence without illumination*: a combination that leaves the soul prey to the arrogance and machinations of the ego-based intellect.

Ash is Grey made manifest; it is symbolic not only of grief and mourning, but also of mortality, repentance and penance. Ash symbolises sin, or spiritual guilt, and is used as a sign of repentance for such guilt. The liturgical use of ash originated in Old Testament times. The ritual of repentance and supplication for forgiveness of sins was enacted by the penitent clothing themselves in coarse sackcloth and bestrewing themselves with ashes. The Church honours this ritual by using ashes to mark the beginning of the penitential season of Lent, when the faithful remember their mortality and mourn for their sins. On Ash Wednesday, the priest blesses ashes made from the burned palm branches distributed on the Palm Sunday of the previous year and 'imposes' them on the forehead of the observant, making the sign of the cross and intoning: 'Remember you are dust and to dust you shall return' or 'Turn away from sin and be faithful to the Gospel.'

These words evoke resonance in the ingenuous, self-effacing, self-denigrating heart and mind of Graphites: willing receptacles for humility and guilt. Assimilated once a year and reinforced through the sacrament of confession, the doctrine of sinful transgression is insinuated not only in the conscious mind, but far more significantly and deleteriously at the unconscious causative level of being. Imbedded belief can defy intellectual refutation, and, when invoked by stress or the passing of years, instil anxiety and contrition in the most logical mind. The delusion of having sinned away their day of grace with no hope of absolution, rests heavily on their conscience; death and its consequences loom before them, large and fearful – the ultimate and 'most horrible' misfortune of Graphites – an anguish voiced by the ghost of Hamlet's father.

> Cut off even in the blossoms of my sin,
> Unhousel'd, disappointed, unanel'd.
> No reckoning made, but sent to my account
> With all my imperfections on my head;
> O, horrible! O, horrible! Most horrible![2]

In the past, Lent was a sombre, stern and bleak period (all grey Graphites words); a time of sobriety and abstinence during which the pleasures of life were abnegated in favour of devotion to repentance, penance and purification. To this day, as a gesture of atonement, various self-imposed restrictions are applied for the forty days prior to Easter: one of the most common being: *refraining from eating sweets*. One of the strange, rare and peculiar characteristics of Graphites is the paradoxical aversion for sweets and deserts in an overweight, insatiably hungry archetype, given to comfort binging! The materia medica unerringly chronicles archetypal ideological behaviour!

Other negative aspects of Grey and Graphites

- The 'little grey man' or the 'plain Jane': insignificant, featureless, colourless, devoid of personality or charisma – overlooked, disregarded, neglected – often passed-over by the homeopath!
- Lack of drive, ambition, motivation, persistence, focus or endurance.
- Unrealised potential.
- Humility, diffidence, self-effacing, self-abnegation.
- Grey lacks enthusiasm and commitment, it symbolises indifference, apathy, boredom, indolence.
- Grey is a simile for *'dull sobriety'*, hence, austerity, asceticism, abstinence, fasting, self-denial, renouncing worldly pleasures.
- Puritanical, moralistic.
- Grey is conventional, straight-laced, 'stick-in-the-mud', prim, prudish, narrow-minded, over-conservative, over-respectable, correct, proper, formal, stuffy, out-of-date.
- The recluse or hermit; the monastic life.
- A bleak perspective – a bleak view of life – life is grey, drab, dreary, colourless, insipid, flat, toneless, without meaning.
- A philosophy of insufficiency: *psoric poverty consciousness* – the belief that there is never going to be enough – 'I won't get it today – I may get it tomorrow – but, tomorrow never comes'.

Grey, neither black nor white, *sits on the fence* between the two, symbolising *indecision, irresolution, hesitancy* (key characteristics of Graphites) – dilemma and quandary – the crossroads in life where critical decisions need to be made and trust, courage and decisiveness waver. Grey lacks a vantage point: lacks a clearly-defined vision of its purpose, direction and goal. Its viewpoint is diffused or split in two: a wavering state between poles. Asked who they support, they cannot give a black or white answer, or they will simply support the underdog, or the side that wins.

Being neither black nor white racially can mean feeling different, inferior, a half-caste, a mongrel, a mutt – not belonging, unwanted and rejected. Where such feelings are expressed or repressed, Graphites must be considered. Grey is the colour of discrimination and rejection; abuses to which the Graphites archetype is frequently exposed.

For the impressionable Graphites archetype with its innate, grey, psoric heritage, growing up in a *'grey environment'* can impinge severely on the psyche. Think of Dickensian London, the world of Oliver Twist: the orphanages, the workhouses and the factories belching grey-black smoke into grey leaden skies and incessant rain drizzling onto grey cobblestones; and today, think of the slums, ghettos and informal townships of the great cities, where life is largely wretched, sordid and impoverished: a fighting-privation, hand-to-mouth existence with little or no opportunity for betterment. This can be the desolate, grey world of Graphites, as it can of Psorinum, Anacardium and Lac caninum. But, take this bleak imagery into a grey, loveless home in an affluent suburb – a home devoid of harmony, care and empathy, where the parents are cold and aloof, or constantly at loggerheads, or where the family is ruled by an autocratic father or mother, who lays down the law and gives children no voice – and, a drear setting, designed to mould a Graphites is in place: a setting from which a blighted psyche, with an inherent fear of men (the male principle), emerges.

References

1   Hering C. *The Guiding Symptoms of our Materia Medica.* Volume 5. New Delhi: B Jain Publishers Pvt. Ltd., 2005. p441.
2   Shakespeare W. *Hamlet.* Oxford: Oxford University Press, 1968. Act I Scene V, lines 76–80. p79.

7

GRAPHITES – 4

Captivity – Anger – Labile Emotions

Captivity

Dark Grey, a shade indicative of Graphites, is a colour associated with *captivity*, actual or metaphorical. It signifies loss of freedom, incarceration and imprisonment or a state of 'clipped wings'. A condition of bondage in which the subject is trapped or 'caged' with no escape, possibly an 'end-of-the-line' scenario in which options no longer exist. Inevitably, the image of a bad marriage or abusive relationship comes to mind; a situation from which Graphites, like Staphysagria, often cannot, or will not, extricate themselves. It can equally apply to a work situation in which, regardless of ability and experience, a 'ceiling' has been reached with no hope of improvement and yet responsibility and accountability remain high. When discrimination – age, gender, looks, race or religion – is the cause of thwarted progress, Graphites may be called for.

The captivity of Graphites may be self-induced. The anxiety generated when confronted by choices and the need for decision-making can be allayed by adopting routines or committing to a system or convention, which they can slavishly follow, rather than having to think, and, especially, rather than having to exercise choice. Graphites easily slips into automaton-mode, moving mindlessly along a predetermined groove furrowed by fear, need and habit. The soul is anaesthetised and pushed aside, at the mercy of the engrained tendencies of a *Psora*-oppressed ego-self. The danger lies in the system they espouse; their need for a haven may submerge them in the doctrines of a cult or religious sect, make them an inflexible tool of bureaucracy, or the pawn of a brutal and repressive regime.

They are captives of habit; habits adopted to enable them to forget themselves and escape from essentials. They can surrender their attention through addiction to alcohol or recreational drugs and by numbing themselves to the realities of life through non-creative activities such as gossip, idle conversation, computer games, internet surfing, trashy novels, escapist entertainment, food, casual sex, excessive sport and specious religious and philosophical notions. They may have a diverse range of means by which they sidestep priorities; some may be intrinsically valid, but in the event, are not authentic, because they are deployed by Graphites with the express motive of easing into automatic mode, blocking out what is central and important and diverting effort into fruitless pastime. Their flight is always away from essentials towards the inessential.

They are captives of the past. They hold onto memories with a determination that lends them a charged existence. Grief, guilt and anger are typical examples of inveterate emotions that so monopolise the mind that they shoulder aside awareness of the present. In like manner, *they are captives of the future,* their minds preoccupied with dread forebodings about what may lie ahead. Cluttered with elements of the past and the future, their minds cannot focus efficiently on the present, which they persistently evade by becoming *captives of the trivial and the inessential.*

They are captives of relationships. Having lost psychic contact with the unconditional, loving nature of the Universe and perceiving themselves as unloved and unlovable, Graphites has a pressing need for a loving, intimate relationship. In their unconscious desire to emulate the Cosmic Concept they are specially attuned to and have lost awareness of, the love they bring to bear on their chosen partner mimics the unconditional nature of universal love. The love of the Universe – the love of the Creator for the created – is pervasive and all encompassing, therefore, in manner true, Graphites wishes to totally merge with their partner: to take on their beloved's life as their own, without desiring to manipulate, dominate or derive profit from them. Typically, they are better able to generate energy and enthusiasm for a partner's needs and interests than for their own. An intimate relationship or loving friendship is often the stimulus needed to encourage Graphites out of their inertia, but, unfortunately, not out of their soul-slumber, which ever-deepens. Their focus is so intensely centred on the other, and away from themselves (*self-forgetting*), that they come to identify fully with their beliefs, opinions and desires, and, in so doing, surrender their own personal point of view and with it: their self-determination. They know their partner far better than they know themselves, and, in such depth, that they sense them as an integral part of themselves. This is the consummation of an ardent, unconscious wish: to find and merge with a 'soul mate', who can become their motive for living. The union is aided by the archetype's fine-attunement to 'others' feelings and emotions: a clairsentience signalled by the electrical and heat conductivity of graphite. The identification with 'the other' can be so complete that they feel their drives, doubts and dilemmas within themselves.

Being subsumed by another's life is a state of abject, invalidating captivity. Despite its seemingly altruistic, egoless guise this self-impoverishment is an intensely ego-driven response to the unrelenting pressure of the superego to sacrifice self and remain low-profile: grey, insignificant and invisible. This is the psychic equivalent of avoiding an imperative – the individuation of the soul, in favour of the non-essential – the destiny of another. Graphites cannot be their 'brother's keeper'!

The stimulating need for such a special, all-encompassing partnership is so crucial to their ego-wellbeing that, without it, they experience psychic numbness – or inertia – which they may mask by moving indiscriminately and promiscuously from one relationship to another or by typically investing their unfulfilled energy in superficial, inconsequential pursuits; disguising from themselves and others their neglect of pressing priorities.

Another dynamic, which, in the light of the above, appears paradoxical, but is true to the grey in-between, fence-teetering posture of Graphites, is the coupling of the intense desire to merge with another with the equally insistent urge to remain independent: to fight against the desire to be subsumed in their partner's identity and to rebel against their preferences and priorities: a push and pull contention that is so characteristic of the ambivalent inner-world of Graphites, yet, most often belied by an outer semblance of calm.

Two serious consequences stem from the Graphites need to merge or bond so dependently with another. Firstly, the inability to let go of such a relationship even in the face of great abuse, suffering and unhappiness and even when being counselled and supported by family and friends. To contemplate breaking free is like thinking of severing off a vital part of their being. This procrastination is aggravated by their characteristic indecisiveness and fear of the future. Secondly, the intense, inconsolable grief they experience when their partner is lost through bereavement, betrayal or abandonment. Graphites must always be remembered when loss of a loved one, human or animal (often a cat), results in protracted grief or when life-changing grief results from disappointed, unrequited or rejected love.

In the Graphites psyche, the *captive* symbolism of Dark Grey and the *control* symbolism of Black are united, indicating the relentless vigour with which the Graphites superego and ego-self repress (incarcerate) all that they cannot accept, resolve or realise into the Shadow of the unconscious. Dark Grey also points to the constitutional inertia of the archetype, which prevents them from fulfilling their considerable potential, and their resigned mediocrity: the grey, indeterminate state between excellence and failure. Sometimes the captive state is not analogous, but frighteningly real. Graphites is a remedy for survivors of imprisonment and for those who have been held hostage and have lived in the chill, grey hinterland between life and death, never knowing whether they will survive. Graphites would have helped heal the emotional wounds of many released from the Nazi concentration camps at the end of World War II.

Graphites has a marked affinity for the feline archetype, both large or small. My visits to London zoo as a youngster were always marred by the distressing sight of the great cats behind bars, pacing restlessly and ceaselessly, back and forth, across the width of their cold, featureless prisons, mindlessly following the same path time and time again. Graphites, captive in their anxiety and fear, like Ars-alb, are driven to constantly move: *anxiety driving from place to place.*

Grey anger

Grey anger is inert anger – *anger that has been repressed, or anger that has 'gone to sleep'* – anger not overtly communicated, but bottled-up or expressed through *passive aggression*!

Repressed anger

Graphites finds making choices difficult, even traumatic, and decisions delayed, or put on hold, may lead to situations deteriorating to crisis proportions. *Graphites knows well enough what they don't want, but not what they do want.* The inherent problems, frustrations and worries resulting from such equivocation and procrastination, often fuelled by the pressure, expectations and impatience of others and their own sense of inadequacy and guilt, may build to such a pitch that an outburst of anger results – *sometimes of violent proportions.* Astonishing, in such a mild, gentle, meek disposition.

Graphites is a very stubborn archetype (Calc-carb) and behind their stubbornness lies *very deep anger*: anger at not being heard and not receiving attention; anger from fear of separation and estrangement; anger at having to follow the dictates of others and anger at being overlooked if they do not comply. To assume a definite position may alienate others and result in their being abandoned or rejected, or, conversely, it may result in their having to submit to the devices and control of others; both, consequences abhorrent to Graphites, hence, they remain stubbornly undecided and uncommitted. Their stubbornness is entwined with their indecisiveness and their inertia. Instead of coming to a decision and working towards a solution that will resolve anger, they stubbornly make no decision, stubbornly hold onto their anger, stubbornly continue to comply while remaining internally divided and nursing resentment (*dwells on past disagreeable occurrences*). Their anger steadily mounts.

Consideration of the Enneagram points to the core of the dichotomy responsible for their anger. Graphites, an Ennea-type Nine personality is positioned at the apex of the inner triangle of the Enneagram with one foot grounded in the terrain of Ennea-type Three: a personality built to achieve an admired image, conform with convention and win approval and the other foot in the terrain of Ennea-type Six, a personality that seeks identity by kicking against authority. Thus, Graphites is caught in an inner conflict of wanting to comply and earn the approval of others and wanting to disobey and break free from control. The conflict is exacerbated by the influence of their wing archetypes: Ennea-type One, exemplified by Arsenicum, the perfectionist puritan; and, Ennea-type Eight, exemplified by Anacardium, the rebellious reprobate. Graphites stands irresolute between the 'goodies' (white) and the 'baddies' (black) of the Enneagram and because of fear, guilt, stubborn indecisiveness and inertia, there it remains, seemingly placid, mild and phlegmatic (grey), but a repository of unexpressed, frustrated emotion (red: Ferrum). Without resolution, the contentious energy pools in anger!

In this state of featureless, emotional stalemate, Graphites must be compared with Alumina, an impressionable archetype that like the clay it composes awaits the conditioning hand of fate to sculpt its identity, rather than forging its own, and, in consequence, unconsciously smoulders with anger and hatred at the imposition: emotions that threaten to break free at the sight of a knife or sharp object that could be used to stab, cut and mutilate!

The anger of Graphites is slow to surface. They tend to hold onto unexpressed anger until a critical level of irritation is reached. When the cause of their anger arises from the behaviour of others, the final outburst is usually the culmination of many years of holding back, bottling-up and repressing their emotions; an internalisation that causes deep-seated stress. Some, will always remain silent with serious repercussions to their physical and emotional health.

Being a typical C-type personality, Graphites first sees mitigating reasons for why the other person has behaved as they have. Not only must they not take up space, make waves or importune others, they deny themselves the right to feel or express anger. By nature, they are impressionable and yielding and can easily be persuaded by the explanations, excuses and arguments of others. Even when deeply offended or hurt, they are more inclined to exonerate the other person's utterances and actions than condone their own anger and resentment. They weigh all aspects of the situation, often placing their own interests last, and it is only after much inner wrestling that they come to full realisation that they have been misused or exploited. Even then, a considerable time, typified by sullen introversion, may elapse before the explosive outburst follows; an outburst that in its violence shocks those who are accustomed to the usually phlegmatic behaviour of Graphites. The showdown and emotional explosion prove cathartic. Like their tears, the release of anger brings great relief to Graphites: the exhilarating satisfaction of an essential need.

- *Angers easily* (2).
- *Anger from interruption.*
- *Anger violent* (2).
- *Rage, fury.*
- *Violence, vehemence – morning.*
- *Anger expressed ameliorates.*

This may be termed *red anger*; its source seated in the iron content of mineral graphite. But, this is a rare occurrence for the Graphites archetype. Their anger is usually expressed indirectly through passive aggression – *grey anger* – which despite its apparent 'inertia' is charged with resentment; it is vindictive and retaliatory.

Passive aggression

While Graphites may not know what they want, they know, well-enough, what others want, therefore, to employ their anger, they simply move into stubborn, resistant mode and either go slow, drop their standard of performance, neglect responsibilities or avoid doing what is expected of them. They become negative, oppositional, obstructive, stubborn and sullen, with intent to frustrate and thwart the other person. This kind of anger is neither black or white; it is *grey anger*! It is roundabout and devious. It may be solely non-assertive, passive resistance, but may also be a carefully veiled vindictive act, that can be termed *catty*: a subtle hostility that stealthily attempts to annoy, hurt or upset. Being catty is being feline and feminine, and Graphites is both: *dreams of cats without number* – a unique archetypal dream that identifies the dreamer! Whereas red anger is '*pistols at dawn*', grey anger is '*handbags at dawn*'. Graphites shares characteristics with both the Lac caninum and Lac felinum archetypes.

Often, those who rely on passive aggression to express their grievances are of an ambivalent nature; like Graphites, tending to waver indecisively between one course of action and another: an uncertain path that leads to clashes with others and frustration and dissatisfaction with themselves. They may hover in a grey area torn between dependency and self-assertion. Such individuals may have grown up in a Graphites environment in which it was not safe to express frustration or anger and forbidden feelings were repressed, denied or channelled through passive aggression. Later in life, this becomes their default way of defending themselves or attacking others, while keeping themselves, and their anger, grey and inconspicuous. To achieve this, Graphites may employ the *silent treatment*: deliberately ignoring the other person by not acknowledging their presence or not responding to their comments. Typical of Graphites is the inconsistency of this behaviour. By keeping the passive aggression random, unpredictable and seemingly 'accidental', Graphites keeps the other person guessing as to whether the snub is deliberate or not. Similarly, Graphites may use *subtle insults* to get at the one they are hostile to. They may offer a compliment and then twist it into a veiled insult by negatively comparing the virtue or achievement they have just extolled with someone else's even superior attainment. Graphites also uses *mocking sarcasm* (3) to undermine the authority or confidence of someone they feel inferior to. When the subject of their sarcasm reacts, the jibe is cushioned by the quick, dismissive rejoinder: "Don't take me seriously, I was only joking".

The inertia and passive aggression of Graphites also manifests as *sullenness*: a subtly grumpy, sulky, sour, moody demeanour that removes them from the general tone of the moment and acts as a damper on proceedings (*peevish irritability* [3]). Comments, remarks or questions are responded to in a somewhat negative vein. Jokes fail to elicit a smile or move them to share the hilarity of the moment. When drinks are offered, they settle for water; when food is served, they have little appetite; when others dance, they sit-out; during conversation, they have little to say – so, they make themselves felt: a heavy presence that weighs on others without them knowing why. They are more inclined to find reason for complaint and criticism than for satisfaction (extremely *censorious and critical* [2], *displeased with everything*). *Stubbornness* is also a sign of Graphites passive aggression; a stubbornness that, even when soundly-based, is deliberately employed to hinder, annoy and punish others. They also express their, otherwise silent, grievance by not helping, neglecting responsibilities, going slow on a job and failing to finish required tasks (*undertakes many things, perseveres in nothing*). A particularly telling way of expressing passive aggression is by withholding sex from their partner; this can be so powerful a motive in a Graphites woman that they utterly extinguish their libido: an implosion that impedes the flow of the Id and must impinge on health.

Philip Bailey provides a graphic picture of the sulky moodiness of the female Graphites, which he likens to that of Pulsatilla.[1] She becomes moody and discontented when she feels unloved or unappreciated, and, like Pulsatilla and many Sepias, she is unable to hide her feelings. She becomes withdrawn, sulky and surly and broods over her grievances, surrounding herself, and others, with a heavy, dark cloud. When approached, she denies that anything is wrong and answers reluctantly in monosyllables. She avoids eye contact, turns away her face and just sits alone, submerged in self-pity and finds solace and relief in tears. Although she is not amenable to sympathy or consolation, if ignored, she may express her seething emotions by noisy activity, petulantly giving voice to her feelings by banging doors, stomping around, clattering utensils and cutlery, until she receives attention or defuses her anger. Such outbursts are like those of Staphysagria, Nat-mur, Sepia and Ignatia.

This behaviour exemplifies their passive aggression, which is typical of a generally timid, gentle nature that is, however, very sensitive, easily offended and frustrated, yet fears conflict and confrontation. They compensate for their unexpressed anger by displacing it into noise production and aggression towards objects (Staphysagria). Anger that she cannot and dare not express directly, she expresses indirectly.

Peevish irritability is the common, overt form of Graphites anger and is attended by a *desire for solitude*. In typical Graphites style, the irritability most often centres around trifles, or is without any obvious cause or reason. Curiously, they can lapse into peevish irritability after sex – as if, for a transient moment, they have been transported away from reality, and, after orgasm, are dumped back into the bleak, grey life they fear; the resentment they feel at the return being directed against their partner. Alternatively, the irritability may be a reaction against the intimacy they have permitted despite unspoken grievances, or an unconscious, attempt to dissuade future overtures.

The peevish irritability of Graphites has certain characteristics:

- *In the morning (when having to face the day).*
- *In children – morose, cross, fretful after eating.*
- *From any disturbance or interruption – would like to be alone – every disturbance irritates them.*
- *When spoken to.*
- *With impatience and intolerance.*
- *Due to being critical and displeased with everything.*
- *During headache.*
- *After eating.*

- *After stool.*
- *After sex.*
- *At trifles.*
- *Causeless.*

Graphites is by nature emotionally sensitive, easily offended and highly critical – all ingredients that can make them abrupt, rude, insolent, quarrelsome, irritable and angry. Most remain passive in their aggression, but those that are quick to anger are just as quick to recover. However, under the surface, they may continue to nurse a grievance.

- *Ailments from anger.*
- *Dwells on past disagreeable occurrences.*
- *Thoughts persistent – haunted by unpleasant subjects.*

Grey – changeable moods

Grey is indeterminate and ill-defined; a colour that is drawn to both black and white or wavers in-between. Graphites, the grey archetype, is emotionally affected by the time of day, particularly the grey transitional hours of dawn and dusk when the world is emerging from or receding into black. Caught between poles and drawn to either one or the other, Graphites experiences different moods in the morning as opposed to the evening.

- *Apprehensive and distressed in the morning; excited even unduly elated in the evening, with extreme activity of the mind, keeping him awake until midnight.*
- *Slow of thought and weakness of the mind with sadness in the morning; excited, hurried and exhilarated in the evening.*
- *Irritable and passionate in the morning; in the evening hypochondriacal.*
- *Inclination to laugh, alternating with despair and grief.*
- *Hysteria.*
- *Aggravation from grief and sorrow, particularly towards evening; timidity and irritability towards morning.*

Their emotions are labile, changeable and alternate between extremes. One moment happy and one moment sad. One moment sure of her course of action, the next in doubt, vacillating and procrastinating and driving herself to despair.

Reference

1 Bailey PM. *Homeopathic Psychology – Personality Profiles of the Major Constitutional Remedies*. Berkeley CA: North Atlantic Books, 1995. pp72–73.

8

GRAPHITES – 5

Soul Somnolence – Hesitancy – The Mundane

The Grey of the 'asleep soul' – loss of unconditional love

In Enneagram terms,[i] Graphites is an Ennea-type Nine, an archetype that has lost the Cosmic Concept of Universal Unconditional Love: the knowledge that all that exists is unconditionally loving and beneficent and that we are all an expression of that love. The loss of this most critical facet of basic trust induces the *specific delusion* that afflicts Graphites: the perception that *love is localised and conditional* rather than boundless and unconditional. Given human behaviour and the relentless processes of the material plane, universal, unconditional love is a concept particularly difficult to hold in consciousness. Hence, all Ennea-types are liable to suffer this limiting misconception, but in Ennea-type Nine archetypes, such as Graphites, Mag-carb and Lac lupinum, it forges the very core of the ego-self or personality. If one does not perceive love everywhere – in everything – always and under all circumstances – then one is disconnected from it and observing reality through subjective filters. One is also disconnected from the love that is the Essence of one's own Being.

Graphites loses what is termed *non-conceptual positivity* by AH Almaas:[ii] happiness derived from suspending all comparisons, judgements and

---

i The Enneagram of Personality, or simply the Enneagram is a description of the human psyche, which is principally understood and taught as a typology of nine interconnected personality types.

For a fuller explanation see Lilley DJ. *The Wolf – A Mythological and Comparative Study*. Glasgow: Saltire Books, 2017. p27–31.

ii AH Almaas is the pen name of A. Hameed Ali, an author and spiritual teacher who writes about and teaches an approach to spiritual development informed by modern psychology and therapy which he calls the Diamond Approach. See: https://www.diamondapproach.org/ Retrieved 14.03.2018.

opinions and perceiving reality to be permeated with Cosmic Consciousness, and, therefore, ever-positive, perfect, loving and good.

The *specific difficulty* arising from Graphites' delusion that love is conditional and localised is the *fixation that who they are is not inherently lovable, valuable, significant or worthwhile*. They experience themselves as disconnected from the unconditional, loving goodness of life. The core of this fixation is an *inferiority complex*: a self-image based on *insufficiency, inadequacy and inferiority*.

Inferiority

Graphites' delusion of personal inferiority, affects not only their concept of self, but also whatever they do or create. They scrutinise themselves with a negative eye, uncompromisingly subjecting themselves to destructive comparison and criticism, and, being Graphites, this self-judgement homes-in on the petty, trivial and inconsequential. They disparage their appearance, their behaviour, their personality and their attributes. Being disconnected from their Essence, they are disconnected from their achievements. Feeling unloved and unlovable, *they cannot love themselves*.

Essence is Cosmic Love; it constitutes the very core of the soul and encompasses spiritual beauty, nobility, radiance and purity. Conviction that one is unlovable is abnegation of the ineffable perfection of Essence and replacing it with a sense of being *a deficient and impoverished soul*. This sense of deficiency and inferiority is common to all ego-based psyches, but for Graphites it is the core issue from which all other psychological difficulties arise.

Central to these difficulties is inertia!

The delusion of unworthiness and inferiority is so imbedded in the Graphites psyche that they are resigned to their mediocre lot and not motivated to work on their weaknesses. Instead, they distract themselves with the superficial and commonplace, as if these possess some intrinsic value that will offset their deficiencies. As always, priorities are neglected in favour of fussing over trifles. In this way, they distract themselves and disassociate from their pervasive feeling of inferiority. This trait of distracting oneself with externals rather than attending to the imperatives of one's inner-life is a central characteristic of the ego-self. Without the quality of Cosmic Love in everyday life, one's activities are relatively empty of meaning.

The knowledge that Cosmic Love exists and pervades every part of the Creation is not sufficient to overcome the delusion of inferiority unless the knowledge is also built into the perception of self. When this is achieved, the life-experience is imbued with lightness, delight, joy and fulfilment. Without it, Graphites experience themselves as dull and heavy. Instead of feelings that are fresh, clean, refined, delicate, exquisite and uplifting, the feelings produced by the Graphites ego-self are akin to a drab, dreary, dismal, 'grey', cold, winter day and induce sadness and despondency. This is life experienced through the ego-self. In contrast, life lived through the soul has clarity, freshness, refinement and the quality of exquisiteness.

The *specific reaction* to loss of Cosmic Love is *inertia*: a state of indolence and resignation that overcomes the soul. Metaphorically, the soul 'goes to sleep', yielding dominion of the psyche to the ego-self. With the soul lapsed into sleep, the Graphites ego-self portrays the inertia in its own inimitable way through apathy, indifference, laziness and disorder; all of which can be summed up in the so-called cardinal sin of '*sloth*'. In spiritual terms, this '*sloth*' is the cessation of the individuation process; the soul is on pause and the ego-perspective of loveless-ness and inferiority commands the psyche. Attempting to escape from and compensate for its diminished sense of self, the Graphites ego-self commits itself to a superficial, material life devoid of spiritual content or goals. This is a turning away from awareness of their painful inner world of want and deficiency and shifting the attention outwards to the external world and its values.

The sense of being unloved and unlovable because of some eradicable flaw or deficiency is intrinsic to the Graphites child; it is inherent in their psoric miasmatic inheritance. Even if they are loved by their parents, the unconscious conclusion of Graphites is that they are loved only for their behaviour, their intelligence, their talents, or their looks: for being bright, good, gifted, cute, etc. and not for the unique preciousness and beauty of their Being, because that is in some inexplicable way flawed, imperfect, 'ugly' and lacking in intrinsic goodness. If, instead of love, they experience neglect, unkindness, harshness or abuse, their conviction of being blemished and worthless will be intensified. As they mature, this sense of inferiority will be associated with some perceived failing: their complexion, their hair, their looks, their weight, their speech, their behaviour, their abilities or their intelligence, etc.

Inferiority projected

An important corollary of this entrenched sense of inferiority is the paradox that no degree of success or accomplishment can ever relieve or resolve it – for it is far too insidious and ingrained. Their fussy preoccupation with trivia and their obsessive attention to detail are signs, not only of attempted compensation for their sense of inferiority, but, especially, of its repression into the Shadow, where it increases in intensity and is further distorted. An inevitable consequence of this repression is the projection of their demeaned self-image outwards, away from their distressed psyche, onto others where it is despised and abhorred. Neither black or white, the greyness of their inferiority may be projected over a wide spectrum and those upon whom it falls will be denigrated and discriminated against. Depending on the intensity of their sense of inferiority and its degree of repression, it can assume such virulent proportions that those upon whom it is focused are dehumanised and demonised.

In Graphites, the most fundamental psoric archetype, the value judgements of superior and inferior that characterise social discrimination are already in place and can be exercised in the areas of race, religion, culture, education and gender. Such discrimination, especially when exaggerated, is always a projection of the discriminating person's own sense of inferiority. Having rejected their inner-self, they reject the other person and what they represent. Such discrimination may lead to scapegoating. This scapegoating explains some of the Graphites character traits that seem out of keeping with the general profile of the archetype, which is perceived as timid, gentle, soft, caring and self-effacing. But, is this contradiction not typical of the manifold nature of the human psyche and is it not to be expected in an impressionable, sensitive and anxious archetype, easily influenced by the prejudices and fears of the society in which it grows up?

With Graphites, the discrimination is manifested in unsympathetic *criticism and censure* of the 'offending' person or the group to which they belong, *insulting, dismissive rudeness, harshness, irritability, impatience and intolerance,* and most characteristic of the archetype: *derogatory, discriminatory humour,* covered by the reprehensible rubric: *mocking sarcasm* (Arsenicum; Carbo-veg; Lachesis; Lycopodium) where it is found in highest degree. The projection demands satisfaction and may precipitate them into heated arguments about those they are prejudiced against. They are very quarrelsome and have no interest in the other person's point of view, giving them no opportunity to voice their feelings (*quarrelsome without waiting for answers*).

Though rage and violence are to be found in Graphites, when vilification becomes hatred and discrimination and scapegoating hardens into aggressive, malicious violence, an archetypal shift has taken place, which, as I described in *The Wolf*, moves characteristically from the Ennea-type Nine archetype (Graphites, Lac lupinum) to either of the Nine's wing Ennea-types: One (Arsenicum: the bigoted perfectionist) or Eight (Anacardium: the sociopathic bully). The archetypal configuration of this triad (see Table 8.1) is apparent and confirmed by Nature's colour code:

TABLE 8.1   The Archetypal configuration of the Enea triad

Ennea-type Eight	Ennea-type Nine	Ennea-type One
Anacardium	Graphites	Arsenicum
Black marking nut	Grey graphite	White arsenic
Anti-social personality	Mediator	Puritanical fanatic

Soul inertia

The *soul inertia* of Graphites is a psychological defence mechanism against the enormity of the absence of Cosmic Love: *a numbing of the psyche* (Carcinosin). With the soul in passive, 'sleep-mode', the ego-self, which always seeks pleasure rather than pain, is free to divert itself with inconsequential activities – the trivialities that so occupy the attention of Graphites. Though this obsessive trait is well-known, in practice, its presence is not always recognised. In its simplest form, it is evidenced in those who, faced with a pressing priority, instead of getting down to the work in hand, busy themselves in tidying their office or with anything other than that which urgently needs to be done. This evasive strategy must also be recognised when the escapist activity, or pastime, is spring cleaning, gardening, being forever in the workshop, compulsively exercising, always reading books or watching DVD's of the same genre, constantly changing TV channels, playing computer games, doing jigsaw or crossword puzzles and engaging in frequent or extended casual conversations. Not that any of these activities are of themselves necessarily negative or bad, but when compulsive and overindulged and when consuming inordinate amounts of time at the expense of more serious and meaningful pursuits, must be recognised as archetypal and indicative of *soul inertia*.

Soul inertia is a dark-grey Graphites state: it is ill-defined, misty, foggy, murky, dense, thick and heavy – a leaden state – associated with lack of vitality and buoyancy – an apathetic, indifferent, bored, languid, ponderous condition. Their eyes give testimony to this jaded lethargy: lifeless, expressionless, dull and vacant. They are burnt-out; there is no fire, no drive or motivation only indolence, laziness, indecision, procrastination and equivocation. The Master of the psyche is on leave and the ego-self is at play. The inner-space is chaotic, disorganised and in disarray and this muddled state may manifest outwardly in uncharacteristic untidiness, dirtiness and clutter. They may neglect their appearance, their hygiene, their diet and forego all custom of exercise. Self-neglect is apparent: they become untidy, unkempt, unfit and overweight (very Sulphur- or Mercurius-like).

- *Dirtiness* (2).

The Graphites indolence, laziness and heedlessness has various shades:

- *Oblivious to what needs attention.*
- *Inability to determine what needs to be done.*
- *Difficulty prioritising.*
- *Losing focus in the details of the task or in over-elaboration.*
- *Inadvertent substitution of less important work for the important task.*
- *Difficulty in discrimination and organisation.*
- *Lack of energy and stamina for the task.*
- *Avoidance and neglect of what needs to be done.*
- *Conveniently forgetting tasks; inadvertent absentmindedness.*

However, paradoxically, some Graphites achieve distraction and loss of self-awareness through committing themselves, often sacrificially, to caring for others; mothering and caring being strong Graphites traits. In doing so, they may be careless of their own welfare and overextend themselves, suffering burn-out or collapse from exhaustion (Carcinosin; Cocculus). It is a characteristic of Graphites that they are not tuned in to their mental or physical limits and fail to learn from previous experience.

Somnolence of the soul is the common cause of the inertia of Graphites; externally, it has two presentations: *passive or active inertia.*

This can best be understood by considering the definition of inertia in physics.

A property of matter by which it continues in its existing state of rest or uniform motion in a straight line unless that state is changed by an external force.

Graphites either remains 'immobile', until forced into action by circumstances, or moves persistently, like an automaton, along a predetermined track or rut.

Graphites has great difficulty initiating action; they are not pro-active, and they are only sluggishly reactive, but once moving, like Silicea, they have difficulty changing direction. With their course determined, routine sets in, and they hold their trajectory with obstinate determination. Their sense of deficiency and inferiority is just as persistent. Their thoughts and habits are deeply ingrained and resistant to modification or change.

The *passive inertia* (state of rest) of Graphites is seen in its indolence, its inactivity and its neglect of priorities.

The *active inertia* (state of uniform motion in a straight line) has three forms.

- Compensatory or inconsequential activity.
- Obsessive compulsive tendencies, especially the obsessive aspect.
- Adherence to the familiar and the known: to custom, tradition, doctrine or system.

The first form of active inertia has already been considered. The obsessive, compulsive form is apparent from a study of Graphites psychopathology and revealed in their tendency to obsess about some aspect of their lives while neglecting important issues. A good example is the overweight Graphites, who is obsessive about using artificial sweeteners and fat-free milk but overeats and regularly binges on fattening foods, or one who takes loads of expensive supplements, yet eats indiscriminately and takes no exercise. Typically, Graphites concentrates on effects (results) and fails to consider affects (causes). This parallels their fussiness over trivia, their focus on the superficial and material aspects of their lives, their neglect of priorities and their shying away from emotional problems.

The third form has all the trappings of austere, formal, sober Grey. *This Graphites is very conservative*; they cling to their conditioning: to the known, the familiar and the trusted. They do not want to stray out of their comfort zone. Like Kali-carb (plant-carbon combusted to its very end-product: ash), they want to maintain the status quo and preserve the establishment, which they believe represents stability and security. They are averse to change and innovation. They are conservative and orthodox, bound to custom, tradition, doctrine or system, which give them a sense of safety; permitting them to relax into their inertia of compliance and conformity. They will obstinately resist change. If their adherence to their chosen ideology casts them in the role of reactionary or activist, they are highly doctrinaire, stubbornly and unswervingly committed to their cause without regard for practical considerations or consequences. They are radical in their conservativism. Trapped by inertia, the Graphites mind is obstinate, dogmatic, pedantic, opinionated and fundamental.

The inert, fettered Graphites strongly resembles Calc-carb, the sessile, anchored oyster, not only in their tendency to be overweight, but in their steadfast disposition. They are stubbornly inflexible in their ways and appear uninspiring, bland and unexciting (grey). Though not vital and dynamic, nonetheless, they are reliable, consistent, persevering and determined. Their disposition is measured and contained, not volatile or explosive. Though at first hesitant, undecided and vacillating, once resolved, they are steady, even rock-like, dependable and predictable. They realise their identity through their work, which, for Graphites, must be the best possible, even to the finest detail. Calc-carb, by comparison, is far more rough and ready, as displayed by the rather coarse, unfinished look of its shell, compared with the artistic refinement achieved by other molluscs.

The placid, gentle, phlegmatic Calc-carb can appear almost bovine in temperament (Tuberculinum bovinum) and Graphites may emulate this; an image fostered by their compliant, affable and non-abrasive natures. This amiability is enhanced by their gentle, caring, empathetic disposition, which is readily occasioned by others' needs. Though not a person to rely upon when quick, decisive action in an emergency is called for, in the aftermath, Graphites comes into her own. Her own anxieties, fears and forebodings put on hold, she willingly and attentively attends to those in distress. Her Earth Mother aspect makes this response natural and spontaneous and she has an intuitive and instinctive feel for what needs to be said and done. Her manner is soothing, calming and healing. *The role of carer is so archetypal and innate to Graphites that it proves beneficial to them emotionally and physically.* It is good counsel to advise the menopausal Graphites to sublimate her libido energy in artistic or caring pursuits.

Part of Graphites inertia is their desire for physical and emotional comfort. Because they are constantly attempting to divert their senses away from their anxiety driven inner-world, their outer-world needs to be inviting, supportive and comfortable and able to provide them with ease and diversion. This is not the love of luxury and opulence of Pulsatilla; it is a practical need for all the material things that reduce the need for effort, ensure security, give pleasure and offer distraction and entertainment.

The inertia and indecisiveness of Graphites are interwoven. They have difficulty formulating their own opinions, viewpoints and values and usually conform unquestioningly to what their parents have told them, the conditioning they receive and the consensus opinion of their society or culture. They are very much people of their times and their situation. Their inertia preserves their conditioned patterns of thinking, perceiving, feeling and conduct – programmed grooves of the ego-self, etched into the psyche from past-experience and imprinting, dictating forward direction – *the past implacably ruling the present* – ego-baggage that weighs them down, dulls their senses and distorts their perception.

- *Dreams – everything distorted.*
- *Delusions*:
  - *Everything is strange.*
  - *Familiar things are strange.*

'Active' inertia

Yet again, significant similarities between Graphites and Kali-carb are discerned and, by extension, with Oak (*Quercus robur*), the archetype that, above all, exemplifies active inertia: an ultraconservative morality that is inflexibly committed to duty and toil in the name of the bureaucracy, religion or tradition that moulded them – a narrow perspective and *unquestioning respect for authority that lands them in a rut,* which they mindlessly and stoically pursue to a point of *exhaustion or burn-out.* In this, Graphites and Oak are as one. The underlying state of inertia gives a mechanical, almost robotic, element to their unthinking compliance and conformity. Numb to their inner-world and obedient to the norms of the outer-world, they become bureaucratic stereotypes, fettered by senseless protocol and deprived of initiative, enterprise and creativity. To distinguish the presence of the archetype, we must recognise that this institutionalised, automaton-like behaviour exemplifies the enigma of *inertia driven over-activity*!

Graphites hates confrontation and dispute and will cling tenaciously to their inconspicuous, 'grey' status. To this end, they are adept at not causing waves. They are ideal corporate cogs, slaves of the system, filling their prescribed niche without complaint. This focussed adherence to order and system, in a person who is otherwise indolent, indecisive and disorganised, is not anomalous in Graphites; it is in keeping with a personality that tends to fixate obsessively on one aspect of their lives (black or white) while the rest is blurred and confused (grey). It is as if their entire emotional investment is in the system they espouse, while all else is side-lined and out of focus.

The building blocks of the biological sphere are giant molecules comprised of carbon, which are, of themselves, faceless, but when aggregated become living entities. The building blocks of a nation are individuals comprised of carbon, who are, of themselves, faceless, but when massed become the populace. In this analogy, the collective role of carbon as a pawn, commandeered and manipulated either by physiological or social convention or protocols, is evident. In these stereotyped alignments, a core facet of the Graphites psyche is fathomed: *a delusion of dependency and inferiority that permits dictators to thrive and become tyrants exploiting the voiceless multitude.* The communism of the former Soviet Union played out this saga of carbon and Graphites to its ultimate end: the subsuming of the needs and aspirations of the individual in the drive of the collective. In this frame, the fundamental position of the Graphites archetype is discerned: as individual – the acquiescent victim; as collective – the subjugated proletariat.

The Graphites superego

The villain behind the scenes, directing the imposter ego-self in its sovereignty of the psyche, is the superego, the stern, demanding inner-bureaucrat, wearing the black robes of judge and inquisitor. The Graphites superego is the coercive henchman of the system and the regime, an inner-voice insistently persuading the ego-self towards passivity (inertia): to self-effacing diffidence, deferring to others and remaining low-profile, invisible and 'grey' – causing no ripples, taking up little space and keeping the peace. It is responsible for the guilt and discomfiture that Graphites feels on having to approach, and possibly importune, someone when seeking help. Although their nature moves them to care for others, it is the superego that makes them feel responsible and imposes guilt if their caring is not self-sacrificing. Through helping others, Graphites sublimates libido energy, but at the level of the ego-self, caring for others eases their feelings of guilt and diminishes their sense of being unloved and unlovable.

The superego keeps the Graphites personality focused on the petty superficialities of the external world and dissuades enquiry into the meaning and purpose of life and exploration of the inner self. It forces the ego-self to minimise the soul's influence upon the psyche. The 'psychic sleep' of the soul is induced by the delusion that love is not universal, but conditional and localised, and by the soul's conclusion that since it is irreparably deficient and inferior, it is not loved and is essentially unlovable. Hence, all the superego needs to do to ensure the continued inertia of the soul is to constantly reinforce the self-denigration and lack of self-love that supports it. This is the default mode of the Graphites superego.

The superego persistently exhorts Graphites not to ruffle feathers, not to upset others, not to speak up for themselves, not to be confrontational, not to promote their own interests, but to always please others and remain nice, accommodating, unobtrusive and unassuming. It immerses them in the inertia and indolence of the typical C-type personality (Carcinosin; Psorinum) – they lose both voice and presence! This repression specifically impairs the function of the fifth chakra, Vishuddha – the chakra of communication and creativity – which becomes blocked or stuck. The level of consciousness of Vishuddha's energy vortex resonates with the frequency of the cancer miasm, *Carcinosis*. Bound by the constraints of consensus reality and conventional norms, the creative, innovative energy of the archetype implodes! Unable to effect constructive, creative change in the external world, the unexpressed revolutionary energy is turned inwards and corrupted, bringing about internal anarchy through carcinogenesis.

Grey – hesitancy, indecisiveness, fear of confrontation, fence-sitting, self-forgetting: the peacemaker

The objective arbiter

Paradoxically out of weakness, uncertainty and inability to stand up for themselves, comes one of the most positive attributes of the Graphites temperament – a quality that accords with their caring, altruistic nature: their *ability to mediate* (Mag-carb). A key characteristic of Graphites is difficulty in deciding: agonising over choices and consequences. This is exacerbated by fear that their choice might inconvenience, displease or offend others. Decision-making becomes painful and onerous and causes great anxiety. They sit on the fence and weigh up all alternatives, considering both sides of every story while discounting their own needs and preferences. Though based on deficiency and self-abnegation, this hovering, self-forgetting stance fosters objectivity, disinterest and dispassion. Their desire to placate others, avoid confrontation and keep the peace at any price, enables them to excel as *facilitator, arbiter, mediator and peacemaker*. They can pour oil on troubled waters. By nature, they are motivated to maintain harmony – a quality analogous to graphite's lubricating function. Originally, this need may have arisen from not wanting to estrange a parent out of fear of losing what little love they seemed to be receiving. But, much of their skill in resolving disputes, bridging differences and promoting consensus stems from seeing all angles and perspectives and appreciating different points of view. What would cause great tension and stress when pertaining to themselves, can be coolly and objectively addressed when the concern of others. In the process of arbitration, they forget self, put bias on hold, remain neutral and disinterestedly evaluate a situation. This makes Graphites a person to be turned to for objective, unprejudiced advice; others feel they can be counted on – and usually they are not mistaken. *In this skill, the grey of indecisiveness and self-effacing diffidence unite and flow into the light-grey of wisdom and peacekeeping.* The propensity to mediate and foster harmony and accord is intensified in the carbonate of magnesium, Mag-carb, the archetype that exemplifies the consciousness of Anahata – the heart or love chakra.

Simulating love

A parallel to this sublimation of deficiency is their archetypal tendency to image themselves in terms of the Cosmic Concept that they are most attuned to, have lost connection with and unconsciously long for: Cosmic Love – the apprehension that the universe is inherently loving and that, being a unique expression of the universe, they are inherently lovable. To compensate for their loss and ease their longing, they simulate the quality they are disconnected from and attempt to be a kind, gentle person, who is unconditionally loving, caring and supporting in an unobtrusive, diffident way. This necessitates ever-discounting themselves and keeping the peace by emotionally retiring into the shadows. They also construct a lifestyle, which makes them feel that their holding environment does, indeed, love, cherish and support them. To maintain this illusion, they get involved in intimate relationships, forge close friendships and become dependent on both; they make their life as easy, comfortable and peaceful as possible; and indulge in pleasure and diversion – preoccupation with the trivial and the superficial. None of these scenarios can solve the underlying problem, which stems from psychic disconnection from the realm of Being and identification with the ego-self. Graphites needs to direct focus away from the shallow and the transient to be able to discriminate the unimportant from the imperative and cultivate authentic action – to recognise what needs to be done and to do it! Obsessing over the passing parade, enriches the ego-self and impoverishes the soul!

Grey of the mundane now

In spiritual terms, the Graphites journey through life is grey and relatively without meaning and purpose. Due to lack of basic trust, the archetype is unable to be fully present in the immaculate, loving 'Now'. Only in the 'Now' can the soul surrender to its destiny and actively and positively participate in the perfection of life's dispensation: a surrender essential to the individuation of the soul. The reality of Graphites lies not in the black and white clarity and authenticity of a vibrant present, but in the grey murkiness of the past and the grey fog of the future. The past clings to them, burdening them with regret, grief and guilt and a sense of having been unlucky and ill-used; and the future haunts them, tormenting them with anxiety, misgiving and foreboding. A 'suffocating' sense of doom and gloom oppresses them. Caught between remorse and dread, they attempt to blur the present by focussing their attention on the greyness of the superficial, the mundane and the trivial.

Intellectual trust

Since, Graphites is the fundamental archetype of the psyche, yielding to distraction is, in some measure, true of all souls that surrender their authority to the repressive and collaborative tyranny of the ego-self and superego. The greater part of most lives would seem to be largely consumed by attention to the routine, the ordinary and the commonplace, without reflection on the esoteric significance and imperatives of life on the material plane. It is a paradox of the human psyche that most of those who earnestly accept the truth of survival after death and fully perceive that life's one-pointed goal is the sublimation of the soul – an ideal achieved by surrender, service, fortitude and trust – nevertheless, hold these high concepts at an intellectual rather than soul level, and in the face of adversity and loss, still succumb to a Graphites-like state of grief, guilt, irresolution, anxiety and foreboding – distracting themselves with trifles – seeking solace in religion – or declining into inertia and despair.

Peculiar characteristics that identify Graphites as an Ennea-type Nine archetype:

- *Substitution of non-essentials for essentials.*
- *Priorities left until last.*
- *Indecisive at every level of functioning.*
- *Habitual, routine, familiar behaviour rather than using initiative, making decisions, being innovative and instituting change.*
- *Difficulty saying "No".*
- *Yielding to others' standpoints rather than asserting their own; deferring constantly to others.*
- *Through constantly surrendering their own position, become uncommonly attuned to the thinking, feeling and needs of others.*
- *Bottling of anger, resentment and humiliation.*
- *Controlling others through passive aggression and stubbornness.*

* * * * *

Grey of the sacred 'Now'

Finally, there is a sublime grey that represents the unconditional love of the Great Mother Goddess: the grey invoked by Mother Theresa, who wore pale-grey, a colour that speaks of caring, helping, serving and sacrificing for the good of all: the grey of peace – the grey of the dove! This is the grey towards which carbon aspires. In the form of graphite, carbon presents its essential archetypal form: Graphites – an archetype that embodies in its multifarious, complex nature both the soul qualities needed to achieve transcendence and the prime ego-characteristics that impede it. Often not recognised, and, therefore, much neglected, Graphites, given on its defining indications, can establish basic trust, depose the ego-self and permit the soul to shed the guilt and grief of the past, dissolve the fears and forebodings of the future and embrace the sacred purity of 'Now'.

* * * * *

The Grey Wolf – an archetypal sibling[iii]

In parallel with graphite's electrical and heat conductivity, the Graphites archetype is *oversensitive to all mental and sensory impressions*. Their sensitivity encompasses psychic awareness, particularly clairsentience. These heightened sensibilities invite comparison with the Wolf (Lac lupinum): an archetype possessing faculties, senses and extra sensory perception far keener than humans. The similarities between Graphites and Lac lupinum are numerous and significant. The animal's common name the Grey Wolf, is a colour connection between the two that is filled with esoteric meaning. Both are of primordial archetypal importance: Graphites being the fundamental building block of sentient life and Wolf the archetype that bears the burden of man's projected iniquities. The similarity extends to the major formative influence that structures the fundamental nature of the Graphites and Wolf ego-self: the loss to consciousness of the pivotal Cosmic Concept – unconditional, universal Cosmic Love – into the Shadow of the psyche. In consequence, both archetypes suffer from the delusion that love is conditional and localised; that they stand outside the loving embrace of the Universe; that they are unloved and unlovable and intrinsically inferior. The ego-self of both archetypes evolves as a compensation for these painful convictions.

Wolf is a warrior archetype, totem of the Nordic and Germanic Gods of War: Odin and Wotan. Wolf is archetypally associated with the metal of war: Ferrum (iron) and the colour red that iron imparts to the blood. As noted, pure graphite always contains at least 4% iron and iron meteorites

---

[iii] For a full discussion of the wolf see Lilley DJ. *The Wolf*. Glasgow: Saltire Books, 2017.

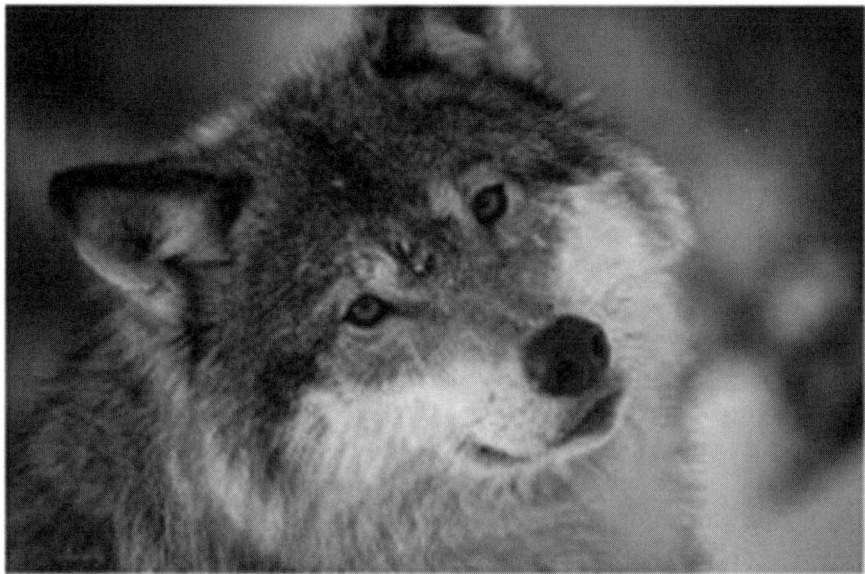

Figure 8.1 *The Grey Wolf (Canis Lupus)*

invariably contain nodules of pure graphite, facts that cosmically signify an esoteric link between the mineral and the animal. Both Wolf and Graphites are indicated for anaemia and adrenal fatigue or burn-out: *the depletion of red.*

The theme of *inferiority* is fundamental to both these great archetypes. In the light of wolf history, it is understandable that Lac lupinum suffers from the delusion that they are looked down upon and that they are the victim of circumstances – dream of social inferiority – fear getting into trouble – desire to please superiors – experience loss of identity – and have a sense of helplessness. Graphites believes similarly that *they are unfortunate and singled out for misfortune* – perceptions that reflect the very real plight of wolves in the world today. Both Graphites and Wolf share *fear of men; fear of the masculine principle; fear of authority figures* and both have *hierarchical and social fears.* This hierarchical sensitivity is expressed in the rubric *ailments from discord between chief and subordinates.* The similar shared rubric: *ailments from discord between family and friends,* underlines the importance of family and friends to both these archetypes and points to their closeness to Mag-carb, another archetype embodying the energy of the Great Mother Goddess and her love of children, animals and nature – a marked characteristic of Graphites and Wolf.

Another link between Graphites and Wolf is provided by Lycopodium, an archetype that shares so much with both – particularly their pervasive sense of inferiority – and provides a bridge between the two. A certain type of Lycopodium walks the same path as the Wolf: a path that in the sexual sphere may lead to Graphites-like erectile problems. All three are motivated by a *desire to escape*!

Lycopodium wants to escape from responsibility, family and children. The Lac lupinum archetype prizes freedom as much as they prize life and *looks for angles to escape* from people and situations that seem to imprison them. Graphites seeks escape from the past, present and future by fleeing from the internal, the profound and the Real onto the diverting, ever-changing surface of life. In their desire to escape introspection and emotional pain, both Graphites and Lac lupinum anaesthetise, or numb, the soul into a state of passivity (Carcinosin), permitting the errant ego-self licence to command their affairs. Characteristic of human nature, they overthrow a benevolent ruler (the feminine principle) and enthrone a tyrant (the masculine principle). In both Graphites and Lac lupinum, the numbing of the soul and the conscience, leads to a feeling of stupefaction or intoxication, experienced especially in waking in the morning. They feel as if they have, in some strange way, been poisoned by sleep. This seeps into and impairs their mental efficiency and their memory.

Graphites and Wolf avoid emotional pain by repression of what they cannot face or resolve into the Shadow. Both are *easily offended, and harbour repressed anger, indignation and resentment.* What characterises both, is the deeply hidden nature of their emotional responses. On the surface, even when grievously hurt, little shows; they avoid sympathy and consolation. They are lone wolves, preferring to be alone, seeking solitude, especially in nature, where they can lick their wounds in peace, without attention or interference. An emotional catharsis is essential to both. In lieu of this, Graphites may externalise emotional pain through a weeping eczema, oozing a sticky liquid that dries to forms honey-like crusts.

9

GRAPHITES – 6

Constitution – Causation – Modalities

Wide archetypal spectrum

To gain some idea of the immense compass of this fundamental archetype, two distinct Graphites types may be contrasted. Despite marked differences, they come from a common mould.

Earthy

At the lower end of the intellectual scale, we have the typical 'labourer' or 'peasant' type, described as coarse, bland, 'thick-skinned', and slow-thinking. A large, heavy-boned, thick-set, fleshy individual – 'simple, basic, earthy and unrefined', with spade-like hands and feet and a broad, full-cheeked peasant's face. A man or woman of the earth, stocky, often corpulent, heavy of mind and body – physically industrious, with hands and nails gnarled, thickened and cracked due to their labours – and due to being Graphites. Gifted with common-sense, physically-skilled, practical, clear-headed, sure-handed, quick-thinking and acting, when faced with intellectual demands, their minds become ponderous, their comprehension tardy and their concentration poor. They are slow to come to a decision, draw up a plan of action and implement it. They dread and avoid mental effort (*dread of mental work*). However, Graphites is also of value for gentleman farmers, blessed with greater acumen than their humbler brethren, who share their love of the earth, their practical competence and often their eczema.

Intellectual

At the upper end of the scale, we find the intellectual, the author, the architect, the artist and the scientist, mentally working to excess, driven by an anxious, conscientious and carefully, meticulous nature, inclined to agonise over the finest and most trifling points of distinction and differentiation. Exhausted by their attention to detail and inability to settle for the broader issues and concepts, their work becomes ever more stressful and a source of anxiety and frustration.

Watching them at work, one is aware of their emotional tension. The more intensely they work, the more anxious, fidgety and restlessly agitated they become. Eventually, they are forced to break off and pace about to relieve their tension. As fatigue increases, so does their anxiety and peevish irritability – everybody and everything irritates them – they may not be spoken to, interrupted or disturbed, otherwise an outburst of anger results. Finally, they find their concentration failing them; they are unable to focus their thoughts, they cannot conceptualise; the mind and memory are dulled. Their work rate slows and finally peters out. They lose confidence, become indecisive and despondent and dread their work. A nervous breakdown is imminent, or they go into 'burn-out'.

- *Mind; prostration of the mind, mental exhaustion, brain-fag* (2).
- *Prostration of the mind after mental exertion – from scientific labour* (unique).
- *Anxiety during mental work.*
- *Aversion to mental work.*
- *Work impossible – after sleep in the afternoon* (unique).
- *Ameliorated in the open air and for taking a walk.*

Hahnemann gives the picture in *Chronic Diseases*:

Anxiety during sedentary work; peevishness; dislike of work; feels as if intoxicated on rising from bed; chaotic feeling in the head; fatigued by scientific work; buzzing in the head. Restless and unsettled; cannot fix thoughts on work, has no pleasure in anything, better after taking a walk.

According to Kent:

The patient becomes very restless when attempting close mental work and there is a marked dread of it.[1]

Causation

From this study of the workings of the Graphites psyche, it is useful to list the causative factors that facilitate the emergence of the Graphites state. Although definite circumstances, situations and events within the holding environment can be identified as causative or provocative, more important is the innate, psoric nature of the Graphites archetype, which distorts their perception of reality. In dealing with the notions, assumptions and persuasions of this most primal of archetypes, it becomes clear that what an individual believes to be true and holds close to their heart, especially when misguided or magnified, is of pivotal importance in determining the means to heal them. This is true of all archetypes, but markedly so of Graphites, whose soul, in 'falling asleep', permits the ego-self to assume full dominion over the psyche. This surrender of authority, warps their reality and catalyses events scripted to startle or jolt the 'hero-soul' out of slumber; a theme common to legend and fairy story.

- *Autocratic, critical, derogatory parents, particularly a dictatorial, forbidding, intimidating father and an aloof, cold, stern mother.*
- *Parental strife, especially an abused mother.*
- *Neglect – being overlooked, ignored, side-lined, minimised.*
- *Rejection.*
- *Ridicule, belittlement.*
- *Mortification, humiliation.*
- *Discrimination, especially racial, religious and ideological.*
- *Love disappointment.*
- *Abusive relationship.*
- *Betrayal of friendship.*
- *Discord between friends; between relatives; between parents.*
- *Discord between superiors and subordinates.*
- *Grief, sorrow, care [2] – bereavement – loss of family, friends, pets.*
- *Fear, fright or anxiety [2].*
- *Guilt (2).*
- *Anger, vexation – anger suppressed.*
- *Indignation, resentment.*
- *Emotional excitement.*
- *Puberty [2].*
- *Menopause [2].*
- *Mental exertion – mental work.*
- *Fine manual work.*
- *Physical exertion – over-lifting.*
- *Suppressed discharges; eruptions; sweat.*
- *Sexual intercourse.*
- *Alcoholism [2].*

Important negative characteristics of the Graphites mental state.
- *Anxiety, apprehension and fear.*
- *Timidity, hesitancy and indecisiveness.*
- *Changeableness.*
- *Slowness, indolence and incapacity.*

- *Doom and gloom.*
- *A sense of depression and foreboding.*
- *Feels unfortunate.*
- *A pessimistic anticipation of misfortune, troubles and failure.*
- *Dejection with great heaviness of the body or of the feet.*
- *Wakes feeling intoxicated.*
- *Discouragement with much weeping.*
- *Sad and melancholic – feels he must weep – with sighing.*
- *Causeless weeping – without provocation.*
- *Weeping – pities himself.*
- *Weeping benefits.*
- *Music makes him weep.*
- *Dwells on past disagreeable occurrences – at night.*
- *A religious depression that he has sinned away his state of grace and is beyond salvation.*
- *Suicidal disposition.*

To round-off the picture of this most fundamental of psoric archetypes, it is of value to consider its modalities of aggravation and amelioration, its food cravings and aversions and the typical skin lesions that are so often the physical trademark of Graphites. However, it must always be remembered that the absence of a history of skin disease must never be taken as an eliminating feature! The Graphites skin can be immaculate and may always have been so!

Aggravations

Graphites is a *chilly remedy* and needs warm clothing and yet dresses for the open air (Carbo-veg, Pulsatilla).

Craving for air is common and marked in the carbons.

A chilly person, who is oversensitive to a warm room and craves the open air – may delight in being warmly wrapped up with the head in a cool draught of air (Ars-alb) – and who becomes easily overheated, which makes them feel ill; cannot tolerate the heat of summer.

Easily chilled and just as easily overheated.

- *Cold aggravates:*
  - Coryzal symptoms; stomach pains; bone pains.
  - Cold air and draughts.
  - Cold, damp weather and getting wet.

- Wet feet:
  - § Getting the feet wet may delay the menses (Pulsatilla).
  - § Causes painful inflammation of the ovaries.
- Cold drinks.
- Worse for bathing and washing.
- *Heat aggravates:*
  - Heat of summer.
  - Warmth of the bed:
    - § Aggravates the itching of the skin.
    - § Scratching aggravates the skin.
  - Warmth aggravates tearing pain in the teeth.
  - Exertion rapidly overheats and aggravates all symptoms.
- Morning on waking – sad, anxious, dull, intoxicated feeling.
- Worse at menses: violent menstrual colic, prostration, morning sickness.
- During and after the menses.
- Light – extreme photophobia (Calc-carb; Conium; Nat-sulph).
- Lying on the left side (Pulsatilla).
- Motion and travelling – sensitive to motion of any kind – they stand travelling very badly.
- Rest: numbness and general feeling of stagnation comes on at rest.
- Full moon – ears feel stuffed.
- Fatty food (Pulsatilla; Carbo-veg).

Ameliorations

- Warmth.
- Warm drinks – especially warm milk for gastric pain.
- Open air – walking in the open air.
- Noise improves hardness of hearing.
- Eating.
- Eructations.
- Touch.

Desires and aversions

Food desires:

- Chicken.
- Bland food.
- Beer.

Food aversions:

- Sweets (candies).
- Salt.
- Fish.
- Meats.
- Cooked food.

Meat/salt/sweet as a combination.
Gastritis or peptic ulcers: pains better by eating or better from drinking warm milk (Ars-alb), or from warm drinks.
Fats aggravate.

Skin and nails

- Internal disorders have a marked tendency to manifest on the skin.
- The skin is dry and harsh and tends to crack, especially on exposure to cold.
- Ailments from suppressed skin eruptions and catarrhal discharges.
- Unhealthy skin – every injury suppurates.
- Itching of the skin all over the body, with or without an eruption.
- Scar tissue is of a low grade – indurating and contracting, breaking open; especially after abscess of the breast; cancer forming upon an old scar.
- Aids the absorption of keloid tissue.
- Eruptions – herpetic, crusted, oozing a thick, glutinous, honey-like fluid.
- Intertrigo.
- Cracks and fissures, worse on exposure to cold: ends of fingers, bends of joints, anus, labia, perineum, nipples, mouth corners, eye corners, behind the ears, under the ear lobe, at the muco-cutaneous junctions.
- Induration and burning in the base of ulcers.
- Recurrent herpes – especially to the anus and genitals.
- Erysipelas spreading from right to left; eradicates tendency to erysipelas.
- Nails – brittle crumbling, deformed, cracked, thickened.

Reference

1 Kent JT. *Lectures on Homoeopathic Materia Medica.* New Delhi: B Jain Publishers Pvt. Ltd., p555.

10

SILICEA – 1

The Crystal Archetype

Stellar alchemy: carbon to silicon

After 600 years of *carbon* burning (fusion), great stars with a mass of about twenty-five suns, run out of fuel and must turn to the next axial element to provide the necessary energy to sustain the star against collapse. At a billion degrees Kelvin, the noble gas *neon* provides this, but in the space of scarcely a year it is exhausted. Heat in the star spirals to 1.5 billion degrees, and, at this intensity, the star switches to *oxygen* as its next life-saving fuel, which, over six months of burning, vitally produces *silicon* and in addition: *sulphur, phosphorus* and the ever-ubiquitous *magnesium*.

The gasses Neon and Oxygen, like all elements, have archetypal profiles, revealed through provings and developed through practice. Neon has been researched by Jeremy Sherr[1] and Clarke[2] provided the first serious consideration of Oxygen, but in terms of treating the human constitution and miasmatic disease, these gaseous elements, like Hydrogen and Helium, both considered by Sherr,[3] are comparatively superficial in their depth of action and it is silicon, in the form of its dioxide: Silicea (SiO_2), that emerges from the creative flow as the second axial archetype of profound stature. Indeed, at this point, it is silicon that is the key ingredient in the creation of matter, for at a core temperature of 3 billion degrees Kelvin, silicon becomes involved in a sequence of multiple nuclear reactions that produce the lighter elements and finally *iron 56*, the element central to the supernova explosion that gives birth to the heavier elements.

Silicea

Silica – silicon dioxide – quartz/rock crystal – SiO_2

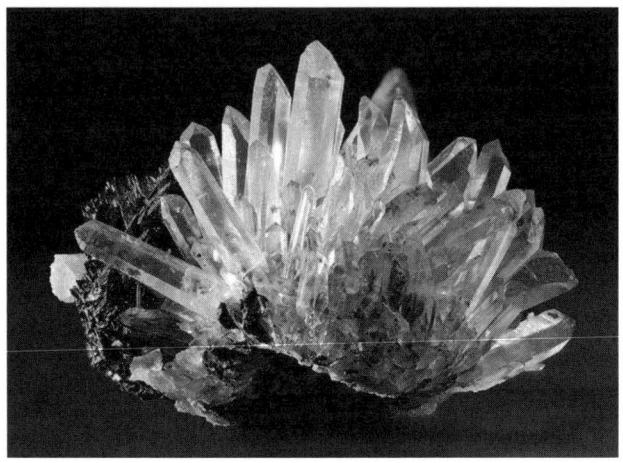

Figure 10.1 *Quartz crystals*

Carbon group (Group IV – modern: Group 14)

As ever, we are persuaded that there is a Divine Artist at work, purposefully preparing a cosmic canvas to be peopled by all the archetypes yet to be created. First, out of the fiery, gaseous furnace, carbon is fabricated, promising life to come, held as a primal thought in the Universal Consciousness while the fabulous setting in which that life will be placed is fabricated. Upon the palate of the Supreme Artist, lie the elements of the *carbon group*, for it is from this highly significant transition point on the periodic table that the first living molecule came into being and the very grandeur of the earthly landscape, which forms the frame and platform for life, took shape. While carbon is the very pillar of organic life, it is silicon, by means of its rigid geometrical patterns and crystal compounds, that is the grand architect of crag and ravine, mountain and valley.

The carbon group elements are: **carbon – silicon** – germanium – stannum (tin) – plumbum (lead).

It is significant that these two singularly important axial elements stand next to one another in the periodic table. Given their key roles in structuring the planet and producing life, it is not surprising that they have proved to be remedies of first importance: Graphites, especially for assimilative, nutritional and metabolic disorders; Silicea, for deficiency of form, structure and resistance and conditions of the rigid, supporting tissues. It was the genius of Hahnemann that conceived a means to release the therapeutic power of these chemically inert substances through trituration and attenuation.

Pure silicon crystallises with isometric symmetry and has the same structure as the carbon crystal: diamond. This is further indication that Graphites and Silicea are therapeutically complementary. Imaging the order of their creation in stellar alchemy, Silicea follows Graphites particularly well and is often called for when Graphites has done all that it can.

Silicea and the halogens

At normal temperature, silicon reacts vigorously with *fluorine* to produce *silicon tetrafluoride* [Si F_4], but will only combine with other elements at very high temperature. Apart from gaseous fluorine, *chlorine* and *hydrofluoric acid* also interact energetically with silicon. These affinities are of great clinical significance, indicating Silicea's close relationship with the halogens, a family of elements that produce syphilis-like pathology. Silicea is indicated for conditions involving the so-called 'lower tissues': bone, connective tissue, teeth, skin and its appendages – and for deep, destructive, inflammatory states that reach to the very bone, e.g. inveterate osteomyelitis – conditions based upon a tuberculo-syphilitic or syphilitic diathesis. Silicea's relationship with Fluoric acid is particularly close. They are complementary: Fluoric acid follows Silicea well and is one of its antidotes. Fluoric acid is similarly suited to deep, destructive, syphilitic processes and, like its salt, *Calcium fluoride* (fluorspar), has a predilection for the bones and the connective tissues. Calcium fluoride is also a remedy for osteomyelitis. The halogen connections of Silicea must always be remembered in clinical situations.

Silicates

Silica is a compound of the two most abundant elements of the earth's crust: oxygen and silicon. It constitutes 60% of the mass of the solid crust of the earth. More than 95% of the earth's rocks contain silica as their principal component. Those composed of pure 'free silica' are classified as *quartz* – sea sand is quartz in the almost pure state (*Silicea marina*) – the rest, made up of silica in combination with other elements, are known as *silicate minerals.*

Feldspar is a name applied to an important group of silicate minerals that are comprised of **silica and aluminium** combined with *potassium, sodium, calcium* or rarely *barium.* In all the silicates, as well as in pure silica, there are groups of four oxygen atoms arranged in space at the corners of a tetra-hedron. There is usually a silicon atom at the centre of the tetrahedron, but it can be replaced, here and there, by *aluminium* (in most cases not to exceed one out of four silicon atoms) and rarely by *beryllium*. At the same time, an occasional tetrahedral corner will be occupied, not by an oxygen atom, but by a *fluorine* atom or an OH pair (hydroxyl). To the homeopath, these configurations point to archetypal closeness and particularly between Silicea and Alumina. Since, every silicon atom is placed in the centre of a tetrahedral arrangement of four oxygen atoms, an archetypal relationship can be anticipated between Silicea and the Number Four archetype.

Four: the number of structure and form

Although now referred to as Group 14, the carbon group elements were originally known as the tetrels (from the Greek *tetra*, which means four) referring to the 4 valence electrons each element holds in its outer orbital. In semiconductor physics, the group is still universally called Group IV, which accords well with their relationship to Number 4.

Four, like all numbers has archetypal meaning. In numerology, four is one of the single digit *destiny numbers*, representing nine distinct arche-types.

As with the creation and the expanding universe, the prime Numbers evolve archetypally, starting with Zero (0) – which denotes *nothing, yet every-thing*: a paradox that encompasses the Void, the Singularity and the *ouroboros*, the snake or dragon eating its own tail: a symbol representing the infinite, eternal cycle of Nature's creation, preservation and destruction – and reaching a zenith in Nine, the number of Odin, the Wolf and the Raven: denoting excellence, attainment and the core qualities of the Creation: Truth (Unity), Perfection (Order, Balance) and Love. The Number archetypes are the dots, which, when connected, denote the soul's path of individuation from the Void to Transcendence.

From Zero (the primal feminine) comes One (primordial unity – the primal masculine). One becomes Two (duality – diversity – differentiation – fecundity – feminine). Three is the creative inspiration and vision that conceives and communicates what may be fashioned out of diversity. Four is what is fashioned and the order necessary to fashion it. Three is the dreamer; four is the organiser! What Three dreams, Four creates, through structure and form.

The structuring power of Four can best be conceived by considering four in its most pure, geometrical form: the square, and, especially, its three-dimensional presentation: the cube – the perfect building block. The organising and structuring competence of the archetype is fully appre-hended when the four interfacing pyramids contained within the cube are perceived: a design that can be replicated into infinity. *Ordered, practical, systematic, persistent, logical, sensible, repetitive and thorough* are important characteristics of Four and of Silicea (silica archetype). The persistence of Four can be likened to the erosion of rock by constantly dripping water or by wind-driven sand: it is *relentless, and inexorable!* Being formally and rigidly structured, Fours are more at ease with the familiar and the tried and are reluctant to change or adapt. The organised nature of the four archetype is reflected in the four limbs of mammals that ground and stabilise; the four seasons; the four cardinal points of the compass; the four elements (earth, water, fire and air); the four essential states (dry, wet, hot, cold); the 4 mathematical operations (addition, subtraction, multiplication, division); and the four temperaments of the human psyche (phlegmatic, melancholic, choleric, sanguine).

Four is the Number of Silicea: the archetype that is the very embodiment of structure and form!

Silicea: the planetary architect

Krystallos is the Greek word for ice. It eventually became the name for quartz and finally the generic designation for all matter that assumes shape out of the gaseous or fluid state. Silicea, quartz, rock crystal has become the very symbol of crystallisation and form; indeed, there is no other mineral to be found in as many different forms as Silicea – the world of Silicea is a world of splendid forms, magnificent shapes and glorious colours.

To attain form, something must be shaped from within and closed off from without and these two, seemingly opposing forces, are inherent in silica, the crystal, and in Silicea, the person! Within the crystal lies the infinite capacity to grow and expand through ever repeated prismatic faces, yet, even as it inexorably creates, this *creative-force* is continuously in contention with the rigid restraints of a strict geometrical design: the *formative-force*, which always achieves the final 'crowning, closing pyramid': the symbol of the soul's ascent towards Self-realisation and spiritual tran-scendence.

The contention between the virtuosity of a free-ranging creative-energy and the constraints of a conservative formative-energy is fundamental to the Silicea psyche. It displays panache and propriety; ambition and diffi-dence; resistance and submission. *The urge to develop and expand is ever-opposed by the need to comply and conform.*

In his last lecture to the Academy of Milan in 1499, Leonardo da Vinci captured this shaping from within and resistance from without, and the struggle it involves, when he stated:

> By the law of the Almighty, the body is the work of the soul, which fashions its outward appearance by hammering it from within, like a goldsmith embossing his material.[4]

The body is the symbol of the soul – it is also the tabernacle of the soul! The form of this tabernacle indicates the aptitudes, tendencies and aspirations animating it. This is particularly true of Silicea: the refined, sensitive crystal being.

What carbon is to the organic world, Silicea is to the inorganic world – the very foundation stone.

The following is attributed to American physician William Gutman (1903–1991), who was President of the American Institute of Homeopathy in 1965:

> The solid structure of the surface of the earth, which supports the whole of organic life is very largely an enormous accumulation of quartz crystals. However, in relation to the earth as a whole, this powerful exo-skeleton is no more than a thin crust: *the earth's skin*; below the crust run the fluid-silicates, penetrating the surface through volcanoes, which open up like *boils and fistulae*. Looking at the geological process: the enclosing of the earth, the shaping of the landscape . . . we perceive again the original tendency of quartz: *its power of formation and solidification.*[5]

This picture captures the formative and strengthening importance of quartz and by analogy underlines the affinity of Silicea for the lymphatic system and its application for deep inflammatory conditions that track to the surface through sinuses and fistulae and for suppurative conditions of the skin.

Quartz properties

In building an archetypal image of a mineral like quartz, much can be learnt from studying its physical and chemical properties and the uses that it has been put to in science, industry and the home. Fused silica is used to make heat-resistant crucibles, flasks and high temperature thermometers. The coefficient of expansion for silica is so slight that it resists fracture over extreme temperature ranges. The thermometers, noted above, for instance, can be heated to incandescence and then plunged into liquid air without damage. Silicon dioxide is resistant to stresses that would destroy other materials. Like a ductile metal, it can be drawn into fine strands that are used in special applications.

The commercial and industrial uses of silica are based on the following properties:

- Heat resistance (refractoriness).
- Negligible thermal expansion.
- Low thermal conductivity.
- High melting point.
- Molten silica recrystallizes slowly.
- Hardness and strength.
- Unusual insolubility in water and acids.
- In its amorphous state: unusual absorptive properties for water, vapour, gases and minute impurities suspended in liquids e.g. diatomaceous earth used as a filtering material.
- The ideal semiconductor: a quality that has made silicon the fundamental unit of the computer world: the 'silicon chip'.

From these qualities, much can be learned about the Silicea archetype. Most categorical is its *resistance and stubbornness*: its resistance to heat and external forces or influences; its stubborn reluctance to melt and its equal unwillingness to return to the solid state. In terms of human behaviour, this points to a disposition that must overcome a state of passive inertia (stubborn and/or fearful recalcitrance) to become productive, but once occupied is liable through active inertia to obstinately persist, even in the face of warning signals and good advice, to the point of exhaustion (compare Graphites). The durability of the substance, its imperviousness to the action of acids and its insolubility, all evidence the innate strength of the archetype, which even when exposed from childhood to the most corrupting society and most sordid circumstances holds true to its principles and its moral convictions. This resilience of character is even more notable when demonstrated in one, who, to all appearances, seems delicate, impressionable and vulnerable; an external fragility, which, as we shall see, is often the presentation of Silicea, both in its natural and human forms. The Silicea archetypal power ('nature') is often proof against a negative environment and an unfortunate upbringing ('nurture').

The hygroscopic pull of amorphous silica has several connotations. In powerfully attracting and absorbing water, silica displays a characteristic, which Grauvogl assigned to his *hydrogenoid constitution*, which, he proposed, was characterised by excess water in the tissues and blood, and heightened sensitivity to cold and damp – according with Hahnemann's sycotic miasm. Silicea must be regarded as even more fundamental to *Sycosis* than Thuja, which is the signature remedy of *Sycosis*. Like Thuja, Silicea counteracts the deleterious effects of vaccination and immunisation, even years after the event – a marked anti-sycotic function. Esoterically, absorption of water (symbolic of emotions), vapours and suspended particles evidences a markedly sensitive nature, open, like Graphites, Nat-carb and Phosphorus, to the emotions of others (clairsentience); intellectually, it signifies outstanding cognitive ability and memory; in terms of the faculties it suggests hypersensitivity to sense impressions, which in Silicea is particularly *to odours* (2) – and, in keeping with the archetype's nature: *to sweet, agreeable odours* (Arg-nit; Aurum; Nit-ac) – and, in highest degree, *to noise* (4): *slightest noise* (4); *painful sensitiveness to noise* (2); *to voices* (2); on a physical level, the hygroscopic quality and filtration capacity of amorphous silica shows the marked affinity of Silicea for the lymphatic circulation, the lymph glands and the functions of the reticulo-endothelial system: defending (combating infection: identifying, removing and destroying pathogens) and healing. Silicea will often be indicated in diseases of the lymphatic system from lymphoedema and lymphadenopathy to lymphoma and leukaemia.

The role of the silicon chip in computer technology suggests the kind of analytical and ordered mind Silicea individuals often have. The archetype is frequently drawn to computer science; a fascination shared by Silicea's dark counterpart, Mercurius, the trickster archetype.

Diatomite

Many varieties of quartz are vibrantly coloured due to the presence of other elements as impurities: rose quartz (pink), amethyst (purple, violet); obsidian (black), onyx (black to white); jasper (red); opal (iridescent due to small inclusions of calcium carbonate). An interesting form of opaline Silicea is the material called diatomite, which consists of the microscopic skeletons of fresh or seawater diatoms. Sponge spicules are also essentially opaline silica.

Here, again, the key importance of Silicea in the hierarchy of homeopathic archetypes is apparent, because diatoms, a major group of micro-algae, the *Bacillariophyceae*, make up the greater part of the phytoplankton, which forms the foundation of the marine food-chain. Not only is all marine life, directly or indirectly, dependent on phytoplankton, these microscopic organisms account for about half of all photosynthetic activity on Earth. A unique feature of diatom cells is that they are enclosed within a cell wall made of silica. This biogenic silica is synthesised intracellularly and then extruded to the cell exterior where it is added to the cell wall, which is called a *frustule*. Not only is this biological synthesis of silica by the diatom unique, it is also highly artistic: the siliceous wall being ornately and symmetrically patterned with a variety of pores, ribs, minute spines, marginal ridges, bossing and lattice-like designs: each, a masterpiece of art by which the different genera and species can be identified. Exquisite delicacy of design points to the sensitive and artistic refinement of the Silicea archetype. The intricacy and perfection of the patterning also reveals a mind that is ordered, meticulously fastidious, attentive to the finest detail and capable of exhaustive repetition.

Diatoms are most abundant in cold latitudes, having a general preference for cold water, and exist in prodigious numbers in the Arctic and Antarctic oceans. Since the siliceous cell walls are virtually imperishable, over millions of years, the unceasing rain of minute valves, onto the bottom of lake or sea, form extensive deposits of diatom skeletal remains, which lithify into friable, light-coloured sedimentary rock called diatomite ('diatomaceous earth'). Diatomite may be of fresh-water or marine origin. Whereas, most deposits are less than a metre thick some are much thicker, even reaching up to 1000 metres. Several million shells are contained in a cubic cm of diatomite.

Such enormous aggregations of 'organic' silica constitute a massive Silicea archetypal statement. It is well to consider the uses to which diatomaceous earth may be put; it provides a signature to the role of silica in the body and indications for Silicea, the remedy.

The properties that contribute to diatomite's usefulness are the following.

- Small particle size.
- High porosity.
- Hygroscopic capacity.
- High surface area.
- Low specific gravity.
- Abrasive quality.
- Chemical inertness.

FILTER MEDIA

The small particle size of diatomite and the open structure of the frustules that compose it, make it a highly absorbent, filtering material. The minute spaces (pores) between frustules trap bacteria and other tiny suspended particles. Diatomite is used to purify drinking and swimming pool water and in breweries and wineries.

ABSORBENT

The hygroscopic capacity (attracting and holding water) of dry diatomite is such that it can attract, absorb and hold water molecules from its surrounding environment to the equivalent of its own weight. This property also enables diatomite powder to absorb skin oils when used in cosmetics and facial masks. It makes a good cat litter.

CEMENT ADDITIVE, FILLER AND ABRASIVE

Diatomite is often used as an additive in the manufacture of Portland cement, being crushed and blended with the shale, limestone and other silicates used in making cement. It can be used as an inert, light-weight filler. Diatomite's small, friable particles of silica are angular and have large surface area; qualities enabling it to act as a mild abrasive in toothpastes, facial scrubs and metal polishes.

FLEA AND TICK CONTROL

Being an abrasive and an absorbent, diatomaceous earth may be used as a dusting powder to control ants, cockroaches, fleas, lice, mites, and ticks. After cleaning bedding and vacuuming carpets, repeated dusting and combing of pets can eradicate flea infestation.

As already considered, the filtering and absorptive properties of diatomite clearly suggest the affinity of Silicea for the reticulo-endothelial system and its defensive and reparative roles. The constructive uses of diatomite point to Silicea's affinity for the formative processes if the body, the skeletal system and the connective tissues that give support, strength and stability to the body.

Its value in getting rid of pests and parasites is of great significance. There is a correlation between the capacity of certain plants and substances to repel insects and their value in the treatment of those who have suffered abuse, especially sexual abuse and rape. Thuja, Cocculus, Staphysagria (louse wort), Cimicifuga (bug bane), Agaricus (fly agaric), Ledum and Anatherum are outstanding examples. When indicated, Silicea can empower a victim to escape abusive situations and stand up to those who bully or harm them. It is a remedy for the chronic psychological consequences of being victimised or parasitised, hence, for the sapping effect that human 'vampires' have upon the emotional life. In addition, like Staphysagria and Ledum, Silicea strengthens the constitution, making it less attractive to biting-insects, and, if bites do occur, Silicea minimises reaction, especially the tendency to fester.

Comparing diatomite's uses and the clinical affinities of Silicea, highlights how the innate pattern of an archetype touches every aspect of its domain, assuring us that nothing is discrete and all is interdependent and subject to law and the will of a Universal Intelligence. This knowledge opens the mind to the symbolic language of the relative sphere and the guiding cues that synchronicity affords the soul on the path to individuation.

The metaphor of glass

Silicea is synonymous with glass, hence, glass symbolises much of the essence of Silicea.

Natural glass

Although man has been manufacturing glass ever since it was invented in Mesopotamia, about 5000 years ago, nature was fabricating natural glass through volcanic activity millions of years ago. This volcanic glass, the most common form being known as *obsidian*, forms when hot lava quickly cools after oozing onto the earth's surface. Another natural form of glass occurs when lightning strikes a sandy beach or a desert surface. This appears in the form of thin, crystalline tubes called *fulgurites* (from the Latin, *fulgar*, meaning thunderbolt). Similarly, *tektites*: small, rounded, cystic bodies of glass, are formed when fiery meteorites violently impact with the earth. The chemical composition of these petrified forms is like granite and they contain a very high percentage of silica, the basic ingredient of glass. The hollow, convoluted, tube of fused quartz that constitutes a fulgurite, typifies the tunnel structure of *fistulae*, and tektites have all the appearance of *cysts* – pathological structures that often yield to the healing influence of Silicea. While many fulgurites are small and fragile and easily disintegrate on contact, others are large, rugged, tubular structures that withstand weathering; while some are rough and crude in appearance, others are the epitome of artistic elegance, resembling complex root systems: patterning in glass, the scattered pathways of electrical power discharged into sand. The natural works of silica exhibit the aesthetic awareness and creative genius of the Silicea archetype.

Deserving attention, is the violence of the forces that forge natural glass. They stand in stark contradiction to the inexorable slowness of most silica/Silicea processes. This seeming incongruity must not be disregarded; it is arresting, and, therefore, relevant! In marked contrast to its common, slow, insidious onset, Silicea psychopathology can be precipitated by *sudden, intense events*, especially *fright*, the shock of *bad news* or some *dreadful, wounding humiliation*.

Manufactured glass

The most commonly manufactured glass e.g. window glass and glass tableware, is called *soda-lime-silica glass* in that its chief ingredients are: sodium oxide (soda) + calcium oxide (lime) + 75% silica (sand) with the addition of small amounts of magnesium oxide and aluminium oxide. This important recipe, a magic mix of molecules, is a pointer to close Silicea archetypal relationships. Since, the fundamental archetypal presentation of sodium, calcium and magnesium is in the form of their carbonate salts – Nat-carb, Calc-carb and Mag-carb must be regarded as central archetypes orbiting round Silicea. Alumina (aluminium oxide) is another; its importance highlighted by its abundance in the earth's crust where it combines with silica and silicates to form clay.

Other significant archetypal connections of Silicea can be made from glass chemistry.

Pyrex (*sodium borosilicate glass*), which stands heat expansion far better than window glass and is much prized in the kitchen, is a combination of silica + boron trioxide + soda (sodium oxide) + alumina. The archetypal representative of boron is Borax (sodium borate). While Silicea is vital to the processes of assimilation, nutrition, growth and development and to the emotional and physical defence systems, Borax, the 5th element in the creation, is vital to the development of self-awareness, self-appraisal, personal uniqueness and the unfolding of purpose, direction and motivation. The two archetypes stand close, sharing many characteristics: hypersensitivity to sound; fear of falling, fear of thunderstorms, easy starting and taking fright; self-effacing diffidence that deprives them of a voice; yielding to the opinion of others; shy and timid, mild and gentle; vulnerable to teasing and bullying; easily taking offence.

As might be expected, other members of the Group IV elements are also employed in glass manufacture.

Germanium dioxide combined with alumina produces *germanium oxide glass*, which is extremely clear glass, used for fibre-optic waveguides in communication networks. Germanium needs to be compared with both Silicea and Alumina. The emotional profile of Germanium demonstrates most clearly the interplay between the archetypes, or complexes, within the psyche (see: *The Wolf*, pp. 150–160).

Lead glass or crystal glass (lead-oxide glass – silica + lead oxide + potassium oxide + soda + zinc oxide – has high density and, hence, a high refractive index, which makes the glassware more brilliant. The price for this aesthetic appeal is less heat resistance and greater fragility; but the glass is easier to cut. Lead is the heaviest of the Group IV elements; it represents the energy of the group taken to its material ultimate. Lead glass exhibits the characteristics of the lead archetype, Plumbum: a highly materialistic person driven to partake of all the pleasures and iniquities of life and to achieve wealth, power and status (brilliance) at the price of moral degeneracy (fragility). Plumbum exaggerates the perversities of *Sycosis* to gross proportions and in its *Syco-syphilitic* mode produces grave pathology involving particularly the neurological and arterial systems.

Zinc, the other important component in crystal glass, is a highly sensitive archetype, intensely sensitive to noise (4) and voices (4), very easily offended, and, like Borax, fears falling and downward movement. Connections made in this way, often reveal unexpected associations, that prove invaluable in practice.

Glass art and technology
There is a fascination in watching a skilled glass blower at work. Their deft technique and refined artistry is mesmerising. Equally spellbinding are the remarkable qualities of the material they are manipulating and moulding.

- It is fluid, clear, yielding, supple and pliant, conforming to every creative whim of the artist.
- Yet, when it sets, it is firm, strong, rigid and inflexible.
- It is transparent, delicate, brittle and fragile.
- Malleable and responsive, exquisite designs of surpassing beauty can be wrought from it.

The slightest blow sharply delivered to a critical spot or a sound wave of critical frequency, can shatter glass, yet the material can resist tremendous forces and sustain a symphony of sound.

These wide-ranging qualities afford insight into the nature and character of the young Silicea. A person who is innocent, impressionable, adaptable and compliant, but gifted with intelligence, intuitive perception and innate morality, by which they weigh and measure people and life. As they mature, cued by what they admire and respect, their impressions, preferences and persuasions set into a framework of values that are proof against the pressures of their environment. They are sincere and honest (transparent), they have integrity and loyalty (firm, strong), they are incorruptible (rigid, inflexible) and one-pointed in their pursuit of excellence (exquisite design). Often, they possess a refined and delicate beauty, which reflects an even greater inner beauty. Though sensitive, emotional and empathetic, they show surprising strength and fortitude in the face of adversity. Outer susceptibility is countered by inner resilience and resolve. Nonetheless, they possess a specific vulnerability and emotional fragility that renders a critical trauma utterly devastating.

Glass embodies colour, light, art and music. The glass prism refracts light, splitting and radiating it into its constituent colours of the spectrum. In this phenomenon, which directly connects quartz with all levels of chakra consciousness, Silicea announces, as in its crowning pyramid, its overriding objective: the individuation of the soul! Glass art is an art form as versatile as the material it uses and as versatile as its mother form: quartz. The cohesive plasticity of the material lends itself to dextrous craftsmanship and delicately refined artistry and the fluid medium infused with splendid, flowing colours, creates art within art. A glass musician can make glass emit celestial music, described as: 'like hearing angels sing'. If a leather-padded wand is repeatedly passed around the brim of a pure quartz bowl, a wondrously, stirring, deep-booming note akin to the holy sound Om, steadily builds to intense amplitude. To Hinduism, Om is the sound representing the Divine, or the power of the Creator. It is the sound-symbol of the Ultimate Reality. All words are said to be forms of this one sound Om, which, expressing all sound, equates with white light, containing all colour.

Glass is surely the most *versatile* of all materials; it can be as imposing and sophisticated as the giant telescope mirrors and lenses of the astronomer, used for penetrating the secrets of the cosmos; as searching as the microscope of the scientist peering into the realm of the minute; or as small and simple as a child's marble. It restores our failing eyesight and projects our vision with clarity to the world about us, but also the world within us, because, as the first mirror after water, it is a sceptre for vanity, permitting us to scrutinise the hidden aspects of our inner nature and ask: "Who am I?" In our homes, it visually maintains our union and communication with the world about us, while secluding, insulating and protecting us, without separating or isolating us.

These observations all portray archetypal qualities that pertain to Silicea. The archetype is as moved by the simple and nondescript as they are by the grand and magnificent. They can contemplate and marvel at the world about them with the same earnest attention they devote to introspection and self-analysis. Whilst participating sensitively and positively in life's parade, the higher Silicea remains detached and dispassionate, removed from the pettiness and superficialities of social intercourse.

The lens of the eye, possessing all the functional attributes of optical lenses, and the eye itself, as the organ of sight, are central to the sphere of Silicea, both physically and metaphorically.

The eye is the window or mirror of the soul.

Silicea, the remedy, brings clarity to the confused mind; it provides an unblemished (unprejudiced ego-free) window to scrutinise life. Silicea, the archetype, has spiritual insight and aspires to Self-enlightenment. The eyes of a Silicea speak volumes, they are truly the mirrors of their souls.

Silica- and silicon-based technology affirms and expands on the exceptional qualities of the Silicea intellect and psyche.

- The lens displays the macro-cosmos – the infinitely vast; glass fibre optics reveals the micro-cosmos – the infinitely small.
- The technology of glass fibre optics permits the human mind to project itself through audio-visual signals across the planet; it extends the power of communication and the dissemination of knowledge.
- In the Silicon chip, the mineral world vies with the organic world in memory and intelligence.
- Tiny quartz crystals provide us with the quintessential timekeeper, precise and accurate regardless of temperature or position.

From these reflections, it is apparent that the Silicea archetype embodies remarkable attributes, traits and potential: *a scientific mind, intelligence, memory, eloquence, refinement, exactitude, precision, punctiliousness, clarity, perspective and the communication and dissemination of knowledge and wisdom.*

Psychic objects
For thousands of years, many cultures have divined that quartz crystals possess both magic and esoteric qualities. The crystal ball focuses the clairvoyant and prophetic powers of the fortune teller; the crystal rod transmits the curative power of the psychic healer; the oscillating crystal orb induces the hypnotic trance of the mesmerist and acts as a responsive indicator in radionics; and the crystal talisman protects the wearer from misfortune and psychic impingement. In keeping with this symbolism, the Silicea archetype is *highly sensitive, empathetic, intuitive and may possess psychic gifts – clairvoyance, clairaudience and clairsentience!*

References

1 Sherr J. *The Noble Gases – Neon.* Glasgow: Saltire Books, 2016.
2 Clarke JH. *Oxygenium. A Dictionary of Practical Materia Medica.* Available online at: http://www.homeoint.org/clarke/o/oxy.htm. (Retrieved 10.03.2018.)
3 Sherr J. *The Noble Gases – Helium.* Glasgow: Saltire Books, 2013.
4 Vannier L. *Homoeopathy Human Medicine.* (trans Clement M.) New Delhi: B. Jain Publishers, Pty Ltd., 1998. p116.
5 Gutman W. *Homoeopathy: The fundamentals of its philosophy: the essence of its remedies.* Mumbai: Homeopathic Medical Publishers, 1986.

11

SILICEA – 2

The Evolution of Science –
Galileo and Sir Isaac Newton

Through glass and the evolution of the lens, Silicea is as closely related to the birth of modern science as Lycopodium is to the birth of the industrial era through coal. In this Chapter the characters of Galileo and Isaac Newton are compared with the profile of Silica.

Galileo (1564–1642)

The birth of science was explosive rather than evolutionary. It occurred when a very simple telescope fell into the hands of a *sandy-haired genius* and he directed his gaze at the heavens. *The year was 1609* and the genius was Galileo. From that moment, Earth and 'man' ceased to be the centre of the universe. It is significant that in 1616, this very practical, unromantic man was precipitated into a *Silicea-like yielding situation* when the Roman

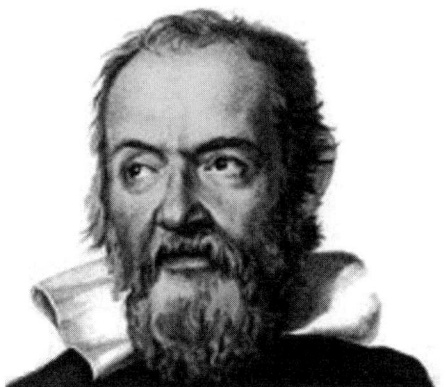

Figure 11.1 *Galileo Galliel (1564–1642)*
(https://bohatala.com/galileo-galilei-biography-and-achievements/)

Inquisition ordered him to recant his strongly averred conviction that the Copernicus theory of *heliocentrism* was correct: namely, that the Sun, not the Earth, was the centre of the solar system. Under threat of torture, though certain of the truth of his observations, he was forced to comply. This was a typical Silicea experience and happening: *enlightenment arrested by ignorance – wisdom blocked by fanaticism.* In 1633, he was tried again and finally sentenced to house arrest for the rest of his life. He died on January 1642, aged 77. Three centuries later, Professor Stephen Hawking was to be born on this very same day.

Archetypal inclination persuades the events of a life and colours the preferences and aptitudes of the individual biased by the archetype. This is apparent in the life of Galileo; evidenced in his trial and recantation, but also in lesser ways.

- Following his father's example, Galileo became an accomplished lutenist. [Silicea is often a *musician, or has a love of music.*]
- He studied *medicine* (a calling of many a Silicea), but his *love of mathematics, especially geometry*, lead him to persuade his father to permit him to change to maths and science (*mathematics – calculus and geometry – either terrify the young Silicea,* or, having a computer-like mind, *they may excel in both*).
- He was *an inventor* (an aptitude shared with Sulphur) – he invented the thermoscope [forerunner of the thermometer]; a hydrostatic balance; and improved the telescope.
- He also studied *fine arts.*
- He *stubbornly refused* to accept Johannes Kepler's belief that the moon caused the tides, and equally stubbornly rejected his concept of the elliptical orbits of the planets, believing implicitly that the circle provided the perfect shape for planetary orbits. Silicea is exceedingly *stubborn* and resistant to persuasion until able to place a new concept in their framework of reality; only then do they graciously adopt it. Silicea is studied and considered, not intellectually impulsive.

Being a fundamental archetype, second only to Graphites, Silicea provides a template upon which the psoric triad, Sulphur – Calc-carb – Lycopodium rests.

- Sulphur/Silicea – the inventor and the theoriser.
- Calc-carb/Silicea – the importance of house, home and family – the insular, self-contained disposition.
- Lycopodium/Silicea – lack of confidence in the presence of great ability – tendency to overdo and burn-out.

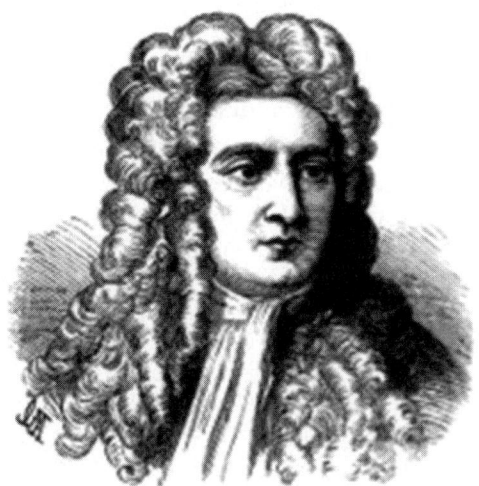

Figure 11.2 *Sir Isaac Newton (1643–1727)*
(Image: Alamy)

Sir Isaac Newton (1643–1727)

The Silicea connection with the evolution of science continued seamlessly with the work of Isaac Newton, who entered the world on Christmas Day, 25 December 1642,[i] in the year of Galileo's death. He was born in the hamlet of Woolsthorpe in the South Kesteven district of Lincolnshire, England. Newton embodied the spirit of Silicea, which, true to its esoteric, archetypal nature, laid, through him, the intellectual foundation and platform upon which the edifice of empirical science would be raised. As colour infuses glass, so the essence of Silicea permeated Isaac Newton, imparting his soaring genius, his singular eccentricity and determining his destiny.

No sooner was he conceived, possibly out of wedlock, to Isaac Newton senior, an illiterate yeoman farmer, and Hannah Ayscough, the daughter of educated, lower gentry, than the archetypal spell of Silicea descended upon Isaac's life! Hannah's thirty-six-year old, newly-wedded husband, sickened and died, leaving her heavily pregnant. By Newton's own account, offered in his later years, the loss (*shock, grief*) brought on labour pains and *he was born prematurely* on Christmas morning, shortly after 2 a.m. – *a typical tiny, frail, weak Silicea baby* that was not expected to survive the week, let alone the 84 years he achieved.

---

[i] According to the Julian calendar in use in England at the time. The gap between it and the Gregorian calendar at that time was 11 days.

Deserted

For three years, deprived of husband and father, mother and child were always together, closely bonded and inseparable. Then, the finger of Silicea destiny turned the page again! Hannah decided to remarry! Her husband, Barnabas Smith, was the sixty-three-year old, well-to-do rector of North Witham, a hamlet just over a mile from Woolsthorpe. Hannah was thirty, or thereabouts. The marriage agreement between the two was coldly business-like and while bringing the two estates equitably together, neglected all thought and consideration for Hannah's three-year-old son. In compliance with terms laid down by Smith, who did not want Hannah's son living with them, Isaac was left with his grandparents James and Margery Ayscough. The married couple moved to the neighbouring village of North Witham and there raised a son and two daughters. Whatever the mother's feelings or regrets might have been at having to leave her father-less, now-motherless, infant son at such an impressionable age, the young-ster must have experienced the enforced separation as *rejection and abandonment* and decided proof of not being loved and, therefore, of being unlovable, due to some blight or inferiority. The absence of a father figure would have deepened Isaac's emotional dependency on his mother, making his sudden isolation more painful and traumatic.

- *Children: dragged on mother's arm* (unique).
- *Children: clinging to mother.*
- *Needs to be held.*
- *Protection: constantly wants mother's protection.*
- *Timidity when alone.*
- *Timidity with other children.*
- *Ailments from separation, abandonment, neglect.*
- *Forsaken feeling; feels not beloved of parents, wife, friends.*

Psychosexual fixation

In this family configuration, another, key Silicea psychic dynamic came into play: the *Oedipus complex* of Freud (to be considered in depth [see Part 2]); a dynamic that underlies much psychopathology, significantly so in young Silicea boys, usually coming into play during the phallic stage of psychosexual development (age 3–6 years: Newton's age at the time of parting from his mother).

In the phallic stage, the young boy directs his libido energy, or sexual desire, upon his mother and directs jealousy and emotional rivalry against his father, because it is he who sleeps with his mother. In the instance of

Isaac Newton, this tortuous interplay was exaggerated, for it was not his own father who was the man sleeping with his mother, but a detested imposter, and it was not the clean finality of death that had effectively deprived him of his mother – *she was willingly taken by another man*, not into remote obscurity, but merely a village away – a metaphorical 'stone's throw'; within reach, but beyond his longing and need. Compounding his exclusion and isolation were the three children the Smith's quickly produced – one of whom was a boy! Adding to the anguish of his hurt was the ever-repeated enactment of desertion. He never knew if, when, or for how long, his mother would visit him; she was unpredictable, ruled by the priorities of her other life; sometimes it would be a mere hour, sometimes an afternoon; and then, there was always the inevitable parting – she, leaving him for that other man: the hated Barnabas Smith and *his* children.

Murderous hatred

Clues contained in his notebooks and personal papers, reveal that Newton loathed and despised his step-father and came to resent his mother for betraying him and placing her affections elsewhere. As a nineteen-year-old undergraduate, Newton kept a notebook in which he wrote down, as a form of confessional purging, an inventory of his transgressions against what he believed the Lord would have expected of him. He drew up two lists: one for sins committed before Whitsunday 1662 and the other for sins committed after that date. Most disturbing are two entries contained in the earlier and much longer list:

- *Threatening my father and mother Smith to burne them and the house over them.*
- *Wishing death and hoping it to some.*

Insights into the twisted complexity of Isaac Newton's psyche startle us for they are at odds with the idealised and sanctified image we spontaneously entertain of the great man – a misapprehension common to his early biographers, who were universally enraptured by his achievements, his prodigious intellect and his celebrity and who graced him with an irreproachable profile, reflecting the faultless persona Newton himself wished posterity to revere. In like manner, many a homeopath holds a glorified image of the Silicea archetype and is startled to find evidence of a convoluted temperament, harbouring bitterness and resentment every bit as keen and malicious as the Nitric acid archetype. One has only to contemplate the inveterate, burrowing destructiveness of a Silicea ulcerative lesion and compare it with the superficial, spreading ulceration of Mercurius, the signature archetype of the syphilitic miasm, to realise that one must not make light of Silicea or its proclivities.

The intensity and violence of Isaac's feelings are apparent in these two lines – understandable in a young boy dispossessed of the mother, who had been exclusively his for three years and to whom he was deeply bonded.

Since Newton never mentions his grandparents in his private papers, it can be presumed that the relationship was not warm; probably aggravated by he, himself, being withdrawn and passively aggressive towards them (Graphites). They could never have hoped to replace Hannah in his affections or compensate for her absence. Fathoming the nature of the child from evidence of his nature as he reached manhood, Isaac cannot have been an easy child for his grandparents to deal with, particularly given the emotions smouldering within.

- *Obstinate, headstrong; children; cry when kindly spoken to.*
- *Averse to being spoken to.*
- *Morose, cross, fretful, ill-humour, peevish: in children.*
- *Mood repulsive.*
- *Looked at; cannot bear to be looked at – anger when looked at.*
- *Irritability in children.*
- *Anger in children.*
- *Anxiety in schoolchildren about their lessons.*
- *Dullness in children.*

However, what is more notable about the anger than its intensity is its festering persistence; the fact that he could recall it so luridly and express it in terms of killing by fire – burning to death not only the hated intruder, but his mother also; and that he 'felt compelled to confess it so many years later, long after the principal object of his hatred (Barnabas Smith) was dead and buried'.[1]

An even more intimate window into Newton's seething, bitter emotions is afforded by his schoolboy exercise book, known to historians as the Morgan notebook. Most illuminating is an alphabetical list of word associations Newton jotted down alongside headings taken from a book by Father Francis Gregory: *Nomenclatura*.

Most pertinent are the following:

- **Father**: Fornicator – Flatterer.
- **Brother**: Bastard – Blasphemer – Brawler – Bedlam – Beggar – Benjamite (Isaac's half-brother was Benjamin).
- **Wife** and **Wedlock**: Whore.

It was eight years later that Hannah, after the death of her second husband, Barnabas Smith, returned with her three younger children to stay at the Newton manor in Woolsthorpe. By then, Isaac was eleven-years-old. The psychological damage he had suffered was ingrained and irreversible. The overwhelming guilt the young boy must have felt on being deserted and kept one apart, would have evolved out of imagining that he must have done something terribly wrong to have been so cruelly and continuously punished. This would have been further compounded by the guilt stemming from his revengeful anger and hatred towards his parents and siblings.

Hannah's return brought further emotional disruption. Was his mother's sudden return a reward: proof that he was guilty of some forgotten crime for which he had now served his time? Isaac had also to face the proximity of his half-siblings: the progeny of his arch-nemesis! There is no extant document that throws definite light on his feelings towards them, other than the derogatory words he chose to write next to 'brother' in his school-book, but given his nature, their association with his betrayal and abandonment and his having to share with them not only his mother's time and attention, but also what had been up until then his private space, he must have harboured considerable resentment against them. He was, by all accounts, a quiet child, not given to emotional outbursts or tantrums. Knowing the intensity of his concealed feelings, declared only in private, *a silent, secretive person is discerned: a closed individual with a deep-seated malicious streak, fed by resentful fires.* Hannah must have been relieved when a year later, in 1654, he left home to attend King's School in Grantham, seven miles away.

Relative to the young Newton, Silicea covers:

- *Desire to kill.*
- *Desires death* (2).
- *Weary of life* (2).
- *Suicidal disposition – by drowning* (2) – throwing himself from a height.
- *Dreams: having been betrayed.*
- *Dreams: of youth time* (3).
- *Anger in children.*
- *Ailments:*
  - *From anger.*
  - *Friendship deceived.*
  - *Humiliation.*
- *Clinging of children to mother.*
- *Constantly wants mother's protection.*

- *Holding or being held ameliorates* (2).
- **Delusion: persecuted.*
- *Delusion: worms or vermin creeping* (invariably implies abuse).
- *Dreams: fire and flood* (2).
- *Dreams: humiliation.*
- *Fear: of being alone.*
- **Forsaken feeling: not beloved by parents.*
- *Offended easily* (2).
- *Precocity.*
- *Intellectual.*
- *Quiet disposition – reserved – mildness* (3) *– timidity* (3).
- *Seriousness.*
- **Thoughts persistent.*
- *Anxiety of conscience* (2).
- *Reproaches himself.*
- *Remorse* (2).
- **Religious affections – sadness.*

The degree to which Newton was emotionally damaged by his childhood trauma was glaringly demonstrated later in life when he began to cross academic swords with his contemporaries in science. But, its insidious effect orchestrated much of his life, forging his eccentric, guarded and reclusive disposition, feeding his insecurities, his obsessive anxieties, his hypochondria, his paranoia and determining his responses to people, women and events.

The Oedipus dynamic, so critical to a Silicea – and, as will be explained later, captured in the highest possible degree (4) in the rubrics: ***fear of pins, of pointed sharp things*** and ***sensitive, oversensitive, to steel points directed towards them*** – points to an immense reservoir of repressed anger held in the Shadow of Newton's psyche: an anger which could be partially sublimated through the intensity and passion with which he wielded his vast, ranging intellect and partially vented vicariously via his driving ambition and supreme egoism; but on a deeper level, nonetheless, subverted his character and left him liable to intemperate rages, inveterate resentment and a malicious desire for revenge.

Grantham

In Grantham, Isaac lodged with the Clarks, the family of the local apothecary. At first, he showed little interest in his studies and his results were mediocre. He was one apart, overlooked by his teachers and generally disliked by the other boys. A book by John Bate: *The Mysteries of Nature and Art* came to hand and captivated him. It contained detailed instructions on how to construct various machines and devices. Having no friends at school, the manual provided him with a welcome pastime and developed his practical skills, which he would later put to good use in the experiments he devised. He was soon designing and building working mechanical models, such as windmills and clocks, that earned him a reputation at school. This new-found enthusiasm took precedence over studying; helped by the fact that he found the formal curriculum uninspiring. His attempts to interest schoolmates in intellectual activities rather than superficial pursuits, such as sport, met with little enthusiasm and distanced him even further from the rest. There was a contradiction in his nature: need for solitude in which he could pursue his obscure interests undisturbed – going where few minds could accompany him – yet yearning for attention and companionship, but unable to bridge the intellectual void between himself and his peers to establish worthwhile communication. Emotionally impoverished, he craved a loving relationship.

He wrote well, composed poetry and all the pictures hanging in his room he had drawn himself, either copied from prints or sketched from life. But, his talent for mathematics and scholastic flare still lay dormant – on hold – waiting their moment!

Several Silicea ineptitudes are listed in the repertory, all of which are, paradoxically, aptitudes Silicea may possess to an advanced degree. Tardy maturing of intellectual ability is common to the Silicea archetype: they are often slow to reach their potential and may at first struggle in the very domains in which they will later excel.

- *Maths, calculating; aversion.*
- *Maths, geometry: inapt for.*
- *Painting; inapt for.*
- *Art; inapt for.*
- *Singing; inapt for.*

Without exception, these are intellectual and creative activities, in which Silicea can be extraordinarily talented. Often, as with the formation of fulgurites and tektites, a catalyst – sometimes dramatic, sometimes violent – may be required to set the Silicea wheels of talent in motion. So, it was with Newton: he was *slow to mature as a scholar* and was regarded by his teachers as *an underachiever.* At Grantham, he remained lacklustre and unexceptional, more interested in constructing devices than in study. In typical Silicea inertia, he needed some external force to fire his genius.

The catalyst

It came in the form of a playground bully! Through time, the bullies of the world have singled out the Silicea archetype for hostile attention. The crystal archetype's quiet, gentle, refined, intellectual nature is like a red rag to a bull, pressing all the buttons of the bully's own disowned 'weakness', which they repress and project onto others. Recognising it in the mild, reserved, timid disposition of the typical Silicea, they attack it to confirm their alpha status.

On the way to school, the bully in question kicked Isaac forcefully in the stomach. The reason for the aggressive attack is not known, but it roused Newton out of his indolence in more ways than one. Enraged, but unable to retaliate immediately, he challenged the offender, a much larger boy, as bullies often are, to a fight after school. They duly met in the church-yard with the schoolmaster's son officiating. Despite their disparity in size and strength, Newton hurled himself upon his foe and fighting like one possessed soon beat his burly opponent into submission. The humiliated bully could never have anticipated the whirlwind of bottled violence and rage that his smaller and weaker adversary wreaked upon him. He was the detested scapegoat marked for all the bitter hatred Isaac nursed against his dead stepfather, Barnabas Smith, and his mother. The fight was cathartic and catalytic!

Even while his bloodied victim struggled to regain his senses, Isaac defiantly declared that he would not rest until he had outstripped the bully academically as thoroughly and completely as he had crushed him physically. He proved as good as his word but setting his sights far higher than above the level of his defeated enemy, he sought top academic honours and soon achieved them. The intellect is the very citadel of Silicea; an edifice erected to provide identity and worth and to compensate for 'being inferior, unworthy of love and unlovable'. Isaac's declaration proclaimed his archetypal intent to methodically build the formidable crystal of his mind until it achieved the supreme pinnacle of Silicea achievement: the crowning, closing pyramid!

Making good from adversity is a common theme of Silicea.

Removal from school

Isaac's newly-awakened academic ability soon came to the attention of the headmaster, Henry Stokes, who, recognising Isaac's unique potential, strongly recommended that on completion of his schooling, he should receive a university education. Yet, it was at this critical point, just when her son was at last coming into his own, that Hannah, without consulting either the headmaster or Isaac, decided to remove him from school. Education was not a priority to Hannah. Isaac Newton senior was illiterate and had farmed successfully and now Hannah needed Isaac's help in managing her not inconsiderable farmlands. Convinced of her standpoint, she disregarded Stokes' consternation and attempts to dissuade her.

Though obedient to his mother's decision, Newton suffered severely from his removal from an environment in which he was blossoming. His schoolbook reflects his anguish at contemplating a life yet again ruined by his mother. As previously, he notes his various 'sins': his peevishness and refusal to complete tasks (*passive aggression*) – and – 'punching my sister' and 'falling out with the servants' (*anger expressed indirectly*) – both, forms of Silicea ire. Instead of watching the cattle, he would recline beneath a tree with a book, and, when assigned tasks in neighbouring Grantham, he would instruct the servant accompanying him to attend to the chores, while he visited Mr Clark, the apothecary with whom he had previously lodged. Clark had acquired a large collection of scientific books. In the back room, behind the shop, Isaac delved into works by Plato, Aristotle, Francis Bacon, René Descartes and other scientific minds, acquiring a wider and more relevant education than he would have achieved through the limited school curriculum. Like many a Silicea, Newton was a notable *autodidact*, capable of self-education without need for formal guidance or instruction. Eventually, it became evident, even to Hannah, that neither the farm or Isaac were benefiting from her thoughtless decision. A second appeal from Stokes for Isaac to return to school, swung the balance and Hannah yielded to common sense and the best interests of her son. At last, the way lay open for Newton to fulfil his pressing need to broaden his knowledge.

These details from Newton's early life, reflect much that is characteristic of Silicea experience and Silicea response to such experience. Typical, is a life dictated by others, without concern for Silicea; slow, but steady unfolding of ability regardless of circumstances – like a crystal, pushing towards excellence; an ability to 'go-it-alone'; stubborn adherence to a self-determined objective, despite obstacles and the dissent or persuasion of others; repressed anger, indignation and resentment stemming from injustice experienced and frustrated objectives; emotions, especially anger, deflected passively or indirectly; anger uncharacteristically vented, suddenly and violently; insular, eccentric nature, content with its own company, seemingly independent, yet longing for a deep, compatible and meaningful friendship; critical intolerance for crudity, stupidity, irresponsibility and inefficiency; an innate morality holding them responsible for their thoughts, emotions and behaviour; convictions differing from mainstream belief without need for debate or proselytising; keeping their opinions to themselves.

Reference

1   White M. *Isaac Newton – The Last Sorcerer*. London: Fourth Estate Ltd, 1997. p17.

12

SILICEA – 3

Trinity College

Solitary and invisible

In 1661, Newton advanced from Grantham to Trinity College, Cambridge. Due to his broken education, he was two years older than other undergraduates. He entered a climate in which the *scientific revolution* was well advanced, and many of the basic works of contemporary science had already appeared.

Newton was now a conscientious and committed student. Initially he remained an inconspicuous member of his group, his remarkable intellect

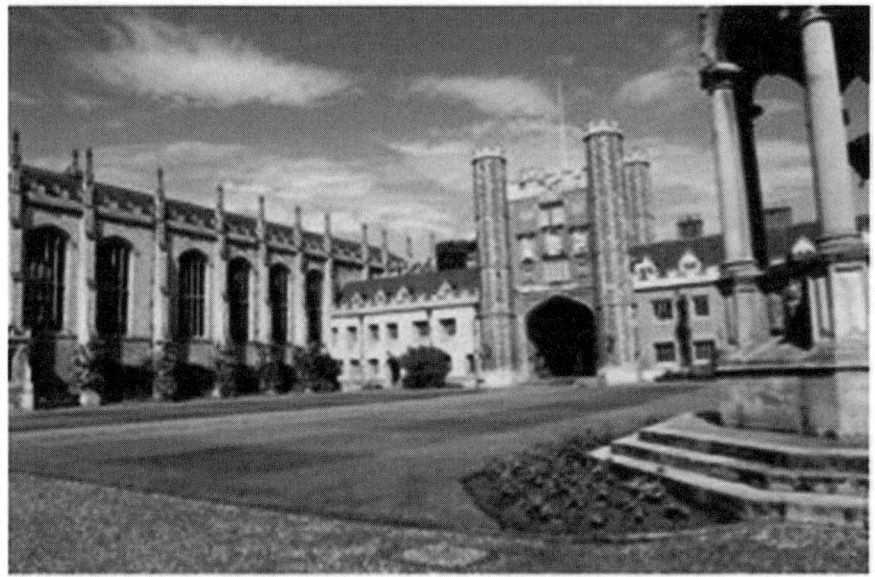

Figure 12.1 *Trinity College, Cambridge*

(Image: Alamy)

quietly imbibing knowledge, causing no ripples to attract the attention of his lecturers. *He was virtually invisible* – a glass archetype!

This 'grey' characteristic, which is typical of psoric Graphites, is also a trait of syphilitic Mercurius, an archetype that can merge with their surroundings and escape detection. The syphilitic organism, the spirochete, Treponema pallidum, *the pale thread*, on gaining entrance to the body, similarly remains inconspicuous (grey), invisible to the body's defences and for years causes no warning ripples. Multi-miasmatic Silicea is both psoric and syphilitic and has an uncanny way of remaining low-profile: the conscientious student, who sits at the back of the class, never asks questions, knows all the answers, yet never volunteers any, always attentive, slips away unnoticed at the close of lectures, does not socialise, is never a source of controversy, always achieves high grades.

This profile certainly applied to Newton. Notable, is the lack of any reference to him by fellow students during his earliest period at Trinity; nor is there the slightest hint of a personal relationship from this time. He was a loner! All we know is that he shared a chamber with a certain Francis Walton whom he thoroughly disliked. Yet again, his 'confessions' provide the window. There are two 'sins' perpetrated against this much-despised individual: 'Using Wilford's towel to spare my own' – and – 'Deceiving my chamber-fellow of the knowledge of him that took him for a sot'.

A characteristic of Silicea entering unfamiliar company is their inability to integrate. They remain aloof, on the outside – not even looking in – because they do little, if anything, to initiate friendship or endear themselves and often find reason why they should not invite familiarity or involve themselves: a defensive indifference or 'looking down' on others to disguise their own hesitancy, timidity and shyness, while displaying an innate egoism. Quartz itself, announces this stand-offish, unapproachable archetypal trait: it is a non-reactive, insoluble substance, immune to impingement by most acids and chemicals and resistant to heat. Other aspects of Silicea that naturally distance them from others are their seriousness, their refined tastes, their deep-thinking, their often-esoteric or obscure philosophy and their inflexible sense of morality and correctness.

Adding to Newton's seclusion would have been the two-year age difference between him and most of his fellows – a significant difference at that time of life – but more alienating was his Puritan faith. Although the restoration had removed the yoke of Catholicism, the great universities were supported and sustained by the orthodoxy of the Anglican Church. Newton's conservative Puritanism was out of step with this central pillar of British society. His first years at Cambridge coincided with his obsessive preoccupation with 'sin', 'confession' and 'repentance', during which time 'his pious detachment from worldly pleasures'[1] would have made him seem a prim, prudish pain-in-the-neck to fun-loving students bent on revelry. Later, he relaxed somewhat, enjoying the odd ale and game of cards, but initially, he lived a solitary life in an alien world, unable to indulge his newly-acquired freedom due to inner reserve and rectitude. His puritanism was not political, nor was it the thin-lipped, sombre, judgemental bigotry of the religious fanatic, who sees Satan lurking behind every bush. It was not a doctrine he wished, or felt he needed, to impose on others. For Newton, worship of God was achieved through industry, the diligent pursuit of knowledge and revealing His glory through unveiling Nature's truths.

Another inaptitude of Silicea, which is given highest grading, is *inaptitude for finance* (3). Many characteristics of Silicea have what seems to be an incongruous mirror image, e.g. fastidious – dirtiness; haughty – servile; obstinately persistent – persists in nothing; and so, it is with finances: the rubric *inaptitude for finance* needs to be balanced by its opposite, but in lesser grade, for with Silicea *necessity is the mother of invention* and need is more likely to dictate Silica's involvement in finance than greed or materialism. Silicea can be very careful and ordered with money or they may *squander from want of order.*

Seeing that he had no popularity to lose and needing to supplement his allowance from Hannah, Newton decided to become a money-lender, a pursuit sure to attract opprobrium. Having no financial base to kick-off from, he must have taken an initial risk (*inaptitude for finance*) that fortunately paid off. He was successful with his venture (*aptitude for finance*), and typically Silicea-like, kept meticulous records of his transactions, as, indeed, he did of his 'sins'. Given his *anxiety of conscience* (2) and *religious affections* there was bound to be an overlap between the two sets of records, and, sure enough, his confessions list notes the cardinal sin: 'setting my heart on money more than God'. The Silicea archetype, more than most, is inclined to such self-scrutiny and critical self-analysis.

John Wilkins – a new room-mate for Newton

Providence was beginning to smile on Newton. His affairs improved. Eighteen months after arriving at Trinity, he managed to contrive the departure of his 'disorderly' room-mate. Early in 1663, John Wilkins, son of the Master of Manchester Grammar School, having also rid himself of a 'very disagreeable' fellow tenant, moved in with Newton and remained for the following twenty years. Despite their long association, little is known of their relationship, apart from their being of similar temperament; that

Wilkins assisted Newton in setting up his experiments; that they parted 'under a cloud'; and that thirty years later, a subtle overture from Wilkins, who had subsequently married and had a family, was curtly brushed-off by Newton.

This last episode, gives commentary on Newton and Silicea's inability to compromise or permit reconciliation after an emotional estrangement, even when a sincere overture is made by the offending person (*averse to being spoken to, even kindly*). The inveterate nature of Silicea's emotions is seen to parallel the inveteracy of its pathology. This inclination to harbour grievance and even malice, approximates the similar persistence of Nitric acid's brooding resentments. When such archetypal similarities go deep, they are often confirmed by superficial markers, which may be quite simple, yet, highly symbolic, and this is true of Silicea and Nitric acid. Both produce sharp, penetrating pains as from a splinter lodged in the skin or deeper tissues: a good analogy for someone who has 'got under one's skin!' Silicea is an excellent remedy for the expulsion of foreign objects such as wood-splinters, glass-slivers, iron-filings and fish-bones. Such objects may fester. Festering expressed emotionally is rancour: revealing the metaphoric connection between splinter pains and imbedded, bitter emotions: those 'thorns that in her bosom lodge, to prick and sting her,'[2] and the shared emotions of Silicea and Nitric acid.

The young scientist

It was in 1663, that Newton's philosophical outlook underwent a major change. He stepped away from the Aristotelian tradition still being taught at Cambridge and turned his mind to the works of Descartes, Robert Boyle, Thomas More, Copernicus, Galileo and others. He also began the mathematical studies that would lead to his becoming the second Lucasian Professor of Mathematics at Cambridge in 1669 and to the development of *the calculus*; heralded by the tract he began in 1669 and completed two years later: *On the Methods of Series and Fluxions*. Within the space of a mere six years (1663–1669), Isaac Newton had become the most advanced mathematician of his time. The foundation was set for the writing of his *Principia* (Mathematical Principles of Natural Philosophy) first published in 1687: his masterpiece and the fundamental work for the whole of modern science.

Though any individual can become greater than the sum of their parts and natural gifts may be bettered by conditioning, education and application, Isaac Newton's phenomenal intellectual development, its largely self-taught origin and the speed with which it came to fruition in an age when science and mathematics were in their infancy, is evidence, not only of his uniqueness, but, as in the precocious, immaculate, musical creativity of Mozart, evidence of *life before birth* – evidence that no one is merely the product of genetic inheritance and the dynamics and events of a single lifetime; that with the experience of many incarnations, the seasoned soul comes into life with destiny defined, aptitudes honed and bearing bounty for all. Newton was born into unfortunate circumstances that blighted his early years and maimed his emotional life; his deceased father was an illiterate farmer; his mother, although from an educated family, favoured farming over learning; he entered a university, still true to the Aristotelean tradition, with only rudimentary mathematical training; his own reserved, insular and independent nature largely insulated him from external mentorship; yet, despite all that was unpropitious in his life and disposition, once ignited, his genius unfurled, as if from within, with a momentum that carried him irresistibly from one discovery to another, inexorably building, like the crystal being he was, an intellectual edifice that made him 'one of the most influential scientists of all time' – 'one of the greatest names in the history of human thought' – his work 'distinctly advancing every branch of mathematics then studied.'

The key role Isaac Newton played in the scientific revolution of the 17th Century and the scope of his influence was archetypal; it may justly be compared with the key role of the silicon atom in stellar alchemy, for when a great star fires silicon to provide its fuel – from a steady, modest, axial progression of hydrogen to helium, helium to carbon, carbon to neon, neon to oxygen and finally oxygen to silicon: a profusion of nuclear reactions take place in which the lighter elements of the universe are fabricated. What silicon was to the universe, Isaac Newton was to science!

The miasms are patently archetypal: *Psora* – the underprivileged; *Sycosis* – the profligate; *Syphilis* – the antisocial. Newton and silicon's roles were not only archetypal, they were miasmatic! Their prolificacy may be compared with the exuberance of the sycotic miasm. Both, were associated with an explosive acceleration in the processes they were key to. Silicon accelerated the fabrication of elements; Isaac Newton galvanised the advance of science.

The Plague

In April 1665, Newton received his bachelor's degree. In the same year, the university was closed to obviate the dangers of the plague (the Black Death) that had struck England in the spring and continued into 1666, until the Great Fire of London destroyed the areas most affected by the disease. For most of the following two years, Newton was forced to remain at home. Without formal guidance, he had sought out and consulted the new philosophy and the new mathematics and made them his own; now, he had time to reflect at leisure on what he had learned. It was during the plague years that he laid the foundation for the calculus, extended earlier insights into the nature of colours and turned his mind to astronomy and the motion of the moon and planets, making deductions that would later prove crucial to the law of universal gravitation. With typical Silicea reticence, he kept all these discoveries to himself.

Light and colour

In 1664, his interest in light and colour led him to experiment with the refraction of light through a prism to view 'the vivid and intense colours produced thereby' and to observe the diffraction of the setting sun's rays through a variety of materials. On one occasion, not realising the danger to his eyes, he observed the sun's rays reflected in a mirror and then, turning his eyes to a dark corner of his chamber, marvelled at the circles of colours that remained impressed on his vision, before dying away. Through repetition, he induced a temporary blindness that necessitated confining himself to a darkened room for three days. But, this indiscretion, pales before the reckless and weirdly archetypal experiment that followed.

'I took a bodkin (a thin dagger or probe) and put it between my eye and the bone, as near to the backside of my eye as I could: and pressing my eye with the end of it (so as to make the curvature in my eye) there appeared several white, dark and coloured circles. Which circles were plainest when I continued to rub my eye with the point of the bodkin, but if I held my eye and the bodkin still, though I continued to press my eye with it, yet, the circles would grow faint or disappear, until I resumed them by moving my eye or the bodkin.'[3]

While striking testimony to his intrepid drive for knowledge, this bizarre experiment, as much as any other happening in this remarkable man's life, points to the presiding influence of the Silicea archetype. Newton's urgent desire to understand all that he possibly could about light and colour, even at risk to himself, is evidence enough of the Silicea connection, but the bodkin inserted into the orbit of his eye is conclusive. The inversion of an archetype's key rubrics is proof and part of the paradoxical nature of the relative plane and of the materia medica (e.g. Nat-mur may be better or worse at the coast; may crave or avoid salt). If destiny demands and certain psychic forces are at play, the archetype may well be drawn to face its fears and do what it fears most.

As already noted, Silicea has, in the very highest grade (4), *fear of pins, of sharp, pointed things* and is *oversensitive to steel points directed towards them.* But, Silicea also has a 'strange, rare and peculiar' symptom: *Fear – pins, pointed, sharp things – hunts for pointed things, although afraid of them.* In this unique rubric, lies the promise of inversion, for though Silicea, seeing ominous portent in sharp-pointed objects, is repelled by them, the archetype, moved by inner compulsion, hunts for them to unconsciously obviate or fulfil what they foreshadow. Such was the dynamic within Newton!

At the level of the Id, the first chakra and the colour red, i.e. at the level of animal survival, the eyes are the organs most vulnerable to the sharp objects that Silicea fears: a danger Lac felinum (the Cat) is well aware of. Yet, Isaac Newton, a Silicea to the core, hunts for a sharp object and in an action, that should be too abhorred to contemplate, inserts a bodkin into his eye socket. Viewed pragmatically: a foolhardy exercise; viewed archetypally: an act motivated from a repressed level of the psyche. Consciously: a rash but focussed searching for knowledge; unconsciously: an urge initiated from the collective unconscious in obedience to dark images laid down by convoluted human emotion: a scenario recognised by Freud, captured in the myth of Oedipus and enacted by Newton (Silicea) in testimony to his unrequited desire for his mother.

The Oedipus complex and its relationship to sharp, pointed objects will be dealt with in Part 2 under Freud's psycho-sexual development stages.

The apple tree incident

It was during the plague years that the famous incident of the apple tree was supposed to have taken place. Newton himself cultivated the story that watching the fall of an apple from a tree had led him to formulate his theory of 'universal gravity'. Whether this was truly how his thought process was first triggered will never be known, but it is far more likely that the development of this vital theory followed the usual pattern of his great discoveries: 'I keep the subject constantly before me, till the first dawnings open slowly, by little and little, into the full and clear light.'[4] This aptly describes how Silicea intuitive and creative thinking unfolds – like the laying down of a crystal structure through the slow, steady accretion of material. As Michael White, Newton's biographer, suggests, the apple anecdote was probably a deliberate fabrication or an elaboration to conceal 'the fact that much of the inspiration for the theory of gravity came from his subsequent alchemical work.'[5] As Hahnemann feared over a century later: to be associated with the much-vilified pursuit of alchemy was to be discredited in the eyes of conventional science. Even later in life, Newton was sensitive to this risk and maintained the deceit of his disinterest in alchemy to 'preserve unsullied his image as the greatest scientist that ever lived.'[5]

Silicea archetype

Every step of his way, this extraordinary man's life is seen to be over-shadowed by his archetype: Silicea. Mysteriously, his life unfolds as would a protracted Silicea proving. The attaining and maintaining of a respected and admired image is central to the strivings and aspirations of Silicea. Well-earned praise and an immaculate reputation are essential to Silicea's self-worth and spur their innate drive for excellence. The all-powerful motivation behind Newton's anxiety-driven need not only to excel, but to be the very best in the world, stemmed from his unconscious desire to be worthy of the love of the mother, who rejected and abandoned him – and – at an even deeper level – to be worthy of the love of the God, whom he unconsciously sensed had repudiated and forsaken him.

Both Lycopodium and Silicea lack self-esteem and suffer from a sense of unworthiness and intrinsic inferiority. Both strive for success, but there are marked differences between the two. Silicea strives for excellence, praise and recognition; Lycopodium craves wealth, power, status and influence. Silicea's compare themselves with their own idealised image and compete against themselves; Lycopodium's compare themselves with others and compete against society. Silicea works within a framework of principles and morals; Lycopodium will set aside both in the pursuit of fame and fortune.

However, despite its virtues, the Silicea archetype is even more fundamental and pivotal to the sycotic miasm than Thuja; it is the very soul of *Sycosis*: the 'Good' aspect of the Tree of Knowledge – Thuja being the tree's 'Bad' aspect. Inevitably, Silicea, for all its 'goodness', like Thuja wears a mask! Though differing hugely from the smooth, cunning duplicity of Thuja, it is, nonetheless, a mask: a persona donned to profit and deceive. Silicea's pretence is an unruffled, calm exterior and an accommodating 'niceness' of disposition: a gentle, sweet, affable nature, concealing feelings of *insecurity, anxiety, impatience and irritability* lying beneath the surface, and, as with Isaac Newton, at a far deeper level, their *repressed anger, rage and resentment*, which may also be disguised and partially allayed by *passive aggression*.

Timidity and quietness may also constitute a Silicea mask: the donning of a low-profile persona, grey and inconspicuous; a shrinking into the background, making themselves invisible so as not to catch attention, invite engagement or arouse expectations. Newton successfully achieved this in his early years at Trinity. At times of stress or challenge, he would characteristically remove himself from society, find sanctuary in isolation and engage himself exclusively in ceaseless, intellectual work: all natural to his Silicea state. While writing his *Principia*, he was so obsessively wrapped-up in his studies, experiments and writing that he neglected himself terribly, scarcely pausing to eat or forgetting to eat at all and rarely getting to bed before 2 or 3 o'clock in the morning, sometimes pushing through till 5 or 6 a.m., when he would give himself four or five hour's repose before returning to his labours. All these efforts were characterised by their stringent exactness and accuracy – in a word – by their Silicea meticulousness.

Hesitancy, indecisiveness and dependency are strategies, hence 'masks', Silicea may employ to gain sympathy and support. By encouraging others to decide for them, take control and shoulder responsibility, they avoid accountability and the risk of failure. Compliance, accommodation and agreement with the views and opinions of others, permit Silicea to avoid friction and confrontation. Even when holding very definite, even ardent, views about a subject under discussion, they rarely express an opinion.

While these limp-wristed traits of Silicea were not typical of Newton, the *avoidance of altercation, confrontation and criticism* certainly was and explains his reluctance to make his ground-breaking discoveries known. His sensitive disposition feared the controversy and criticism they would evoke. Often, it was only the pleading and pressure of friends that moved him to publish his findings.

The wounded child within his psyche demanded that the image of superiority and unsurpassed brilliance that gave him self-esteem and worth, and unconsciously made him feel loveable, should be irreproachable. Hence, his gentle deceit about the falling apple to conceal the fact that it was his exotic, alchemical explorations rather than his strictly scientific work that had first revealed to him the power of attraction and repulsion and that all matter attracts matter. When this peerless image was subjected to derogatory criticism and he was accused of plagiarism, the raw wound of his abandonment was exposed, and his mask of reticence fell away, revealing a seething wrath that could not be contained and knew no bounds.

Silicea is a major omission from the pivotal rubric *ailments from anger suppressed*, which I regard as *the Wolf rubric*: a rubric representing the archetypes closest to the primal Wolf archetype. It is an Isaac Newton rubric – in highest grade. He was a lone, scientific Wolf!

Crimson

A notable eccentricity of Newton's was his passion for the colour crimson. He surrounded himself with the colour. One of his biographers, Richard de Villamil remarked that Newton 'lived in an atmosphere of crimson.'[6] It was a fixation that began in youth and persisted into old age. As a teenager, in 1659, he recorded in his Morgan Notebook some three dozen recipes for the formulation of coloured dyes, and most of these were for different shades of red. One gave instructions on how crimson could best be prepared from the 'clearest blood of a sheep' hung up in a punctured bladder to dry in the sun and later, according to need, used after dissolving it in alum water. He had crimson curtains, a crimson mohair bed, a crimson settee, a crimson easy chair and crimson cushions. Michael White writes in his biography of Newton: 'Rather than revealing deep insights into his motivations or neuroses, a fascination with crimson probably demonstrates little more than an odd quirk of personality.'[7] He may be excused this dismissive assumption, for it is only in the light of archetypal analysis that this 'odd quirk' can be elucidated.

In terms of the archetype, a fascination for any colour is of prime significance. Colour is Nature's most fundamental code, used to disclose the arcane energy concealed within her symbols. Much can be read into Newton's obsession with crimson, which, more than any other shade of red, represents the colour of blood: a symbol of the very life force itself and thus of vitality and animal power, or, as with all symbols, the opposite: loss of vigour, assertiveness and drive. Red embodies the spirit or consciousness of the first, or root, chakra, Muladhara: consciousness at the level of self-preservation. Crimson red is the colour of the Id, the universal vital force that drives the basic instincts of personal survival through aggression and species survival through reproduction. Aggression, modified by circumstances and need, incorporates the survival strategies: 'fight, flight or freeze'; reproduction incorporates the all-important libido principle, which is expressed via the sexual, creative or devotional drives.

Red, especially crimson red, is powerful and intense; it has great emotional impact, denoting desire, passion, lust, rage and explosive violence and issues a strident warning of life-threatening danger. Red is the colour representing the action of adrenaline, the flight or fight hormone; it signifies the adrenaline rush that amplifies the senses, fires the emotions, flushes the cheeks and galvanises action. Along with cortisol, adrenaline sustains a state of vigilance and arousal – a heightened readiness to respond defensively – and primes the organism to react decisively and aggressively to challenge or threat.

Even this cursory evaluation of crimson evidences profound connotations from which its significance in the life of Isaac Newton can be deduced. From the moment of birth, his emotional and physical survival depended solely on his single mother. She was his *everything*: the source of sustenance and love and the focal point of his own affections and stirring, puerile sexuality. His entire being was bonded to her when, at 3-years-of-age (the commencement of the *phallic phase* of psychosexual development), a Hades-like being appeared, usurped his position in his mother's affections and forced her to desert him. He was abandoned, his very survival threatened. In psychosexual terms, he was *castrated* – robbed of his masculine power – impotent! The raw, primitive aggression of the Id, as ever focussed on survival, held the anger and drive to kill the intruder, his hated adversary for the affections of his mother, and to punish her. Unrequited, the primordial infantile rage was repressed into the Shadow of the psyche: a resident force that in later years announced its seething presence in a seemingly innocent fascination for the colour crimson.

Attracted or charmed by the colour red is common to a small group of archetypes centred on the Wolf (Lac-lupinum) archetype: Raven (Corvas corax), the perennial companion of the wolf; Lycosa tarantula, the wolf spider; and two outstanding warrior archetypes: Ferrum metallicum (iron) – the metal of war; and Agaricus (fly agaric or scarlet cap) – the psychotropic mushroom reputed to have been used by the Vikings to arouse their Berserker, fighting ardour; and the archetype essential for the wounded warrior who has lost much blood (lost much red): China (Cinchona officinalis), an archetype that fears wolves and dogs more than any other. At the opposite pole, *aversion to the colour red* and *fear of red* feature Alumina, an archetype so intimately related to Silicea (aluminium oxide and silicon dioxide being the major constituents of clay) that it spotlights a link between Silicea and red: a connection further evidenced by Silicea being the inspiring archetype of Newton: a man charmed by crimson. The relationship is also stressed by Silicea and Alumina having similar obsessive fears and impulses provoked by seeing sharp-pointed objects: Alumina, specifically for knives (*fear at the sight of blood and knives*) and Silicea for pins, needles and open scissors – promptings that can be linked to the Oedipus complex and the upbringing of Silicea.

Since, repression is operative in Newton's being *charmed by the colour red,* the idiosyncrasy is essentially morbid: a compensation for unexpressed emotions. Negative-red signals repressed, imploded or congested energy (Ferrum), or, conversely, 'bled-away' energy (China). In the instance of Isaac Newton, as with Wolf, the attraction to red in its negative presentation signals unexpressed, choked-off, unrequited anger, humiliation, indignation and resentment; emotions that unconsciously pushed him away from society, made him a scientific recluse and fired his relentless pursuit of knowledge. The passion, intensity and focus invested in his exacting explorations and the enormous pride derived from his discoveries and from the celebrity he achieved were all Red, compensatory survival emotions. They made him painfully vulnerable to contradiction or any criticism of his concepts (*easily offended* [2]; *ailments from contradiction; ailments from humiliation* [2]) and, given the wicked wit of fate, in equal measure, ensured that he would, indeed, be criticised and rebutted – since, what we transmit, we will undoubtedly receive – a psychic boomerang as sure as night follows day.

Optics

Newton's first scientific endeavour after receiving his professorship was to return to optics: the subject of his first studies. His work on the properties of light and his sophisticated theory of colour based on the observation that a prism decomposes white light into the colours of the visible spectrum and that the spectrum when passed through a focused lens can be reconstituted as white light, clearly define Newton as a Silicea. His experimental method using a few pieces of card, a couple of glass prisms and lenses was as beautiful in its simplicity as it was in its ingenuity and efficacy: all testimony to the refined elegance of the penetrating Silicea intellect. Newton's intimate archetypal relationship to Silicea is demonstrated in that, wishing to better understand the nature of light, he ground his own lenses. Indeed, Newton himself was a lens: the focussing glass for all that had gone before and all that was yet to come.

Reflecting telescope

Despite this critical, ground-breaking success, Newton shared his findings with only those closest to him, notably, the mathematician, Isaac Barrow, who was influential in Newton's early education. Although, he could have gained professional publicity through Barrow's affiliation to the Royal Society, Newton *misanthropically* preferred to remain silent and turned his attention to developing a new and superior kind of telescope, which would use a reflecting mirror rather than a combination of lenses.

With typical Silicea application and craftsmanship, he worked on the project entirely alone. He cast and ground the mirror from an alloy of his own formulation (tin and copper), polished the mirror and made the tube and the mount and fittings.[8] He even created the tools he would require for constructing the telescope. Where others before him had failed, he fashioned an optic device that was of great technological significance and of unsurpassed quality and power at that time. It was little more than six inches long, but of exquisite design.

By using a mirror to focus light, Newton's refined, reflecting telescope produced sharp images devoid of the *chromatic aberration* that blemished the lens-produced images of refracting telescopes. At Barrow's insistence, towards the end of 1671, Newton reluctantly agreed to let him show the telescope to a small group of associates at a meeting of the Royal Society.[9] John Flamsteed (soon to be appointed Astronomer Royal) was delighted with it and within a few days it was demonstrated to Charles II.

Such was the enthusiastic response to the telescope, that on 11 January of the following year, 1672, Newton was voted in as a member of the Royal Society (he would become its president in 1703 and hold the position until his death in 1727). Newton was delighted by the acclaim he received; *recognition of worth and praise for achievement* are of infinite importance to the Silicea ego-self. His appointment emboldened Newton to put forward to the Royal Society the optical theory linked to the creation of the telescope in a lengthy document that has become known as the *Theory of Light and Colour*. Surely, no title could better capture Newton's Silicea orientation? Like any Silicea in such a situation, Newton was hugely anxious about the Royal Society's response to the submission of what he himself judged to be: 'the oddest, if not the most considerable, detection which has hitherto been made in the operations of nature.' To his relief, he was informed by the Secretary of the Royal Society, Henry Oldenberg, that it had been 'exceptionally well received.'

Newton's acceptance into the Royal Society, propelled him out of cloistered academic and physical seclusion onto the larger scientific platform and very soon brought him into contact and conflict with the individual whom destiny had appointed his nemesis – his psychic boomerang – Robert Hooke.

References

1   White M. *Isaac Newton – The Last Sorcerer*. London: Fourth Estate Ltd, 1997. p50.
2   Shakespeare W. *Hamlet*. Oxford: Oxford University Press, 1968. Act 1 Scene V, lines 87–88. p79.
3   White M. *Isaac Newton – The Last Sorcerer*. London: Fourth Estate Ltd, 1997. p61.
4   *Ibid.*, p85.
5   *Ibid.*, p87.
6   *Ibid.*, p296.

7   *Ibid.*, p97.
8   *Ibid.*, p168.
9   *Ibid.*, p169.

13

SILICEA – 4

Confrontation

Robert Hooke (1635–1703)

Robert Hooke was born in 1635, in Freshwater on the Isle of Wight, some seven years before Isaac Newton. He too had a traumatic childhood; his father hanging himself in 1648 when Robert was thirteen. He received his adult education at Christ College Oxford. He was a frail child and of indifferent health, but from an early age showed intense and wide-ranging interest in the world about him; his curious, investigative mind making him one of the leading polymaths of his time. He was a mathematician, scientist, natural philosopher, surveyor and architect. For forty years, he was the curator of experiments at the Royal Society.

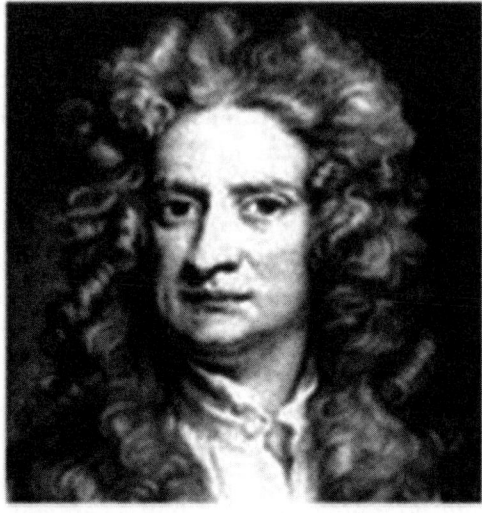

Figure 13.1 *Robert Hooke (1635–1703)*

From a common fatherless adolescence, two more divergent personalities than Newton and Hooke cannot be imagined. Whereas, Newton was an oversensitive, timid, secretive introvert, who shunned society, Hook was outgoing, assertive, abrasive and 'gregarious in the extreme.' Both had brilliant minds, but they operated in an entirely different manner.

While Newton could assiduously and methodically concentrate on a single problem or concept for decades, Hooke was driven by a roving, impatient energy that caused him to restlessly flit from one enthusiasm to another. He could never devote undivided attention to any subject for very long. Even his greatest work *Micrographia*, ostensibly a treatise on microscopy, evidences his capriciousness, the text wandering off course to contemplate several highly original theories concerning the nature of light. Published in 1665, the treatise was well known to Newton, who secretly admired it.

Antagonistic archetypes

In comparing Newton and Hooke, we face two antipathetic, incompatible archetypes emerging not only from life experience and events, but from the universal patterns indelibly woven into the boundless tapestry of the collective unconscious; archetypes eternally destined to confront one another, mutually hostile and deprecating, across an irreconcilable divide. The homeopathic materia medica is the textual counterpart of the collective unconscious, documenting the idiosyncrasies and traits, loves and hates, preferences and prejudices, imaginings and dreams of the archetypes, thus, providing a map into the darkest recesses of the human psyche. Knowing Newton to be archetypally Silicea, the homeopath can be certain that Hooke, his inveterate adversary, must be Silicea's nemesis: Mercurius! The plot is scripted in the collective unconscious; it is inescapable!

The feud was portended from birth: both infants were frail and sickly, but the one was oversensitive, timid and gentle: a typical Pulsatilla child; the other, was restless, active and irascible: a typical Chamomilla child. How often in the nursery do these two polar-opposite, infantile archetypes confront one another: the wimp and the tyrant, the victim and the bully, the beta and the alpha individual? Pulsatilla (meadow anemone) often matures into a Silicea adolescent and adult and Chamomilla, though most often maturing into a Mag-carb (magnesium carbonate), may prove to be a young version of Mercurius.

From reports and portraits painted of him as an adult, we know that Newton was of good height, held himself well and had an elongated, angular face with pointed features, a long sharp nose, dark piercing eyes and wore a serious, solemn, stern expression that seldom yielded a smile. Hooke, grew from childhood proving that the cause of his infant frailty and ill-health stemmed from constitutional blighting. He has been described as 'crooked' and 'pale-faced' and as a man who 'is the most and promises the least of any man in the world I ever saw.'[1] His crookedness was due to spinal curvature that severely stooped him and reduced his height.

There is no extant portrait of Hook; unusual for those times when men of eminence, or those deeming themselves eminent – both true of Hooke – regularly had portraits painted of themselves. Newton, as President of the Royal Society, did much to obscure Hooke and erase memory of him, including, it is said, destroying (or failing to preserve) the only known portrait of him. Given Hooke's nature, we can anticipate that his features readily displayed the feelings and emotions of his spontaneous, impatient, aggressive, extrovert nature, in marked contrast to the rare emotions evinced by the inscrutable, stay-out-of-my-space countenance of the intro-verted, secretive Newton.

It was in their lifestyles that the men deviated most. Hooke's life was multifaceted: he loved frequenting the coffee-houses, gossiping with friends, drinking port and indulging in sexual exploits, the details of which he committed to his diary, even noting the quality of his orgasms. Newton's life was spent in isolation, within the walls of Trinity College, Cambridge; an austere, ascetic, celibate existence obsessively devoted to unravelling the laws of the Universe. Hooke, the libertine, would have derided Newton as a desiccated, prudish, self-opinionated zealot, while Newton, the puritan, would have dismissed Hooke as an undisciplined, loud-mouthed dilettante: a conceited, superficial dabbler in science. White graphically describes Newton's attitude to fellow scientists: 'Newton had only contempt for anyone who merely dipped into learning and did not drain it of blood or throttle it into intellectual submission.'[2] In their respective attitudes, values, and behaviour Newton and Hooke gift us insight into how Silicea and Mercurius perceive and judge one another. Both have huge egos and neither gives the other credit.

Silicea and Mercurius are profoundly syphilitic in their energy yet, stand at opposing poles in the syphilitic miasmatic framework: Silicea oversensi-tive, refined, elegant, principled and aloof; Mercurius, sensitive and deeply emotional, but coarse, warped, devious, and mercurial. The syphilitic miasm is typified by ulceration and Silicea and Mercurius produce ulcera-tive lesions that in their specificity perfectly image the contrasting mental processes of Newton and Hooke. Silicea is slow moving and chronic, its ulcers single, inveterate and deeply penetrating; Mercury is quick acting and acute, ulcerating rapidly, producing numerous satellite ulcers that coalesce and spread superficially. In temperament, Silicea and Newton are measured, dogged, persevering, stubborn, profound and relentless; Mercurius and Hooke are spontaneous, hurried, capricious, distractible, shallow and virtuoso. In keeping with these differences, the Silicea ulcer is deep, regular and symmetrical, whereas, the Mercurius ulcer is shallow and has an irregular, even zig-zag outer margin.

From the outset, Newton and Hooke instinctively disliked one another and this aversion matured into a hatred that persisted after Hooke's death and remained with Newton till the end of his long life. This intense antipathy is born out in the interaction of Silicea and Mercurius homeopathically. The remedies are highly inimical. They may not be used before or after one another; such incorrect use leads to aggravation that can prove distressing to the patient and difficult to resolve. Any shift from one to the other must be achieved through the mediation of Hepar-sulph, an outstanding anti-syphilitic, which must be interposed before giving Silicea after the use of Mercurius, and vice versa.

These significant similarities between substance and subject reveal the archetype as an energy field bringing into coincidence events, life, matter, disturbed function and tissue change falling within the compass of its frequency, thus, composing a unique narrative, themed in the collective unconscious and touching all levels of existence. So, it is with Silicea and Mercurius and so it was with Newton and Hooke, their living counterparts: by their very nature, archetypes inescapably cast as adversaries and drawn into conflict for the edification of both and the realisation of destined objectives.

Intolerant of contradiction

Newton's paper on the *Theory of Light and Colour* that he volunteered for consideration by the Royal Society in 1672, though generally well-received, met with dissent from Robert Hooke, who was by then a leader among the members, and, as Curator of Experiments, was required to analyse and comment on scientific work submitted to the Royal Society. Considering himself a master of optics, he wrote a rather condescending and cursory critique of the little-known, younger man's paper. Its dismissive and self-promoting tone, casting the writer as a presumptuous, unseasoned upstart, threw Newton into a towering rage. To be faced by trivialising criticism on the first occasion of sharing with his peers the conclusions of his years of painstaking work was intolerable and brought out all the anger and paranoia he had nursed since childhood. He was unable to confront criticism, contradiction or correction in a measured or rational manner. The disparaging attitude of Hooke threatened the immaculate all-transcending model of achievement that Newton had to maintain to justify his lovability and draw to him the 'conditional' love of God. He had a burning desire to bring Hooke down and humiliate him before his peers.

Lest these emotional reactions and motivations be thought excessive and out of character for Silicea, consideration of the archetype's profile is revealing.

- *Contradiction*: *intolerant of contradiction* (2) – *has to restrain himself to keep from violence.*
- *Ailments from:*
  - *Contradiction* (2).
  - *Egotism.*
  - *Humiliation.*
  - *Excitement*: *mental and emotional symptoms from excitement* (3).
- *Violence, vehemence – when crossed* (2).
- *Offended easily* (2).
- *Temperament choleric* (2).
- *Loss of self-control.*
- *Abusive, insulting.*
- *Censorious, critical.*
- *Egotism, self-esteem* (2).
- *Haughty.*
- *Contemptuous.*
- *Defiant.*
- *Delusions:*
  - *Persecuted – that he is persecuted.*
  - *Pursued by enemies.*
- *Mistrustfulness.*

The Trickster

Hooke, unlike Newton, did not have the financial resources to exclusively devote himself to research, he was forced to keep himself busy to make ends meet, especially when he, with two other surveyors, was appointed by the City of London to initiate the rebuilding programme after the Great Fire. In consequence, many of the original ideas born of his inventive mind could not be developed for want of time, or, were abandoned because he was unable to profit from them. In an age of rapid scientific progress in which new ideas were born to different minds almost simultaneously,

Hooke was fated to see many of his own theories brought to fruition by other researchers. Ill-graced physically and lacking funds to gain the scientific recognition he longed for, Hooke desperately needed prestige to allay his feelings of inferiority and bolster his compensatory egoism and bluster. He did what the Mercurius archetype has always done: he played the scheming *trickster*!

There is evidence that Hooke assumed credit for many of the ideas that he appraised on behalf of the Royal Society and made claims regarding inventions that he could not later substantiate. He complained when Newton was lauded for creating the first reflecting telescope, affirming that as early as 1664, he had made a similar, inch-long device, far superior to any 50-foot-long refractive telescope, but had been hindered in developing it through the intervening 'plague happenings' and the fire.

It is intriguing to note how critics of Newton and Hooke and critics of Silicea and Mercury have tended to show similar patterns of preference and prejudice. Early biographers invariably eulogised Newton and demonised Hooke, turning a blind eye to Newton's histrionic rages, unforgiving resentment and spiteful vindictiveness and ignoring Hooke's staunch loyalty to friends and the royalist cause, his brilliant mind and his very real contribution to science. Likewise, Silicea has always been thought of as the refined and virtuous one: the 'goody two-shoes' of the materia medica – pure, innocent and angelic, while Mercury is the ne'er-do-well and out-and-out 'baddy': a reprobate given to subterfuge and malice – dark, corrupt and diabolical. Small wonder the two are so incompatible! However, like all of us, the archetype has both a light and dark side – often starkly contrasting. In personifying the Silicea archetype to a marked degree, Newton provides a window through which both the exemplary and less wholesome qualities of Silicea can be viewed.

Enmity

The first crossing of swords between these egotistical men set the tone for their future correspondence, which in accord with the custom of the times was conducted with excessive, often obsequious courtesy thinly disguising undertones of mutual loathing and mistrust. Silicea testifies to this ambivalence and the inner conflict it triggers.

- *Will: contradiction of will* (2).
- *Suppression by will of natural inclinations in order to be proper* (unique).
- *Antagonism with self* (2).

At every opportunity, Hooke sought means to challenge and discomfort Newton. At one point, he accused Newton of having stolen content from his own work *Micrographia*. Like Mercurius, Hooke thrived on intrigue and gossip. Instead of making his complaint through official channels, he used informal meetings with his friends in London coffee houses to express his grievance, knowing that news of the accusation would filter back to Newton, and, being public, would rile him even more. He was not disappointed.

Adding to Newton's emotional reaction was the niggling awareness that although he had not plagiarised any content, he had omitted giving Hooke credit for a concept in *Micrographia* that had originally inspired him in his own experimental work. Newton was never a man to give credit unless absolutely necessary and *once crossed he never forgave*.[3] Add *anxiety of conscience* (guilt) to *intolerance of contradiction or criticism* in a proud, paranoid man with a chip on his shoulder and one can be certain that the level of resentment and protective anger will rise exponentially.

Replying to a letter from Hooke, in which his enemy implied that Newton's work merely rested on 'notions' that he, Hooke, had 'long since began' and were 'sentiments of my younger studies,' Newton, following much 'false flattery', wrote a sentence that has become famous, but remains generally misunderstood as a testimony to his modesty.

"If I have seen further, it is by standing on ye shoulders of Giants."

In one line, he tacitly acknowledges the 'notion' in *Micrographia* that inspired him, thus discharging his debt to Hooke, and in a backhanded compliment calls Hooke a giant, thereby, cruelly mocking Hooke's dwarfed stature and conferring on him a similarly 'dwarfed' scientific status – supportive not pivotal! Furthermore, Newton tells Hooke that from his elevated perspective, he has access to knowledge beyond Hooke's vision.

This exposes a typical and telling Silicea offensive strategy: *indirect, devious, two-faced, double-edged, clever and nasty* (all markedly sycotic). Newton reveals here, in full, the spiteful, uncompromising and razor-sharp viciousness of his character.

* * * * *

Stephen Hawking (1942–2018)

It is of archetypal significance that another outstanding scientific mind chose to use this famous line from Newton as the title of his book: *On the Shoulders of Giants*: *the Great Works of Physics and Astronomy*, published in

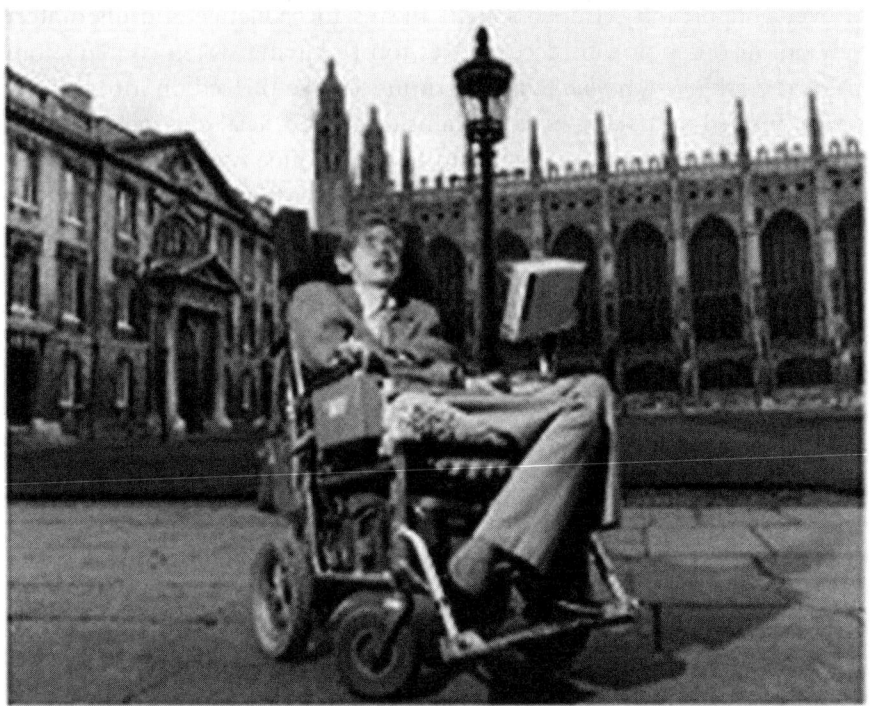

Figure 13.2 Professor Stephen Hawking (1942–2018)

(Image: Alamy)

2002.⁴ The author is Stephen Hawking, the world-renowned theoretical physicist and cosmologist, who, was born in Oxford, England on 8th January 1942, on the 300th anniversary of the death of Galileo, and died on 14th March 2018, the day on which Einstein was born in 1879. An interesting historical link and profoundly archetypal!

Like Newton before him, Hawking was Lucasian Professor of Mathematics at the University of Cambridge (1979–2009). His fame as a scientist is matched by his heroic fight against a rare, early-onset, slowly-progressive form of amyotrophic lateral sclerosis (ALS – also known as motor neurone disease) that gradually paralysed him. Conventional medicine considers ALS to be due to genetic abnormality, and moderate to severe head injury has been identified as a precipitating risk-factor.[i]

The defining feature of ALS is the death of both upper and lower motor neurones in the motor cortex of the brain, the brain stem and the spinal

---

[i] Head injury and the long-term effects of concussion are often met by Nat-sulph, a major anti-sycotic remedy. Silicea has the same causative and miasmatic affinity as Nat-sulph and in addition enjoys a close relationship with Carcinosin, a major remedy for the chronic effects of head injury.

cord. Other than supportive therapy, there is no successful orthodox treatment known for the disease.

Reflecting on Stephen Hawking's case hypothetically and considering his achievements and his links to Newton, is there a homeopathic remedy, possessing the necessary specificity and depth of action, that could have been given to Hawking, at the time his condition was first observed, with some hope of curing, arresting, or at least modifying, or slowing, its intractable and inexorable progress? Silicea is a strong contender – it has the credentials!

Evaluating Hawking archetypally, in the light of his connection to Isaac Newton and Newton's connection to the Silicea archetype, a definite pattern is discerned. Hawking and Newton belong to a distinct archetypal mould: *the scientist* – at an accentuated level – their brilliance transcending that of their peers – traversing unchartered terrain and lighting beacons for others to follow. In the sphere of science, their genius attains the archetypal status of *seer* or *mage*. Newton's intellectual prowess was fostered by seclusion: reaching out to rarefied realms from behind the cloistering walls of Trinity College; Hawking's untrammelled mind soared above the confines of his creeping paralysis to probe the mysteries of the 'overhanging firmament'. Neither were initially successful academically and each came into their own over time; both had a passion for and excelled at mathematics; both neglected their formal studies; both were autodidacts, able to teach themselves without formal instruction; both, despite exceptional ability had doubts about themselves and suffered anticipation anxiety before examinations or peer review; both were very secretive about their private lives – and both image Silicea!

The mantle of the archetype is pervasive; it touches every facet of a person's life, determining the situations and events they are exposed to; the constellation of family, friends, colleagues, teachers and adversaries that accompany and surround them on their life journey; the perspectives, prejudices, principles and enthusiasms that motivate, distract or impede them; their emotional, intellectual, and physical attributes; and the diseases that afflict them.

> A combination and a form indeed,
> Where every god did seem to set his seal,
> To give the world assurance of a man.[5]

Knowledge of the general archetype (scientist, warrior, king, queen, trickster, etc.) provides a blueprint to the patterns of destiny that will impinge, mould and temper the individual and affords clues to identifying the specific archetype that can restore and heal them. So, it is with Isaac

Newton and Stephen Hawking: scientists both and both at the top of their game; great minds that have propagated and disseminated knowledge for the understanding and benefit of others: a function that parallels the cascade of nuclear reactions sourced from the axial element silicon in the process of stellar alchemy.

The Cosmos cues the curious, alert mind by presenting signposts and landmarks. Those relating to the evolution of modern science were loud and clear. Galileo was central to the initiation of the scientific revolution and he was a Silicea archetype; Isaac Newton was born in the year of Galileo's death and he too was a Silicea; Stephen Hawking was born in Oxford, England, on January 8, 1942, the 300th anniversary of the death of Galileo: a startling 'coincidence' of which the great physicist was always proud, and he died on the same day of the same month that Einstein was born. Such indicators are not to be ignored and passed off as chance, since chance does not exist: the universe is governed by laws set by the Universal Consciousness. The Silicea baton is passed from one great mind to another: an indication of Divine Intent. Faced by this background and gifted knowledge of what his patient was destined to achieve against the severest odds, the hypothetical physician, searching for a curative remedy for Stephen Hawking during his final year at Oxford, would have been well advised to place Silicea at the top of his list.

The hierarchy of Group 14 of the periodic chart commences with carbon and with increasing atomic weight advances through silicon, germanium and stannum (tin) to end in plumbum (lead). Chronic lead poisoning selectively attacks the central nervous system causing neuromuscular and neurological symptoms. Family and thematic connections tend to entwine, therefore, lead's propensity to produce neuromuscular paralysis adds weight to the consideration of Silicea at the onset of ALS and Plumbum will follow it well. In similar vein, for those sufferers from ALS who have difficulty breathing and run the risk of serious respiratory infections, Stannum is a remedy to be kept in mind.

Hawking was often asked questions about the fate of the universe and life on Earth; whether life could exist on other planets and in other galaxies or other universes; and the likelihood of aliens being able to visit Earth from out of space. Of special interest to many, personally wrestling with their own beliefs in the ever-widening gulf between religion and science, is what this exceptional mind thought about the existence of God and the possibility of life after death. Probably much to their disappointment, and, such being their respect for the opinion of the renowned scientist, even dismay, Hawking made it clear that he did not believe in a creative intelligence called God and that he considered heaven, or an afterlife, a myth –

a 'fairy story for people afraid of the dark' – 'no one created the universe, and no one directs our fate.' In September 2014, he put it bluntly when he declared in an interview with *El Mundo*, the second largest printed daily newspaper in Spain: 'I'm an atheist!'

This cold, pragmatic, utilitarian view of the creation, though warmed by his deep appreciation of the grand design of the universe, might seem to point away from Silicea as Hawking's remedy, but many a crystal person is persuaded and informed by the marvels and mastery of external phenomena and fails to search beyond what can be weighed and measured – just as silicon, silica and the silicates pertain especially to the Earth's crust and not its depths. It is a paradox of the relative dimension that high intelligence can unseat wisdom and that wisdom often flourishes best in the unsophisticated, uncluttered mind.

Turning to the repertory, we find Silicea in the rubrics:

- *Godless*: *want of religious feeling* (1) – along with *Anacardium* (2), *Lachesis (3), *Lycopodium* and *Sulphur* (both 2).
- *Indifference to religion.*

* * * * *

Self-imposed seclusion

After Newton's malicious letter to Hooke, the discord between them was, for a time, laid to rest, but various disagreements and arguments with other members of the Royal Society continued and when on the death of Henry Oldenburg, Robert Hooke became Secretary of the Royal Society, the oversensitive Newton felt that circumstances had become intolerably unsympathetic. After his brief excursion into the scientific community, he withdrew once more to Cambridge and lapsed into silence. The death of his mother the following year completed his isolation. For six years, he maintained a brooding silence, resisting all attempts to coax him out of his self-imposed seclusion. But, within the walls of Trinity, against a background of continuous alchemical experimentation, his fertile mind was formalising the theoretical ideas that would be brought together and elucidated in his *Principia*, a work that would immediately make him an international figure.

Exacting work ethic

His work regimen during this time was intense, tireless and unceasing and his correspondence, largely exchanged with the Astronomer Royal, John

Flamsteed, was exclusively dedicated to his work. The capacity to one-pointedly address an intellectual or creative endeavour to the exclusion of all else in life is a marked characteristic of the Silicea archetype. It images the incremental growth of the quartz crystal, inexorable building from itself, of itself, to itself in its relentless advance towards the realisation of the final, crowning pyramid of its crystalline structure. Not only was Newton's commitment to his undertaking totally absorbed, it was strict, exacting and meticulously precise and accurate.

His biographer, Frank Manuel, wrote of him:

> To force everything in heaven and earth into one rigid, tight frame from which the most miniscule detail would not be allowed to escape free and random was an underlying need of this anxiety-ridden man.[6]

Like a metaphysician rather than a scientist, he seemed to be able to understand nothing unless he understood everything. The fact that he ground his own lenses is homeopathically significant – he would not merely reason his way to the truth, he would physically manipulate the world into revealing its nature.

Fixity of purpose and devotion to the pursuit of the finest detail is characteristic of Silicea.

The inevitable danger emanating from such uncompromising, concentrated labour, no matter how fulfilling and goal-driven, is physical, emotional or intellectual breakdown. This is the usual sequence in Silicea: first, a draining away of physical energy, an enervated state that demands rationing of physical output; then, comes increased emotional vulnerability, making the least care, worry or stress traumatic and exhausting, forcing them to ration their emotions by avoiding certain people and situations; finally, when emotional withdrawal fails to stem their decline, the very bastion of Silicea, the intellect, is assailed and loses competence.

Just as is found with Ferrum, a large proportion of the characteristics and symptoms of Silicea that have emerged from provings, reflect the physically enervated, emotionally weakened and intellectually impaired state of the archetype: a picture that can be misleading if considered fundamental. Comparing this biased picture with the nature and habits of Newton could lead to Silicea being side-lined or even overlooked as his archetype.

Silicea appears under *indolence, aversion to work; aversion to thinking (2); aversion to reading (2); aversion to mental work (2); mental work fatigues; writing fatigues (2); ailments from mental work: writing, reading; weakness of will; persists in nothing (2); postpones everything to the next day; indifference, apathy (2)* and, as previously noted, *aversion to mathematics; inapt for painting* (unique); *incapacity for business; financial inaptitude; woman: inapt for housekeeping.*

We must rather be guided by the peculiar idiosyncrasy that often predisposes the Silicea archetype to extend themselves to the limit and decline into enervation. Silicea tends to become *obsessively fixated* in the pursuit of an interest, enthusiasm or duty (*monomania*). The fixation is characterised by *obstinate adherence* to the task and *exacting perfectionism* that demands the very best of them. The fixation may lead to physical and mental exhaustion. Often, they need the encouragement, direction or example of someone they respect to get them started. A request or instruction may initiate their endeavours, but once committed, they apply themselves with unremitting conscientiousness. As with Newton, their labours may be driven by a compensatory need to *achieve and excel.*

Silicea does not know when to compromise or stop. Although they may procrastinate and waver before making a start, once involved, they turn a deaf ear to those who warn them that they will burn themselves out. They are obsessively committed to work and achieving their objective. In this respect, Allen highlights an important characteristic of the dedicated Silicea: 'although exhausted from hard work and close confinement, *he will overcome his nervous disability by force of will.'* They show determination and tenacity of will under extreme duress! Often a nature mild, gentle and yielding, lacking self-assurance and self-confidence, yet tempered by inner strength and moral resolve.

Just as the science of lenses reveals the majestic and the miniscule, the Silicea mind can range over concepts and philosophies of great scope and magnitude or become entranced with the infinitely small – and to far greater effect than Sulphur. These abilities link Silicea to Isaac Newton, as does their fear of confrontation and their intolerance of criticism and contradiction. Their reaction to these impingements is passive aggressive, but severe provocation can precipitate an angry outburst. This can be delivered in a cold, controlled and cutting way or with an explosive, resentful violence that appears totally out of character and shocks those against whom it is directed.

Obsessive traits

Some Siliceas' display the archetype's tendency to become fixated through obsessive fastidiousness: *the frequent need to wash hands* and a *mania for cleanliness.*

Always washing her/his hands.

Agaricus, Arsenicum, Coca, *Lac caninum, Medorrhinum,* Mercurius, *Natmur,* Platina, Psorinum, Sepia, Silicea, *Sulphur,* Syphilinum, Thuja, Tuberculinum (also Curare and Oscillococcinum).

Silicea, being the apex archetype of this important obsessive-compulsive group is closely related to the other hand-washing archetypes. Sufficient to note here:

- The four miasmatic nosodes: Psorinum, Medorrhinum, Syphilinum and Tuberculinum, pointing to Silicea's multi-miasmatic nature and flagging the conspicuous omission of Carcinosin from the rubric (it should be included).
- Thuja: emphasising its closeness to Silicea and confirming Silicea's very strong anti-sycotic power.
- Lac-can: indicating the victim role of Silicea.
- Mercury: Silicea's nemesis; always close by!

Siliceas' know what they want and know what they don't want! Although they may at first hesitate and equivocate, once committed they will not be swayed; they are impervious to external pressure. In choosing, they are cautious, exacting and extremely fussy and this critical eye applies to possessions, friends and the choice of a partner! Their philosophy and opinions develop in the same way, taking form over time and resolving into a crystal-clear conviction that stands firm against the persuasion of others. Nor do they need to impose their thoughts or beliefs on others

Attention to the finest detail was of prime importance to Isaac Newton: no stone could be left unturned; the lenses and mirrors he fashioned were of the highest order and his telescope an exquisite work of art. This exacting dedication illustrates the spread of a key trait across adjoining archetypes – in this instance: Graphites and Silicea. Expressed negatively, it is *obsession with trivia*; expressed positively, it is *attention to the finest detail*. In the negative sense, both archetypes may compensate for lack of confidence and a sense of inefficiency by concentrating on inconsequential trivia rather than committing themselves to the 'meat of the matter' or to an endeavour that tasks their abilities.

Silicea, like Graphites has:

- *Conscientious about trifles* (3).
- *Too pedantic about trifles.*
- *Aggravation from trifles.*
- *Trifles seem important* (2) – *Graphites, Hepar-sulph, Nit-ac, Nux-vom.*
- *Starting at trifles* (2).
- *Irritability from trifles.*
- *Anger at trifles.*
- *Anger, irascibility, at trifles – from extreme nervous weakness* (unique).

- *Anxiety about trifles* (2) which extends to *anxiety of conscience*: feeling guilty about small, trivial matters unworthy of consideration.
- *Remorse about trifles* (unique).
- *Weeping at trifles.*

As much as Newton's sacrificial commitment to research laid the foundation for modern science, his burning need to know everything, his intense penetrating focus and his unswerving perseverance were intellectual feats compensating for a deeply injured psyche. His need to surround himself with crimson was testimony to this and to the deep anger pent up within him.

Repressed sexual desire

As noted, crimson is the colour of the first or survival chakra, hence the colour of the Id, the universal vital force and the basic instincts. It is the colour of the aggressive force essential to personal survival and equally the colour of the libido desire essential to species survival. The powerful libido energy may be expressed not only sexually, but also creatively, religiously or spiritually. For many reasons: physical, physiological, emotional, moral, religious or spiritual, the sexual urge may be thwarted. For health and emotional balance to be maintained, the withdrawn or repressed sexual energy needs to be expended physically through exercise, especially dancing, or sublimated creatively or spiritually. When this fails, the frustrated sexuality, like all repressed energy, is corrupted, impacting negatively on the physical and emotional health of the individual, and, through perversion and projection, impinging, often destructively, on others.

The entwined nature of sexual, creative and devotional energy needs to be comprehended when appraising human behaviour and human psychopathology. Contention between these libido energies, especially, between religious morality and sexuality, is often an underlying factor in much personal and collective suffering. Misogyny thrives on such conflict; as was cruelly demonstrated in the atrocities of the Inquisition. Here, the miasmatic influence, though primarily psoric (original sin), is manifestly sycotic (duality: good and evil) but moves to the syco-syphilitic in its destructive mode. The first intimation of the conflict between morality and sexuality emerges in Pulsatilla, the archetype representing the infantile and immature psyche. The archetype may entertain strange notions that sex is somehow unseemly and sinful. In consequence, they suppress their sexual desire and become prudishly critical and condemning of what they perceive as laxity in others. Along with Apis, Camphor, Conium and Staphysagria,

Pulsatilla appears in highest grade in the rubric: *aggravation from suppression of sexual desire* (male and female). A serious omission in the rubric, in both sexes, is Silicea, the archetype that is the mature counterpart of the immature Pulsatilla and is also inclined to repressive prudery and puritanism. A subtle indication of underlying sexual/religious conflict is evidenced by Phos-ac, which experiences *sadness after masturbation*, indicating self-reproach after self-pleasuring, a sentiment common to previous generations still affected by Victorian inhibition. Silicea experiences the same sadness after masturbation, but can react more outwardly: *irritability after sexual intercourse* (3) – showing a greater degree of moral contention (Calc-carb (3) and Sepia (3) and Graphites in lowest grade.)

Hindrance to the flow of the Id is a fundamental factor in the evolution of disease; it disturbs the harmonious function of the governing vital force. The repression can affect either the aggressive or the sexual limb of the Id, or both, in varying degree. Two rubrics are of cardinal importance in this regard: *ailments from suppressed anger* and *ailments from suppressed sexual desire*. Both rubrics pertain to the repression of red or crimson.

Isaac Newton's impoverished emotional life and the ever-seething anger, waiting to explode at the least criticism of his work or accusation of plagiarism, demonstrate that he suffered from marked repression of both limbs of the Id: a state characteristic of the Silicea archetype.

Abandonment

The prenatal death of Newton's father predisposed Isaac to bond with Oedipus-like intensity to his mother and experience murderous anger and hatred toward Barnabas Smith when his rival for his mother's affections usurped his position of favour and won Hannah's attentions. This destructive anger extended to his mother when she abandoned him. Neither anger could be vented, both were repressed and consigned to the Shadow of the psyche, where they fulminated silently and insidiously. The act of betrayal left him *emasculated, alienated, isolated, humiliated, indignant, resentful and enraged*. His physical and sexual survival were imperilled. At three years of age, his utter impotence would have induced *a primal fear of annihilation*, a fear inherent in the colour red, and, especially, blood-crimson.

The following rubrics are relevant:

• *Ailments from friendship deceived – friendship betrayed*:
  Aurum, Ignatia, Mag-carb, Mag-mur, Nux-vom, Phos-ac, Silicea, Sulphur.
  For the young child, the most important friendship that can be betrayed is that between mother and child. This aspect of the rubric is confirmed

by the presence of Mag-carb and Mag-mur, which represent Mother Nature, magnesium being central to the chlorophyll molecule.

- *Forsaken*: feels as if not beloved by parents, wife, friends:
  Arsenicum, Calc-carb, Lycopodium, *Mag-carb,* Sepia, Silicea, Sulphur.

Abandonment is a major aetiological factor in the psychopathology of Pulsatilla and Silicea. It may lie at the root of both emotional constitutions, but it is particularly Silicea that develops deep-seated fear, sadness, *guilt and anger*. Though averse to sympathy and consolation, because of feelings of emptiness and abandonment, Silicea is *ameliorated by being held*.

No one held Isaac Newton!

- *Forsaken feeling.*
  Pulsatilla is in highest grade among the archetypes that feel abandoned. Pulsatilla often grows up to become a Silicea.
- *Ailments from indignation.*
  Pulsatilla (3) and Staphysagria (4) have the highest grading. This is relevant to Silicea, for the three feminine archetypes of the *Ranunucu-laceae* family of plants: Pulsatilla – Staphysagria – Cimicufuga are the more superficial counterparts of the deeper-acting Silicea.
- *Ailments from humiliation.*
  Staphysagria is given the highest grading (4); Pulsatilla and Silicea are graded (2).
- *Anger with silent grief.*
  Staphysagria (3), Pulsatilla (1).
- *Anger with reserved displeasure.*
- *Anger suppressed.*

References

1   White M. *Isaac Newton – The Last Sorcerer*. London: Fourth Estate Ltd, 1997. p187.
2   *Ibid.*, p176.
3   *Ibid.*, pp185.
4   Hawking S. *On the Shoulders of Giants: The Great Works of Physics and Astronomy* Philadelphia PA: Running Press, 2002.
5   Shakespeare W. *Hamlet* Oxford: Oxford University Press, 1968. Act III Scene IV, lines 60–62. p137.
6   Manuel FE. *A Portrait of Isaac Newton*. Cambridge MA: Belknap Press of Harvard University Press, 1968.

14

SILICEA – 5

Breakdown and revenge

Celibacy

Isaac Newton never married. His only close contacts with women were his unfulfilled relationship with his mother, whom he perceived to have abandoned him, and his later guardianship of his half-niece, the beautiful, clever and witty, Catherine Barton, of whom he was very fond. There was a wide-spread belief that Newton died a virgin. Voltaire, the French Enlightenment author, historian and philosopher, happening to be in London at the time of Newton's funeral, commented on the great scientist, saying that 'he was never sensible to any passion, was not subject to the common frailties of mankind, nor had any commerce with women. . . .'[1] This fanciful and lofty appraisal shows with what undiscerning deference the great scientist was viewed by his contemporaries. It would, indeed, seem that Newton had no commerce with women, but that he was passionless and devoid of common frailties was a patent misconception encouraged by Newton's inscrutable countenance, rigid reserve, paranoid secrecy and the inflexible will that focussed his entire being upon whatever project consumed him. Behind the pensive, introspective gaze and dour, unsmiling, elongated features, lay a repository of powerful, long-constrained emotions. Without doubt, despite the intense channelling of the libido energy into intellectual creativity, repressed sexuality must have strained for a vent. At once, at the height of Oedipus-sexual-fixation and jealous rage against Barnabas Smith, he had been emasculated and the aggressive and libido power of the Id thrust back upon itself. The implosion of unrequited energy provided his genius with the fuel and impetus required to break through into rarefied, unchartered realms, but left him sexually rudderless.

The only rebuttal to the notion of immaculate celibacy averred by Voltaire possibly lies in the close relationships Newton had with two men.

The first was his long association with John Wilkins, his chamber-companion at Trinity College. This lasted twenty years and came to an abrupt and acrimonious end. While the sudden finality of the breakup would suggest an intense, emotional rift, there is no substantial evidence that they had a physical relationship.

Fatio de Dullier

Newton's second friendship, however, with a young Swiss mathematician, Nicolas Fatio de Dullier, may well have been sexual. Fatio entered Newton's life during the warm afterglow of the international recognition of the *Principia*, when Newton, at his most relaxed, felt free to set aside his paranoid defences and was most vulnerable to the opportunistic charms of this self-promoting, precocious, scientific firefly. They first met at the Royal Society on 12 June 1689 and the friendship blossomed almost immediately. Fatio had much to gain from his association with Newton.

He had a reputation for currying favour with distinguished and influential people. His seductive charisma soon worked on the reclusive, introverted Newton, who had been starved of young, intelligent company and of someone close with whom he could safely share his thoughts without the threat of criticism or competition. He very soon became infatuated with

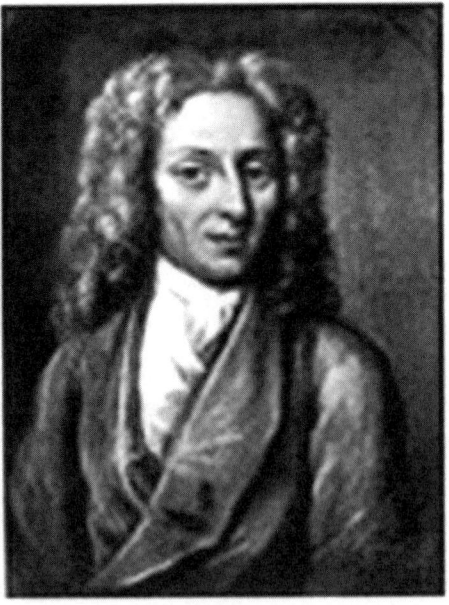

Figure 14.1 Nicholas Fatio de Dullier (1664–1753)

the young man. For his part, Fatio, undoubtedly conscious of the nascent sexuality of the older man's interest, used his intelligence and nimble wit to captivate Newton with flattery and adulation. Although others in Newton's scientific circle were soon disenchanted with the facile, but academically lightweight, Swiss, Newton clung to the relationship for fully four years. Deeply enamoured, he needed to believe in Fatio. His *dreadful loneliness*, denied for so long, was naked and exposed, and engulfed him. When Fatio was taken seriously ill and family and financial difficulties threatened to force him to return to Switzerland, Newton was distraught.

He proposed that Fatio take lodgings with him in Cambridge, so that he could support him. This, apparently, did not fit in with the young man's plans, because nothing came of it. During the first months of 1693, the emotional urgency of Newton's letters to Fatio steadily increased, then, suddenly, in early summer, all correspondence between the two ceased and was never resumed. What finally opened Newton's eyes to the self-serving duplicity of Fatio is not clear, but the intense relationship came to an abrupt and unexplained end. Newton was fortunate to escape its parasitic hold, but 'within weeks his caged emotions overflowed into temporary insanity.'[2]

As fascinating as any recounting of Newton's history must be – relating as it does to the genius, who embodied the scientific revolution commenced by Nicolaus Copernicus (1473–1543), and, whose 'grand synthesis,' *Principia* (1687), formulating the laws of motion and universal gravitation, provided its *closing crowning-pyramid* – this narrative is given with the express purpose of displaying the all-encompassing sway of the archetype: touching every aspect of a person's life; colouring and orchestrating the events that impinge upon them; prompting their emotions, their perspectives and their drives. The archetype is also a force field of universal and esoteric compass. Acting through Newton, the archetype accelerated scientific progress (formative phase: *Psora*), paving the way for modern technology (proliferative phase: *Sycosis*); now, in its destructive phase (*Syphilis*), it is deleteriously impacting on the ecology of the planet and eroding humanity's faith in a spirit dimension. The perspective of Newtonian physics has unseated God, destroyed heaven and reduced 'man' to dust and ashes (*Godless, lack of religious feeling; indifference to his religion*).

The archetype here in question is Silicea, and, the man, quintessentially a Silicea, is Newton: a genius – 'so great an ornament of the human race'[3] – and yet, a man exhibiting all the idiosyncrasies, strengths and frailties of his presiding archetype, which, for a time, unhinged his mind!

Relevant Silicea rubrics relating to this period in Newton's life:

- *Quiet disposition.*
- *Reserved.*
- *Seriousness.*
- *Impressionable.*
- *Yielding disposition.*
- *Servile, obsequious, submissive.*
- *Spineless.*
- *Dependent.*
- *Character – lack of character.*
- *Will – weakness of will.*
- *Self-control – loss of self-control.*
  - *Wants to control himself.*
- **Magnetised – desires to be magnetised* (3) = vulnerable to magnetic, charismatic persons.
  - **Mesmerism ameliorates* (3) – surrendering self-determination to the will of another.
- *Sexual fancies* (2):
  - *Frequent, involuntary* (unique).
- *Thoughts – sexual.*
- *Dreams amorous – with erections – with orgasm.*
- *Lasciviousness, lustfulness – sexuality.*
- *Affectionate.*
- *Amorous disposition* (3).
- *Ecstasy.*
- *Company: desire for company.*
  - *Aggravation being alone.*
- *Holding – being held ameliorates.*
- *Effeminate* – a rubric that can be related to homosexuality.
- *Love sick – with person of own sex* – Pulsatilla, Staphysagria, *Thuja* – hence, Silicea.
- *Sadness from masturbation* – the Puritan!
- *Irritability after sexual intercourse* (3) – the Puritan!
- *Ailments from*:
  - *Abandonment, desertion* (2).
  - *Friendship deceived* (2).
  - *Humiliation.*
  - *Bad news* (2).
  - *Fear, fright, shock* (3).
  - *Unrequited, disappointed love* – Staphysagria (4) – hence, Silicea.

○ *Excitement – emotional, mental symptoms from excitement* (3).
○ *Sexual excesses* (2).
• *Being beside oneself –* distraught!
• *Delusion – persecuted.*
○ *Pursued by enemies.*
• *Insanity, madness.*
• *Mania, madness.*

Mental 'distemper'

Isaac Newton's emotional breakdown first came to light in the content of a letter written on 13 September 1693 addressed to Samuel Pepys, the famous English diarist, a personal friend of Newton. Without reason or context, Newton informed Pepys: 'I must withdraw from your acquaintance and see neither you nor the rest of my friends anymore.' He also confided: 'I am extremely troubled at the embroilment I am in and have neither ate nor slept well this twelve month nor have my former consistency of mind.' His paranoia – friends had become enemies to be avoided – and his deranged state were clearly evident and prompted the alarmed Pepys to ask John Millington, a Cambridge colleague of Newton, with some haste, to call upon him. Though only days had elapsed, Millington found Newton lucid and restored, and, he himself, marvelling at the 'very odd letter', which he confessed had been due to a 'distemper that much seized his head.' During this 'distemper', a second letter, written in a shaky, uneven hand, had been posted to John Locke, another close friend. Its content was far more disturbing. Newton asked Locke's forgiveness for thinking Locke had 'endeavoured to embroil me with women'; for having declared, on hearing Locke was ill: 'it was better you were dead'; and for taking Locke for a Hobbist (a follower of Thomas Hobbes, the political philosopher, whom Newton despised as an atheist).[2]

As brief as this mental and emotional unhinging was – coming hot on the heels of the sudden rupture of his intense relationship with Fatio de Dullier, and expressing through these discordant letters, his resident paranoia, his sexual repression and his tender, religious sensibilities – it was of both clinical and archetypal significance. 'It was as though all the fiends that Newton had ever harboured were let loose at once.'[2]

The need to write the letters, in which emotions eclipsed intelligence, hearkened back to his adolescent need for a confession book (*anxiety of conscience* (2); *religious affections – sadness*). Though most probably occasioned by the pain of unrequited or betrayed love, their content reveals that they relate to fixations dating from the past. The speed with which the 'distemper' subsided, seemingly without trace, far from indicating resolution, demonstrates the facility with which Newton could re-secure his sycotic mask, even when struck to the very core of his being, and the efficiency with which the archetype closed vents that were releasing psychic pressure, restored superficial, nervous equilibrium and re-imposed its relentless repression of painful emotions. Silicea, comprising the major part of the Earth's crust, is metaphorically and archetypally well-placed to achieve these ends; they are innate qualities of the substance, the subject and the archetype.

The completion of the *Principia* and its presentation to the world, brought Isaac Newton's scientific mission to a close; ahead, lay thirty years of contention with the 'fiends' dwelling in the Shadow of his psyche. The Fatio saga was the beginning of this new chapter. It initiated his search for a position in London rather than Cambridge and resulted in his being appointed Warden of the Royal Mint. After the emotional crisis resulting from his split with Fatio, only briefly did he ever return to sustained scientific work. The move to London effectively concluded his creative activity.

Psychic dynamics

It is of value to reflect on the dynamics that prevailed in Isaac Newton's psyche during this vital transition period in his life. The international recognition, acclaim and fame he received for *Principia*, lowered the protective level of his innate paranoia. This dropping of his guard invited the advent of Fatio – who, cued by the archetypal siren call, duly made his entrance – and it opened Newton to the overtures of the younger man. The ardent nature of their intellectual intercourse and the younger man's manipulative charms quickened the dormant sexual aspect of the older man's libido force, which had remained morbidly inhibited ever since the 'psychological castration' suffered through his mother's rejection of him in favour of the 'sexual' rival he so detested. Throughout his formative and Cambridge years, the libido, robbed of sexual expression, had been channelled through creative activity (model building; scientific and alchemical research) and fired to genius level by the choked-off rage he harboured against Barnabas Smith and his mother. Small wonder that any criticism, contradiction or disparagement of the fruit of this creative work – so critical to his image, identity, worth and 'lovability' – caused inordinate rage. On an unconscious level, attacks on his mental prowess and morality jeopardised Newton's 'survival'; they threatened the 'annihilation' of the wounded child within.

Although the original intent of 'The Great Work' of the medieval and Renaissance alchemists was the transmutation of base metals, such as iron, copper and lead into the noble metals, silver and gold, the process became likened to man's spiritual growth and ascent from a crude, primitive, 'base' state to a refined, enlightened, 'noble' state: a process of internal alchemy, which can be equated with the individuation or Self-realisation of the human soul. Thus, a mystical component, compounded of astrological and religious influences, vested the practical techniques of alchemy with esoteric significance. Newton was heir to this legacy; the arcane permeated the extensive alchemical experimentation that provided the inspirational background to his conventional scientific research. Newton was one of the last mystic scientists, who could at once perceive the majesty of the creation in all its scientific detail and still retain a reverence for God and believe in the spiritual destiny of man. He was a theist rather than a deist, believing in the continuing participation of the creator in the workings of the creation. He warned against considering the Universe a mere machine, akin to a great clock. He saw God as the Master Creator whose existence could not be denied in the face of the grandeur of all creation.

In alchemy, the devotional and creative aspects of the Id come together: 'religion' and 'science' merge. This was a psychic imperative for Newton in whom the primal sexual instinct had been stifled. Pure science can be a cold, heartless discipline, which, because of its very nature, slays the arcane and exalts matter to sovereign status. Although the scientific atheist may claim to be enraptured by cosmic vistas and subatomic phenomena, in psychic terms these ardent avowals are specious: intellectual intonations or mantras to appease their own unconscious despair at being 'disconnected' from the Divine. Alchemy sustained the sexually impoverished Newton; it permitted the repressed crimson of the Id to drive his intense intellectual and emotional creativity and bless it with reverence. Reciprocally, this invoked the inspiration needed to illuminate his scientific endeavours. For all the unremitting effort he put into science, the lifetime he expended on alchemical experimentation suggests that the quest for the *philosopher's stone* was his dearest objective – a striving far more philosophical (devotional) than scientific.

With the *Principia* lauded, his paranoia allayed and the *mesmeric influence* of Fatio impinging on him, the creative (scientific), devotional (alchemical) tide of the libido, which had dominated his psyche since childhood, ebbed, and the sexual tide, so long repressed, began at last to swell, charged with the redirected force of repressed crimson. Wisdom and intelligence were set aside as infatuation gained momentum, propelling the love-starved Newton into a sexually charged relationship that over four years gained possession of him. Its powerful sway is evidenced in the mounting emotional intensity of his correspondence over the final months of the liaison. What brought this expanded coda to a crescendo followed by a sudden divisive finale will never be known, but the Silicea dynamic is starkly portrayed. In getting started, Silicea often wavers and delays until a critical point is reached, sometimes a crisis, sometimes the proverbial straw, sometimes a realisation, which galvanises them into action. Once committed they persist: often far beyond the expected, the necessary or the wise – then – the converse applies: a crisis, a final straw or a sudden realis-ation halts them, and when it does, the break is uncompromising and decisive. Newton dealt with both Wilkins, his lodger, and Fatio, his paramour, in this Silicea-like manner. The end was final, unequivocal and irrevocable.

One of the greatest problems facing the Pulsatilla, Staphysagria or Cimicifuga archetype is the inability to terminate an abusive, toxic or irretrievably damaged relationship. Silicea, the archetype that stands behind all three, achieves this with its usual precision. Just as it can success-fully extrude a festering splinter, so it can abort an imbedded, destructive relationship. Inter-current doses of Silicea can assist any one of these three *Ranunculaceae* archetypes achieve emotional freedom.

Newton's sudden break with Fatio was a classic Silicea act. At the time, he would certainly have benefited from a timely dose of dynamised Silicea in high potency. In the event, he was exposed to the full force of the psychic turbulence that ensued. During the relationship, the potent creative and devotional aspects of his libido-driven energy were withdrawn and fully invested in his sexual infatuation. Then, at its height, Newton abruptly choked it off. The sexual energy imploded psychically, unhinging his sanity and flooding his emotions with all the paranoia, gender-fear and religious prejudice that had pursued him since childhood. For a brief period, Newton was out of control, at the mercy of wild, directionless forces.

Certain fears, dreams and delusions of Silicea are relevant to Newton's 'distemper.'

- *Fears animals:*
  - *Cats.*
  - *Dogs.*
- *Dreams:*
  - *Pursued by dogs* (2).
  - *Pursued by cats.*
  - *Pursued by wild animals.*

- *Delusions:*
  - *Sees dogs.*
  - *Sees vermin.*
  - *Sees worms creeping.*

The Silicea archetype troubled by gender uncertainty or sex-related diffi-culties may have dreams of being pursued by cats or dogs or may fear cats or dogs: cats being lunar and feminine; dogs, solar and masculine. In rare instances, these dreams and fears may relate to sexual dysphoria from dissatisfaction regarding biological gender and the desire to undergo gender reassignment (Calc-carb – sees cats and dogs). More often, as with Newton, they relate to psychosexual difficulties derived from the disrupting inter-play between inherited constitution and traumatic events. *Delusions: vermin and worms creeping* may be indicative of abuse and of being victimised: a warning from the higher self to avoid or escape from a damaging situation or bad relationship e.g. not to become embroiled with someone like Fatio. Dreaming of cats and dogs is also characteristic of Graphites, an archetype that frequently overlaps with Silicea e.g. obsessing over trivia.

Newton's workaday mental state soon returned to normal. Considering the extreme signs of emotional imbalance evidenced by the letters he wrote; the recovery was remarkably swift. The very nature of Silicea is order and structure, not chaos: the rigid exactitude of the crystal archetype soon restored balance: the mental turbulence settling back into the long-estab-lished grooves laid-down in childhood. In the depths, however, the stresses had mounted, for energy must find expression. Whatever the final cause of the rupture with Fatio may have been, the consequence was even greater repression of Newton's sexuality: a recoiling of injured energy into the darkness of the Shadow: a zone where that which is repressed is perverted. Whereas, theological deliberations and study of the hermetic tradition partially compensated for reduced scientific output, nothing, other than inflation of the aggressive aspect of the Id, could possibly counterbalance the puritanical stifling of the sexual instinct. To give this resident rage recti-tude and offer it a sacrificial scapegoat on which to vent its fury, the uncom-promising, bigoted bureaucrat of the psyche, *the superego*, stepped into the breach.

Warden of the Mint

Newton's post of Warden of the Royal Mint, assumed in 1696 through the patronage of Charles Montagu, 1st Earl of Halifax, and held for the last 30 years of his life, afforded his superego full opportunity to exercise its authority and direct him, without conscience, to vicariously sate his desire for revenge in the most bloodthirsty manner. Bringing to his responsibility as Master of the Mint all the conscientiousness that characterised his labours of the past, he set himself the task of tracking down and punishing the many counterfeiters, who, at the time, were severely damaging the coinage. Counterfeiting was high treason, punishable by death through being hanged, drawn and quartered: a particularly gruesome end. Unlike previous Wardens or Masters of the Royal Mint, Newton, like a blood-hound, went into the City disguised as a frequenter of bars and taverns and sniffed out evidence himself. Extending his bureaucratic reach, he had himself made a justice of the peace in all the home counties under his juris-diction. In this role, he personally conducted cross-examinations and in the 18 months between June 1698 and December 1699 successfully prose-cuted 28 counterfeiters.[4] The assiduous, hands-on attention Newton devoted to his detective work and the bringing of offenders to justice, conviction and a harrowing death, suggests a fixated rage, ravening serially for satisfaction, yet beyond gratification (*desire to kill*). The close relation-ship between Silicea and Alumina is chillingly evident.

Hatred

Newton's need to vengefully and vindictively strike back at those who crossed him, indicated that something more than rage was operative. Red is the colour of repressed anger, but the colour that enchanted Newton most was *crimson*: a deep, intensification of red – red redolent of hatred – hence, *hate-red*! It drove him to expunge, wherever possible, all record of his arch-tormentor, Robert Hooke, even his portrait, a goal that came within his reach once he became president of the Royal Society in 1703 and assumed the mantle of patriarch of English science. In 1705, Queen Anne knighted him, the first scientist to be so honoured, and his inflated ego took on the crimson hue of overweening pride. He ruled the Royal Society with the authority of a dictator and, at times, that of a tyrant. His dealings with the Astronomer Royal, John Flamsteed, were particularly arrogant and condescending. On one occasion, to suit his own ends, he demanded the immediate release of Flamsteed's research data before the Astronomer Royal was ready to publish. Not willing to comply with the president's self-centred whim, Flamsteed ousted him by a court order. In revenge, Newton eliminated all reference to the invaluable help he had received from the astronomer in later editions of the *Principia*.

Calculus controversy

During the later years of his life, Newton's greatest wrath was reserved for Gottfried Wilhelm Leibniz, the brilliant German polymath, philosopher and mathematician, who developed differential and integral calculus quite independently of Newton. Through refining the binary number system, Leibniz also laid the foundation for virtually all digital computers. As ever, the Silicea connection holds true!

Newton developed his method of fluxions some time before Leibniz began his own serious delving into mathematics, but due to his reticence and fear of contention and criticism, he did not publish his findings; hence, in 1684, it was Leibniz, who published the paper that first made the calculus common knowledge. From this, a *priority controversy* arose between opposing factions each claiming precedence for one or other of the two mathematicians. Blatant charges of plagiarism were levelled by both sides. Inevitably, the chief protagonists themselves were drawn into the fray. Whereas, Leibniz's attitude, though assertive, remained moderate and considered, the invidious nature of the contention, roused Newton from anger (red) to fury (crimson). At the height of the dispute, he anonymously wrote, under the names of co-operative young supporters, most of the letters published in his defence. As president of the Royal Society, he appointed an 'impartial' committee to weigh the rival arguments; clandestinely wrote the official, published report of the committee's deliberations in his favour; and, then, to crown his manipulations, anonymously gave the review a positive critique in the scientific journal: *Philosophical Transactions of the Royal Society.*

Though he knew, beyond doubt, that he had discovered the calculus first, the accusations of dishonesty made against him and the knowledge that Leibniz, and many others in the scientific world, would always choose to believe that the German had crossed the line first, gnawed at his peace of mind for the rest of his life. His impeccable image had been publically assailed and the cutting edge of his peerless intellect challenged by another: insupportable blows to the 'wounded child' within a man, who had unconsciously spent the better part of his life assiduously striving for the unsurpassed excellence that would make him lovable in the eyes of his mother and his God. Even Leibniz's death could not allay Newton's wrath; his anger and resentment pursued his rival beyond the grave. The unresolved dispute consumed him during the final 25 years of his life. No matter the subject, almost every paper he wrote during those years, would digress at some point to level accusations against the German philosopher, revealing the unremitting rancour that raged within him.

Despite these psychic storms, Isaac Newton's passage to the next life was a peaceful one. He died in his sleep in London on 31 March 1727 at the age of 84 and was buried in Westminster Abbey.

In his alchemical experimentations, Newton was inevitably exposed to mercury vapours. After his death, his hair was examined and found to contain a significant amount of mercury. It has been conjectured that mercury poisoning might explain the eccentricity of his later years. Certainly, being a Silicea, would have rendered him singularly sensitive to mercury, but his life story reveals that he was an eccentric from his earliest years. Mercury may well have exaggerated the vindictive traits that later became so conspicuous. It is clear that the two elements are ever-fated to meet antagonistically.

A gentler, contemplative, more modest Newton lay concealed within his anxiety-driven, hypersensitive, egotistical nature and this was reflected in a whimsical memoir he wrote:

> I do not know what I may appear to the world, but to myself I seem to have been only like a little boy playing on the seashore and diverting myself in now and then finding a smoother pebble or a prettier shell than ordinary, while the great ocean of truth lay all undiscovered before me.[5]

These are Silicea words written by a Silicea man describing a Silicea scene – finding pebbles and shells on a sandy seashore!

Dark Silicea

These episodes from Newton's life cast light upon aspects of the Silicea archetype that might otherwise be overlooked or marginalised. Who would in a spontaneous, knee-jerk response think of Silicea for a person demonstrating such Platina-like dictatorial arrogance, such Thuja-like manipulative duplicity, such Staphysagria- and Nit-ac-like vengeful resentment, such Mercurius-like obsessive paranoia, such Hepar-sulph-like murderous rage and such an Alumina-like perversity: desire to mutilate. Yet, all these characteristics are present or potential in the materia medica of Silicea as they were in the nature of Isaac Newton. Indeed, the very pathology of Silicea possesses all the relentless, rancorous, destructive elements exhibited by Newton. No case history could better document the dark side of Silicea and verify the acute/chronic relationship of Staphysagria and Silicea and Nitric acid and Silicea.

As always, the profile of the archetype overshadows all, encompassing destiny, disposition, intellect, physical makeup and the diseases the body is heir to.

Just as the study of Graphites through the colour grey provides a many-layered appraisal of the archetype that the memory can hold, so studying Silicea via the complex personality and extraordinary life of Isaac Newton, gifts insights into the Shadow of the great archetype and highlights aspects of its nature that might otherwise be missed. Vivified by Newton, these facts can be readily recalled in a clinical encounter.

Matching Silicea rubrics related to the Leibniz episode:

- *Ailments from:*
  - *Contradiction* (2).
  - *Egotism.*
  - *Humiliation.*
  - *Anger suppressed* (2) – my addition.
  - *Indignation.*
- *Ambition – much ambition.*
- *Contemptuous.*
- *Egotism, self-esteem* (2).
- *Haughty.*
- *Selfishness.*
- *Offended easily* (2).
- *Suspiciousness.*
- *Intolerant of contradiction* (2) – *has to restrain himself from violence.*
- *Deceitful, Sly.*
- *Liar.*
- *Defiant.*
- *Audacity.*
- *Anger:*
  - *From contradiction* (2).
  - *When looked at* – in the adult this becomes: when scrutinised; when subject to appraisal; when criticised; when accused.
  - *When aroused.*
  - *Temper tantrums* – child or adult.
  - *Violent.*
- *Loss of self-control.*
- *Abusive, insulting.*
- *Temperament choleric* (2).
- *Quarrelsomeness, scolding* (2).
- *Violence, vehemence* – *when crossed* (2).
- *Monomania* (2).

References

1   Voltaire (1894). '14'. *Letters on England*. In: Wikipedia: *Isaac Newton*. Personal relations, ref. 98.

2   White M. *Isaac Newton – The Last Sorcerer*. London: Fourth Estate Ltd, 1997. pp247–249.

3   Smyth GL. *The Monuments and Genii of St Paul's Cathedral and Westminster Abbey* (translation). pp703–704.

4   Westfall, R.S. *Force in Newton's Physics: The Science of Dynamics in the Seventeenth Century*. London: Macdonald, 2007. p73.

5   Brewster D. *Memoirs of the Life, Writings, and Discoveries of Sir Isaac Newton* (1855) (Volume II, Chapter 27). Wikipedia: *Isaac Newton. After death – Fame*.

15

SILICEA – 6

Guiding characteristics

Causation – aetiological factors – *'ailments from'*:

- *Severe fright or grave, emotional shock* (3).
- *In childhood: fright, abuse, neglect and abandonment.*
- *Abandonment – adult (forsaken feeling; feels not loved by parents, spouse, friends).*
- *Betrayed friendship (friendship deceived).*
- *Over-study and close confinement – sedentary life* (2).
- *Mental exertion – writing and reading* (2 unique).
- *Anxiety* (3).
- *Fright, fear or anxiety* (3).
- *Emotional excitement* (3).
- *Alone – being alone – solitude – loneliness.*
- *Anticipation, foreboding, presentiment.*
  - *Stage-fright* (2).
- *Bad news* (2).
- *Anger, vexation.*
- *Anger suppressed* (2).
- *Confrontation* (2).
- *Contradiction – criticism* (2).
- *Sympathy, consolation* (2).
- *Egotism.*
- *Mortification, humiliation, chagrin* (2).
- *Sexual desire suppressed* (2).
- *Masturbation* (2).
- *Sexual excesses* (2).
- *Menopause.*
- *During thunderstorms* (2).
- *Moon phases: during the increasing moon* (2) *and during full moon* (3).

The Mouse

Edward Whitmont described Silicea thus:

The mouse – a timid, delicate, white mouse that will fiercely defend its own small territory.

This 'white' Silicea does not show the archetype's Shadow aspects.

- *Shy timorousness.*
- *Self-protectiveness.*
- *Anxiously restricted outlook on life.*
- *Apprehensive of the unknown.*
- *Self-limiting existence, locked into unchanging and insignificant routine.*
- *Work and endure is their philosophy* (Calc-carb; Psorinum).
- *Retiring, easily intimidated.*
- *Would rather pass unnoticed; averse being spoken to.*
- *Apologetic manner – people pleaser.*
- *Avoids attention, but anxiously protects his rights, principles and privacy.*

The emotions of a certain Silicea 'white mouse' provide a good picture of the nervous, tense, self-effacing nature of this gentle type, but, hints of a more difficult Silicea are discernible.

- *Hair pulling and nail biting; talking and walking in sleep.*
- *Worse from criticism or contradiction.*
- *Worse for noise.*
- *Worse in situations where they feel out of control.*
- *Never competitive in sport.*
- *Introverted.*
- *Highly-strung.*
- *Prone to immense anger, which they do not have the confidence to voice.*
- *Insecure and self-conscious.*
- However: *very assertive.*
- *Stubborn.*
- *Sulks easily.*
- *Passive aggressive.*
- *Bad communicator about important issues.*
- *Cannot handle criticism or flattery.*
- *Sense of great responsibility and duty regarding work and raising a family successfully.*
- *Does not enjoy small-talk and parties.*
- *Hates crowds.*
- *A good listener.*

- *By nature, not a warm type of personality.*
- *Overdeveloped sense of not hurting people even when it is necessary to be forthright.*
- *Sometimes sense of dishonesty at being unable to say what they feel and think.*
- *Cannot reprimand or criticise subordinates, hence, cannot accept managerial responsibility.*
- *Uneasy speaking on the telephone.*

Marked characteristics

- *Anxiety driven – difficulty feeling safe – lack of basic trust.*
- *Difficulty, or inability, trusting people.*
- *Problems with intimacy.*
- *Poor self-image.*
- *Perfectionistic expectations – of self and others.*
- *Difficulty with spontaneity.*
- *Fear of being out of control.*
- *Inflexible opinions.*
- *Secretiveness.*
- *Rigidity.*
- *Intellectual – intellectually pedantic.*

Fears

- *Lifelong fears* (festering fears).
- *Pins, Pointed, Sharp Things* (4).
- *Injections* (4).
- *Pins, pointed sharp things, hunts for pointed things, although afraid of them* (unique).
- *Night – at night.*
- *Suffocation – at night – cannot lie down.*
- *Of not waking from sleep* (fear of dying in sleep).
- *While lying in bed* (2).
- *Dark.*
- *Being alone.*
- *Robbers – on waking.*
- *Noise* (2).
- *Fear because of noise in ear.*

- *Animals:*
  - *Cats.*
  - *Dogs.*
- *Emotional breakdown.*
- *Killing her child.*
- *In a crowd.*
- *People.*
- *Strangers.*
- *Disease – of impending contagious, epidemic disease – e.g. AIDS.*
- *Fear drives them from place to place.*
- *Pursued by enemies.*
- *Evil.*
- *Anticipatory fear before examinations or public speaking or meeting a friend (2)*
- *Timidity about appearing in public; about talking in public (2).*
- *Anything new or unfamiliar (2).*
- *Undertaking anything.*
  - *Undertaking a new enterprise (2).*
- *Failure – examinations – public address – business or in work or in what they attempt – despite great natural ability – undertakes nothing lest he should fail (2).*
- *Occupation.*
- *Work – dread of work – dread of literary work (2).*
- *Responsibility (2).*
- *Falling.*
- *Downward movement.*
- *Claustrophobia.*
- *Thunderstorm.*
- *Lightening.*
- *Misfortune.*

Anxiety

Newman was an 'anxiety-ridden man' and Silicea is a very anxious remedy. Anxiety is more constant than fear.

- *Exaggerated – out of proportion to circumstances.*
- *With sleeplessness.*
- *In bed at the full moon.*
- *On waking from frightful dreams.*

- *At midnight, ameliorated on rising* (unique) – *at midnight on waking* (unique).
- *On waking, ameliorated on rising* – *after 3 a.m.*
- *While lying; better on rising* (2).
- *While sitting.*
- *While standing.*
- *Driving from place to place* (Ars-alb, Graphites).
- *Ameliorated by motion* – *better walking.*
- *Anxiety of conscience* (2) – i.e. guilt.
  ○ *Anxiety of conscience about trifles* (unique).
- *Anxiety about trifles* (2).
  ○ *Anxiety about trifles due to extreme nervous weakness* (2).
- *With debility* – *with weakness.*
- *After eating.*
- *Experienced in the stomach* (2) – *in pit of stomach.*
- *In the stomach, worse during the menses* (unique).
- *In the chest or heart region* – *during menses* (2).
- *With palpitation* – *with perspiration* – *with hot head.*
- *During the menses* (3).
- *Anticipating an engagement* (2).
- *In schoolchildren* – *about their lessons.*
- *About the future* (2).
- *After fright* (2) – *remaining for a long time.*
- *With fear.*
- *With biting of the nails.*
- *About himself* (2).
- *From pains in the anus* (2).
- *About health* – *especially during menopause.*
- *With weariness of life.*

Delusions – fancies, imaginings, assumptions

- *Swallowing pins and needles* (2 – unique but compare Mercurius).
- *About pins and needles* (2).
- Left half of the body does not belong to her – she did not own her left side.
- Body divided.
- Divided into two parts.
- He is double (remember Silicea has: *two trains of thoughts* and *contradiction of the will*).

- *Being in different places at a time* (2).
- Someone walks beside him.
- Elevated in the air.
- Injury – will receive injury.
- Persecuted.
- Pursued – by enemies.
- Sees thieves, robbers – in the house.
- Head enlarged – head is too large.
- Water.
- Animals:
  - Sees dogs.
  - Sees vermin crawl about.
  - Creeping worms.
- Criminals.
- He is a criminal – he has done wrong.
- Die – he is about to die.
- Dead – he is dead.
- Dead persons.
- Insane – will become insane.
- Fail – everything will fail.
- Faintness.
- Fancy.
- House full of people.
- *Horrible visions* (2).
- Sees phantoms – night – *all over* (2) – *on closing the eyes* (2) – dwells upon delusion of phantoms – frightful, while trying to sleep at night.
- Sees ghosts.
- On a journey.
- Lascivious.

Dreams

Silicea, like Mag-carb and Emerald, has 'dream-catcher' ability. In the Silicea sensitive person, it encourages dreaming and the retention of dreams – often promoting dreams that assist in understanding the psychic dynamics of the analysand, assessing progress and supplying clues to the next remedy.

- *Many (3) – crowding one upon another* (2 – Kali-carb, Sepia, Thuja).
- *Vivid (3) – lucid.*
- *Before midnight.*

- *On first going to sleep.*
- *Rousing the patient.*
- *Dream continues after waking.*
- *Half waking.*
- *While awake (2).*
- *Nightmare.*
- *Unable to shriek when desiring to during frightful dream.*
- *Frightful (3) – followed by fear.*
- *Disgusting.*
- *Amorous (2) – morning – evening.*
  - *With erections.*
  - *With ejaculation (2).*
  - *Breaking sleep (2).*
- *Sexual intercourse.*
- *Lewd, lascivious, voluptuous.*
- *Carousing.*
- *Things desired.*
- *Anger.*
- *Animals:*
  - *Anxious (2).*
  - *Cats pursuing him.*
  - *Dogs (2) – pursued by dogs – a large dog following him* (unique).
  - *Pursued by wild animals.*
  - *Snakes.*
  - *Vermin.*
  - *Worms creeping.*
- *Crystal; ice; mirrors.*
- *Cobwebs.*
- *Sand criss-crossed with sticks.*
- *Anxious – anxiety alleviated on waking (2).*
- *Heavy, anxious (2).*
- *Business (2) – of the day – neglected.*
- *Dreams about things heard, read, talked or thought about.*
- *Confused.*
- *Disconnected.*
- *Vertigo (2).*
- *Disease.*
- *Epilepsy – he had a fit.*
- *Earthquake.*
- *Events long past forgotten (3) – historic (2) – previous events (3) – the time of youth (3)* [unique] *– events of the day.*

- *Falling.*
- *Fantastic.*
- *Fire.*
- *Flood* (2).
- *Boat foundering* (Alumina; Lycopodium).
- *Drowning – of a man drowning* (2).
- *Storms* (2) *– at sea.*
- *Frightful storms* (unique).
- *Accidents.*
- *Treason* [unique].
- *Murder* (2).
- *Being murdered.*
- *Being strangled.*
- *Being pursued* (2).
- *Being betrayed* (unique).
- *Humiliation* (2).
- *Wrongful accusations of having committed a crime* (Galileo!).
- *Robbers* (2) *– fighting with robbers.*
- *Ghosts* (2) *fighting with ghosts – pursued by ghosts.*
- *Battles – fights.*
- *Quarrels.*
- *Dead bodies.*
- *Dead people.*
- *Death – approaching – that he is to die.*
- *Cruelty.*
- *Persistent* (2).
- *Pleasant* (2).
- *Restless* (2).
- *Journey* (2).
- *Foreign country – a country far off* [unique].
- *A desert* [unique].
- *Visionary; prophetic; clairvoyant* (2).
- *Somnambulistic.*
- *Intellectual.*
- *Weeping.*

The advanced Silicea

- The combination of rigidity and resilience, strength and flexibility, give stability to the Silicea character as it develops.

- They are unpretentious, unassuming and humble and their humility and diffidence are honest and sincere.
- Honest and face up to the truth.
- Free from egotism, boastfulness or any need to dominate.
- They neither introvert their emotions nor hurt others by emotional behaviour.
- Considerate and kind even at their own expense.
- Always willing to stand down in favour of another.
- Open and transparent, not devious or secretive.
- Tolerant, understanding, concerned and helpful.
- Empathetic.
- No desire to dominate or manipulate.
- Equable disposition; even tempered.
- Reliable, conscientious, honest and responsible.
- Sense of duty, responsibility, integrity.
- Sensitive and intuitive, always willing to see the other persons point of view and to put the best interpretation on their motives without being gullible or naive.
- Good judges of character, but exercise patience and tolerance towards others' weaknesses.
- They have high morals and principles but are never self-righteous (*c.f.* Kali-carb).
- They aspire to excellence and perfection; honest search for self-growth.
- Their friendship and love are unqualified.
- They live harmlessly.
- They are detached, dispassionate and selfless.

Causative influences

- *Exposure to cold winds and draughts.*
- *Cold exposure to the uncovered head, neck, spine and feet.*
- *Cold, damp weather.*
- *Cold changes in weather – from warm to cold and from dry to wet.*
- *Getting the feet wet.*
- *Overheating.*
- *Thunderstorms.*
- *Physical exertion – straining – over-lifting – injury (ligaments and tendons).*
- *Sexual intercourse – orgasm – sexual excesses.*
- *Loss of vital fluids – blood, semen, diarrhoea, lactation. etc.*
- *Suppression of foot sweat and of the menses.*

- *Vaccination – immunisations.*
- *Splinters and foreign bodies in the tissues.*
- *Mining — inhalation of small particles, stone dust – gold miner's and stone cutter's silicosis.*
- *Milk + lactose.*
- *Gluten.*

Aggravations:

- **Emotional stress.*
- **Nervous excitement.*
- **Fright.*
- **Criticism.*
- **Contradiction.*
- **Consolation.*
- **Mental exertion.*
- Silicea is a *chilly remedy* and catches cold especially when the head or feet are uncovered.
- *Cold and becoming cold.*
- *Cold air; cold draughts.*
- Uncovering (especially the head, neck, spine and feet).
- *Damp; cold, damp weather;* worse at the approach of winter.
- Drinking cold water = dry cough; loss of consciousness [warm drinks relieve cough].
- Change of weather (especially from warm-dry to cold-damp).
- Before and during a thunderstorm (in contrast, the Sepia patient feels worse before a thunderstorm, but better when the storm breaks and then quite enjoys it).
- Becoming overheated.
- Averse to warm food [gastric symptoms better for cold food].
- After eating.
- Milk (averse to mother's milk = vomiting and diarrhoea).
- Bathing.
- Light; Noise.
- Touch; Pressure.
- Jarring (especially the spine); walking <; every step is painfully felt (incarcerated flatus).
- Combing the hair.
- Suppressed sweat (especially of the feet).

- Moon changes; *during the new or full moon* – nightmares, somnambulism, talking in sleep, headaches, epilepsy, emotions.
- Night.
- During menses.
- Intercourse – masturbation.
- Lying on the left side; lying on the painful side (lying down may aggravate asthma and headache).
- Standing.

Ameliorations

- *Warmth.*
- *Summer.*
- *Wrapping up* (especially the head).
- Warm room.
- Warm drinks relieve the cough.
- Wet, humid weather (Causticum).
- Sometimes symptoms are relieved by cold, dry air.
- Repose.
- Lying down relieves debility, exhaustion (Psorinum).
- Lying on the painless side.
- Desire to be magnetised which relieves.
- Profuse urination (headache).

Desires and Aversions

Craves:

- Only cold things.
- Ice cream and ice water – feels comfortable when it is in the stomach (Phosphorus).
- Sweets.
- Eggs.
- Rarely milk.
- *Loves fruit, raw vegetables, salads.*

Averse:

- *Disgust for meat and warm food.*
- *Fat.*
- *Milk: aversion to mother's milk; child vomits as soon as it nurses* [Aethusa].
- Meat.
- Salt.
- Warm food.

Milk brings on vomiting, colic and diarrhoea.
    Child nurses well, but food passes through undigested.
    Canine hunger, but sudden disgust for food on attempting to eat.

Sphere of Action

- Mental, emotional and physical exhaustion and debility.
- Malassimilation – defective nutrition.
- Affections of:
    - Nervous system.
    - Reticulo-endothelial system and lymphatic glands.
    - Connective tissues.
    - Skin and its appendages – hair, nails.
    - Teeth.
    - Skeletal system.
- Indurations – skin, nails, glands, fibroid growths, exostoses – Silicea makes the soft tissues hard and the hard tissues harder.
- Suppuration.
- Sweat of single parts, especially head, neck, axillae, feet.
- Offensive sweat.
- Aggravation from suppression of sweat, especially foot sweat.
- Chilliness with aggravation from cold; amelioration from heat.
- Discharges – chronic, purulent, thin, acrid and offensive.

16

OTHER ARCHETYPAL FORMS AND SYSTEMS

Mathematical forms

To Pythagoras and Plato, the most immaculate and fundamental of the archetypal principles underlying the manifest world were *the mathematical forms of geometric shapes and numbers.*

These forms become symbols when viewed archetypally: metaphors for something more profound and universal. They can be used to communicate hidden levels of meaning and transcendent realities. This is particularly true when the image presents in the context of a vivid or lucid archetypal dream.

Behind the external appearance of things, a higher reality, a more radiant beauty and a greater wisdom exists, whose transcendence can only be comprehended in symbolic form. Myth and symbol possess the power to reveal the deeper meaning with a clarity and richness that can evoke both intellectual and emotional response. They bring together aspects of the conscious and the unconscious, the rational and the intuitive, providing a portal into a finer dimension.

On examining the significance of symbols, we discover that they can be compared to homeopathic remedies. They direct us to something beyond themselves, to that which would otherwise remain unknown, intangible and indefinable. The symbol is the portal to a spiritual realm; its energy is continuous with its ethereal counterpart and inseparable from that which it symbolises. The potentised remedy is the portal to a mysterious archetypal world of healing power with which it is confluent. In contemplating a physical image or a remedy archetype, we are in the presence of its invisible essence, for it is the epiphany of a hidden force. Every object and every remedy is a unique revelation of the mystical and expresses specific archetypal attributes, intimating another more potent reality that informs and energises it.

Geometric shapes

The Circle

The circle is one of humanity's oldest, most revered and celestial symbols, perceived as embodying the Creator, the uncircumscribed centre of the cosmos: a circle whose centre is everywhere, and whose circumference is nowhere – hence, *the circle is the symbol of that which cannot be symbolised*: the boundlessness of infinity, the omnipresence of the Absolute. The circle is understood to image perfection, unity, indivisibility, eternity, totality, infinity and wholeness – all of which are facets of the highest Reality.

In the form of the *ouroboros*, the circular image of a snake swallowing its own tail, the circle symbolises the cyclic and eternal nature of existence through incarnation, death and reincarnation; the self-renewing seasons of Nature perpetually recreating herself; the unity of duality; and the Oneness of all. It is also a primal metaphor of the Divine Feminine, the Womb of Creation: all encompassing, gestating the thoughts, energy and forms of the creation. *This symbolism links the circle to the blackness of the Void* – the blackness of the Deep – and the colour Black (see Graphites).

The Snake archetype relates to the most profound aspects of the circle: to the spiritual ascent of the human soul achieved through progressively shedding the many 'skins' of the ego-self that constrict it and prevent transcendence.

The coiled snake clearly represents the circle in amplified form. When drawn out, the coils become *the spiral: the fundamental symbol of the Universe*: the spiralling circle of life energy that flows through every aspect of existence. It symbolises the cyclic, rhythmic forces that produce and maintain the material universe and the wave-form of the energy fields that pervade it. These connections and connotations are indicative of the primordial importance of the snake as archetype, as symbol and as remedy – particularly Lachesis (Brazilian pit-viper, bushmaster) and Naja (cobra): the former representing the Viperine snakes and the latter the Elapidae, the two major venomous snake families.

Other creatures participate in the symbolism of the circle and each stands high in the archetypal hierarchy of the materia medica. The Wolf (Lac lupinum) stands out in this regard, as does the Dolphin (Lac delphinum). On returning from a successful hunt, the wolf runs in wide circles as if to trace the image of the moon in the snow; Wolf provers dream of whirlpools, seals circling, a polar bear chasing in circles, a whale turning on a spit; and during proving trials found themselves doodling circles. Dolphins swim in ever-tightening circles to trap a shoal of fish; provers dreamed of walking in a circle clockwise, of being on a merry-go-round turning clockwise, horses racing clockwise. Belladonna (deadly night-shade), Stramonium (poison apple) and Thuja (northern white cedar) need to walk in circles. The Amerindians, ran whooping round their Thuja totem poles to arouse their battle frenzy and, similarly, Norse warriors in the Viking-age, after taking Agaricus, worked themselves into a berserk fury before battle. The autistic Thuja child perseverates by endless spinning movements of the hands, while the Agaricus child runs and dances and makes involuntary movements with the hands as if winding a ball of wool. The Spider is a circle archetype, spinning its silk in circles to form a web and the hyperactive Lycosa child runs around and around in circles. The flower stems of Cyclamen (sow-bread), unfurl and re-furl spirally, in a circle; Cyclamen is a remedy which cures severe vertigo in which objects seem to spin around the sufferer in a circle. The colonies of Bovista (puffball), a mushroom-like fungus, form fairy-circles in meadows; Bovista is an arche-type associated with the psychic forces of Hekate: necromancy: prophecy and communication with the spirits of the so-called 'dead'.

The celestial symbolism of the circle is represented by the sun and the moon. However, it is the moon, with its ever-changing face that represents in full all that the circle implies, for while the sun is hot, fiery and mascu-line, the moon, like the circle in its highest form, the ouroboros, is cool, mellow, feminine, enigmatic, mysterious and related to the deepest levels of the unconscious. The archetypes most responsive to the influence of the full moon are all under the thrall of the circle in its most powerful lunar form: Argentum (silver: metal of the moon), Arg-nit (violated silver), Arsenicum (the murderer in the night), Calc-carb (the oyster: the pearl – 'teardrops of the moon'), Luna (the moon), Lycopodium (werewolf), Phosphorus (night-light), Pulsatilla (the moon maiden), Silicea (mature moon maiden – mother – crone) and the two outstanding, Gothic arche-types synonymous with the power and mystery of the moon: Wolf and Raven!

The pearl is the 'quintessential symbol of light and femininity – its pale iridescence associated with the luminous moon, its watery origins with fertility, its secret life in the shell with the miracle of birth and rebirth.'[1] The mysterious light emanating from the pearl made it a symbol of wisdom, esoteric knowledge and spiritual enlightenment. The pearl is an emblem of sexuality and fecundity, being associated with the love-goddess Aphrodite, who emerged from the sea and blew to shore on a scallop shell; yet also of innocence, purity, virginity (maidenhood), celibacy and perfection. The Romans valued the pearl above all other gems as a protective talisman, significantly, against the attacks of *rabid dogs* (Belladonna, Stramonium) and to prevent *lunacy*. In its supreme symbolism, the pearl represents the soul's journey towards Self-realisation and the ineffable virtue that marks its attainment.

In contrast, pearls, like diamonds, have been associated with ill-luck and misfortune, as they carry a legacy from their past. Whether the 'pearl with a past' proves a blessing or a curse depends on the traits resident in the wearer. A pearl can carry the contagion of malice or the promise of love, but resonance will be the attractive or protective force. The same psychometric power is characteristic of quartz crystals. As seen in the example of Isaac Newton, the tenacious holding onto old grievances is a marked characteristic of the Silicea archetype; the same tendency must be recognised in Calc-carb. The cleansing of newly-acquired crystals and pearls is wise and can best be achieved by soaking them in sea water or water mixed with sea salt – at the time of the full moon! Knowing the natural history and symbolism of the pearl, this 'treatment' is homeopathic. All forms of psychism relate to *Sycosis*, as does the duality of the pearl's legacy and its watery origin. The full moon presides over the ocean and the watery domain and Nat-mur, the salt and sea remedy, is a key sycotic remedy for the elimination of deeply-imbedded emotions that may be nurtured and harboured for a lifetime. Salt cleanses the soul, just as it can cleanse the crystal or the pearl.

As *zero*, the circle is the feminine progenitor: Creatrix of the mathematical numbers and provides a link between the symbolism of shapes and forms (ouroboros/sphere = zero; obelisk = 1; triangle/pyramid = 3; square/cube = 4).

The Square

In contrast to the dynamism of the circle, *the square* and its three-dimensional form, the cube, are the most static of the graphic, symbolic shapes, and both became the ancient sign for the earth. A circle surrounding a square, stands for heaven enclosing the earth, and, conversely, the image of a circle within a square symbolises the divine spark within the material body. The stable, ordered, grounded configuration of the square provides a symbol of permanence, security, balance, soundness, moral rectitude and good faith (a 'square deal'). It is, however, also a symbol for over-conservatism – a rigid, inflexible, traditional attitude (a 'square') – and for an earthbound state of materialism and lack of spiritual values. In this latter context, our attention alights upon the cuboid, crystal formation of feldspar, Calc-fluor (calcium fluoride), and finds confirmation of these observations in the remedy's love of the good things of life, its acquisitive, miserly nature and the substance's affinity for the lower, grosser tissues of the body: the teeth, bones and connective tissue.

The Triangle

Like the circle, *the triangle* is a dynamic and powerful symbol. It shares the symbolic meaning of the number three, and, hence, of all things triple, in triad, or in trinity. Its alignment defines its meaning.

The equilateral triangle resting on its base with its apex pointing upwards is masculine and solar and represents ascent, prosperity and harmony. It is the alchemical symbol for fire and represents the passions, or fiery emotions, but also the fervour of spiritual aspiration and endeavour.

The reversed triangle depicted with its apex pointing downwards is feminine, and lunar and represents the Great Mother Goddess, water, rain, fecundity and heavenly grace. The two interpenetrating to form a hexagon, known as the Seal of Solomon (a mythical and magic signet ring, said to have been possessed by King Solomon, which gave the wearer psychic powers), represent the combination of fire and water, the merging of masculine and feminine and therefore the union of opposites; a process intrinsic to the evolution of the soul.

In its Christian symbolism, the triangle denotes the holy trinity of Father, Son and Holy Spirit, uniting the three in a single godhead; hence a sign for God.

Silicea, is an archetype closely aligned with the symbolism of the triangle and the pyramid. Quartz or rock crystal, forms beautiful crystal structures all of which are crowned with a closing pyramid of triangular facets. All the mountains of our planet, with the exception of limestone and dolomite formations, are largely vast aggregations of silica crystals; a fact that defines Silicea's archetypal pre-eminence. Silicea is a morally and aesthetically refined archetype moved by an innate urge to grow, develop and improve and ultimately to attain spiritual excellence. This is the aspiration of the triangle!

Numbers

Numbers, like the geometric shapes, are mathematical forms bearing powerful symbolic and archetypal meaning. Numerology, the study of the mystical significance of numbers, and the art of numerological divination, are of ancient origin and were of particular interest to the Chinese and the Greeks.

A great deal of invention and legend surround the life and teachings of the Greek philosopher and mathematician, Pythagoras (570–495 BCE). Today, he is only remembered for his geometric theorem, nonetheless, during his life he developed philosophical theories, which not only lead to his devout adherents, the Pythogoreans, forming a religious sect to pursue his concepts and practices, but also exerted a marked influence on the thinking of Plato. To Pythagoras, the laws of mathematics underpinned the fabric of creation; everything was related to its principles, and numbers represented the ultimate reality. Today, on a more superficial level, the binary numeral system implemented in digital electronic circuitry and used internally by almost all modern computers provides us with evidence of how by the symbolic use of numbers, visual and auditory images of physical reality can be captured and encoded. From this technology, the ability to create computer-simulated environments, replete with visual, auditory and tactile sensory simulation, has been developed. Life-like environments and experiences known as *virtual reality* can be generated giving further proof of the imaging power of numbers and providing practical evidence of what Pythagoras postulated.

Plato interpreted the immaculate elegance and eternal, transcendental quality of numbers as being absolute and archetypal.

The archetypal forms are of importance in homeopathic practice because their images are intrinsic to the unique nature, qualities and action of each remedy; to the aspirations, aptitudes, beliefs and behaviour of each patient; and to the dynamics of their dreams. Recognition of the presence of the archetype and its influence is invaluable in matching remedy and personality at a deep, curative level. Archetypal thinking and knowledge is of inestimable value in understanding and interpreting Nature's code, which is particularly expressed through the signatures of shape, number and colour, all of which are archetypal. We discover that through the wisdom of archetypal philosophy, we are able to apprehend the interconnectedness of all things and of all knowledge and the indissoluble unity of the Cosmos. The art of homeopathy is largely the harmonising of archetypal energy between patient and remedy. By revisiting the fantasy world of our childhood, returning to the time when we still dwelt in the realm of the archetype and recapturing its magic mystery, this faculty can be reawakened. The homeopath needs to have the intuitive, imaginative and uncluttered mind of a shaman to walk with confidence in the hallowed halls of fable and fantasy where the inner mysteries of life are revealed.

Number One archetype

[handwritten margin note: remedies in MM intro]

Viewing the materia medica archetypally, we discern that some of its remedies stand out large and bold, projecting their nature assertively, even monumentally; others, while mighty, are reserved and withdrawn; some, by any definition, remain small and inconspicuous. Like the human characters on the stage of life, all remedies are not equal. Equality, like Beauty, is an absolute, eternal principle of Reality and pertains to the Spirit not the soul. It is not the Spirit that requires healing, it is the soul, and equality is not the frame of the soul. From the moment of creation, the relative universe arrayed itself in hierarchies. From their primitive, animal-like beginning, human troops and eventually tribes were ruled by hierarchical behaviour essential for survival. Modern communities are constructed on hierarchical principles; even the path of human life is subject to the hierarchy of age. Equality pertains to the Essential state of Being. The very act of incarnation constitutes loss of both freedom and equality. All men and women are equal in Essence, but not in reality; a glance in the mirror is proof enough. Likewise, all remedies are not equal and the materia medica reflects this inequality; it has hierarchical structure. The homeopathic practitioner needs to know which remedies are primary and fundamental, and why that is so. Such remedies must be of critical importance and frequently called for.

A good starting point is the study of the ancient, symbolic interpretations of the Number One archetype and to relate these to homeopathic remedies. To achieve this, we need to think in myth – as we do when interpreting the dreams of our patients. However, in doing so, we soon discover that it is not necessary to set aside science – myth and science walk hand in hand.

Being singular, the Pythagoreans did not consider 1 to be a number, which means plurality, but rather as the source of all other numbers; it was *the point*, the common basis for all calculation (see the symbolism of *pin* in Part 2). They considered odd numbers to represent the masculine principle and even numbers the feminine. 1, however, was deemed to hold both masculine and feminine principles in potential form, and when added to either even or odd numbers changed their respective gender principle to the opposite. Missing from this concept is the primordial precedence of *zero*: the numerical mother symbol from which all numbers derive, just as all manifestation is born from the womb of the Void and all colours emerge from black.

The understanding of the Pythagoreans is similar to the science of the Chakras. The first, third, fifth and seventh chakras are primarily masculine and the second, fourth and sixth chakras are primarily feminine. Although the first chakra is masculine, at its base the power of *Shakti* (feminine) and *Shiva* (masculine) is expressed dynamically through *Ida* and *Pingala*, the feminine and masculine *nadis*, or energy channels, that spiral upwards, imparting spin to the chakras and from these energy foci suffusing the entire body. The masculine and feminine principles are, themselves, archetypes of major importance.

In Western tradition, Number One possesses a phallic and aggressive symbolism, which corresponds to the basic instincts rooted in the primordial functions of the first chakra: procreative sex and the fight and flight response. Knowledge of the chakra system is essential to all forms of 'energy medicine.' The understanding provides a template against which archetype and patient can be evaluated with regard to consciousness, emotions, organ affinities, miasmatic predominance and clinical progress.

If we contemplate the Number One esoterically, as through the eyes of Pythagoras, Plato, or a mystic; its meaning expands infinitely. The Arabic numeral 1 stands erect, proud, single, majestic; embodying the origin and the outcome, alpha and omega, the beginning and the end; a mystic centre from which all else radiates. By the addition of itself to itself, all positive, whole-numbers are created; it is the essence of all things, indissoluble and indivisible; the symbol of the first principle and thus of the unique, the universal and the sublime; an image of primordial unity, of the universe and of the Creative Essence; Number One symbolises God and the universe. It is also the symbol of the Self, which ultimately stands alone, splendid, complete and realised; one with the Oneness to which it must return. This was presaged millions of years ago when a primitive hominid, *Austrilopithecus*, first adopted an upright bipedal stance, in the manner of 1, and established the distinguishing characteristic, which eventually made *Homo erectus*, and finally, *Homo sapiens*, the paragon – the first among animals.

It is not within the scope of this introductory work on archetypes to systematically define the nature and elaborate the characteristics of the nine single-digit numbers and the seven colours of the spectrum. Each system deserves a work of its own. However, for the most part, these profiles will emerge much as black and grey have in the study of Graphites and as red has in the study of Wolf. As an example, however, it is of value to consider the characteristics of the Number One Archetype.

Number One

Being archetypal, Number One is associated with a definite personality profile. Study of the ancient lore of numerology and the arcane symbolism of the Tarot, provides us with revealing insights into the mythology and traits of the primary number. The exercise evidences the common conclusions of different esoteric systems and demonstrates that invaluable insights into archetypal nature can be derived from sources outside homeopathic provings.

The physical delineation of 1 in the Arabic form provides valuable clues. It may be likened to a focal point; an arrow; a straight, narrow path; a staff; a sword; a spear; a spear-shaped tree; a tall tree branching at its crown; a stone pillar; an erect phallus: all metaphors that are full of meaning – images conjured from the collective unconscious – the material of dreams.

The review of the Number One personality that follows is garnered from the intuitive imaging of numerology and the Tarot. The result of intuition, insight, observation and experience without recourse to provings, the portrait is a revelation to the homeopathic physician. Two very familiar archetypes emerge – similar, yet different, but closely related.

The One symbol pertains to origin and beginnings, hence, to innovation, discovery, invention, construction, creation: first-man, primitive man, stone-age man, hunter-gatherer, farmer, explorer, pioneer, artisan, inventor, technician, engineer, scientist. Whatever the gender of the individual, the energy, drive and focus of One are distinctly masculine. They possess an uninhibited, unselfconscious freedom of action and thought, untroubled by self-doubt, need for the good opinion of others or anxiety of conscience. Whatever their intelligence, even brilliance, they retain an unsophisticated roughness and guileless spontaneity, which, though refreshing, can be crude and startlingly free of delicacy or concern for the sentiments of others. They do not pussy foot around issues, but boldly state their opinion. Diplomacy is foreign to them; they are blunt and forthright and intolerant of double-dealing. A rough diamond!

This is a curious and creative intellect. A pioneering, independent, fertile and inventive spirit, blessed with initiative, enterprise and ambition. Their perspective is markedly left-cerebral, gifting them with an aptitude for mathematics, science and technology and an inquiring intellect, functioning with clarity, objectivity, penetrating vision and an insatiable appetite for observation, investigation and analysis. A penchant for speculation and theorising, which may reach obsessive proportions, permits them to push back the shadows of ignorance. This single-mindedness and total preoccupation with a current fascination can so narrow their focus that they neglect all else, including their environment and themselves. Always at the cutting edge, their explorations, experimentations and inventions lead them into uncharted territory, opening up new vistas of opportunity and development. Their originality, innovativeness, novel ideas and entrepreneurial drive often bring them into contention with the established order and the mores and conventions of traditionalists.

They are practical and physically skilled and possess a love of the earth and the outdoors, but in their trailblazing and drive to penetrate, explore and master the wilderness, they have desecrated nature with club, arrow, spear, scythe and rifle. Like the archer who aims the arrow that the number resembles, they set their eyes on distant targets and have a remarkable ability to maintain their focus amid distractions and confusion. Decisions are made with ease and once an enthusiasm takes root, or an objective is visualised, they pursue either with passion, one-pointedness and resolute determination. This may lead to obstinacy and a stubborn inability to compromise or change direction.

The archetype is clever and shrewd; many are cunning, wily and highly opportunistic, ever ready to take the gap or seize the advantage. Their self-confidence, efficiency and competence move others to lean on them for guidance, support and solutions to their problems. They are able to motivate others to initiate and bring about change. Leadership comes naturally to them; they have a need to take over and take charge and are not comfortable in a subordinate role. They love to be the one who is the focus of attention, in the limelight and commanding centre-stage, flourishing in the warmth of applause, praise and adulation. Their bearing and behaviour may be assertive, officious and domineering, a trait which tends to isolate them from others, who experience them as overbearing and intimidating. Always upward moving and striving for superiority and the pinnacle of success, for Number One, second best is never good enough; they must be in control and wear the crown. This may bring the loneliness of the one at the top, aloof, secluded and solitary. They are competitive and push others aside in their drive for achievement and success. The careers they tend to choose are sport, the military, big corporations, politics, scientific research and computer science, or they become inventors, designers, engineers or explorers.

At their best, they shine and shed light about them like the sun, the first among stars; but at their worst, their ascendency inflates their egos, and puffed with self-importance, they see themselves as being above error, authority or temperance; those about them would then rather extricate themselves from their company and seek the comfort of the shade. These arrogant Number One's are intensely egocentric, intolerant of the frailties of others, judgemental and disparaging and do not suffer fools gladly. Domestically, they are often tyrants, bullies and patriarchal chauvinists, lording it over the women in their lives. At their lowest, they are the alpha male with all his selfish, swaggering, posturing and chest-beating conceit, establishing and defending a territory. Andy Capp belongs to the netherworld of the archetype, the shadow form of the successful, driven achiever.

For all this, Number One possesses the drive and the will to achieve greatness both creatively and spiritually. Their recessive feminine nature inevitable finds some expression in their love of fantasy and theorising, which, coming to the fore, may bring pause, permitting them to ponder the purpose of life and their own inner nature. Their potential is infinite and once their goal aligns with their spiritual destiny, their purpose and mission overshadow the demands of the ego-self and they become congruent with their archetype in its highest form, achieving at onement with the Divinity within.

This description of the Number One personality profile derived from numerology and the Tarot has an authentic ring to it. In fact, speaking in Number One terms and language, it feels 'spot-on.'

However, it is homeopathic appraisal and analysis that incontrovertibly proves, not only that Pythagoras and Plato were correct in recognising the archetypal status of each primal number, but also the accuracy of this intuited description of the Number One archetype. The art and science of homeopathy gives access to the deepest and most remote regions of the unconscious. The homeopathic potency, especially when given in a dilution in excess of the 30CH, has the depth of action to reach into the realm of archetype and myth – the collective unconscious – and in a subject constitutionally sensitive to its action cause its own archetypal picture to surface in emotions, dreams and physical symptoms. The Number One picture described above is closely related to one of the most fundamental homeopathic archetypes: Sulphur; or its more sophisticated relative: Nux vomica. Being the more basic of the two, let us look more closely at Sulphur's Number One credentials

Sulphur

Hahnemann, himself was the first to define the *Number One* status of Sulphur among the other leading archetypes of the materia medica. In his Paris years, Sulphur was most often the first remedy the Master would give to stir up reaction and prepare the way. Sulphur was soon recognised as the prime archetype of the psoric triad: Sulphur – Calc-carb – Lycopodium: a sequence often followed in practice. Relating to the volcanic, pre-biotic period of planetary evolution, Sulphur is more primordial than oceanic Calc-carb and terrestrial Lycopodium.

If a patient, male or female, should present with the personality traits described above, the homeopath would immediately place Sulphur at the top of the list of likely remedies. From proving trials and over two hundred years of experience, Sulphur has been found well-suited to individuals of this emotional type. Its energy is most similar and the emotional symptoms it evokes closely match the personality described. When thus indicated, Sulphur can elicit a healing response irrespective of the nature of the patient's ailment.

The typical Sulphur individual, has no doubt that they are, indeed, *'numero uno.'* The archetype is not troubled by modesty and is convinced of its pre-eminence even in the absence of evidence (*rags are riches*). However, in archetypal terms, Sulphur's instinctive hubris is not misplaced.

In the evolution of our planet, Sulphur played a predominant role, being the element most associated with the period of intense volcanic activity that fashioned and shaped the planet. Its odour is prevalent wherever volcanic gases emit; it is abundant near hot springs; and rich deposits of the element occur in all volcanic regions. In biblical times, it was referred to as *"brimstone"* (burn stone), which in religious myth was paired with fire as the devil's preferred torture for fallen souls. The ongoing role of volcanism in shaping the grand architecture of the planet and fostering biodiversity, continues to this day. Characteristic of Number One, is the ability to recognise potential in the new, the raw, the wild, and the untilled and bring it to fruition. Number One and Sulphur are the archetypal pioneers, initiators and entrepreneurs.

Sulphur is a remedy for childhood when assimilation, nutrition, growth and elimination are disturbed; for the formative period of life, analogous to the volcanic period of planetary evolution. The volcano child, like Number One, is hyperactive, always on the move, headstrong, self-willed, unruly, inquisitive, into everything, adventurous, daring, playful, full of mischief and very difficult to control. Both archetypes are related to the new horizons and changes of direction that present at the transition points of life: puberty, adolescence, adulthood, midlife and old age.

Rune tablets

Like the Tarot, rune tablets, bearing the symbols of ancient Germanic alphabets, when used for divination purposes, exemplify images bearing esoteric meaning and linked to unseen influences. When chosen at random with sincere intent, they proffer advice intrinsic to their symbolic content, which invariably proves appropriate to the circumstances and concerns of the one seeking help; proving that nothing is truly random. The name *rune* itself, means 'secret, something hidden' and the rune letters are now regarded as a mystic text.

Colour

Colours are generally more evocative of symbolic meaning and arouse more immediate emotional response than do shapes, numbers and letters. The fiery passion and ardour of red, the cowardliness of yellow, the jealousy of the green-eyed monster, the melancholy of 'the blues,' the black-hearted villain, the pomp and nobility of purple, the virginal purity of white and the golden halo of the saint, become part of our idiomatic thinking from an early age, and most of us are drawn to certain colours and may feel an instinctive aversion to others. Colours are connected to emotion, personality and morality; they are vibrations and expressions of energy; they are powerfully archetypal. When white light passes through a prism it splits into the full spectrum of colours; hence all colours are contained and realised in white, which is symbolic of illumination and self-enlightenment. But, the colour within which all other colours are hidden and held in potential, unrealised form, is black, which is synonymous with the Void and Cosmic Darkness before the first stars brought light to the creation; its potential is infinite; it is mysterious and connected to the mystic, the enigmatic, the dark and the occult, to that which is private, secret and hidden. It is the undifferentiated force from which the colours of the chakra energy system emerge: firstly, the warm, magnetic colours with the longest wavelengths and lowest frequency – red, orange and yellow – then green, symbolising balance between warm and cool, the colour at the *heart* of the spectrum and at the *heart* of the chakras – and finally, the three cool, electric colours with the shortest wavelength and highest frequency – blue, indigo and violet. As Dr Letari and my father successfully put into practice, colours prove wonderful remedies, especially today when they can be administered in homeopathic potency and when so much more is known about their archetypal characteristics. The colour archetypes of the spectrum will be considered as independent remedies, in conjunction with associated archetypes and when studying the major chakras.

Music

Music is another archetypal energy possessing healing power; it has been used therapeutically since classical times. Hippocrates played music to his emotionally disturbed patients and Aristotle described music as a force that purified the emotions. The effect of music upon disposition and wellbeing is well known. As with colour, depending on the mood of the music and the sensibility of the audience, the response will range from euphoria to dysphoria. Being energy frequencies musical notes can be captured by exposing a carrier medium (medicinal alcohol) to the desired note for a predetermined time; the note-saturated medium can then be potentised to produce a remedy. I have no experience with these music remedies, but I am certain that once the psychological profile of a note has been determined, appropriate selection will prove rewarding. In homeopathic consultation, it is always of value to ask regarding the importance of music in a patient's life, what kind of music they prefer and how they respond to it. This knowledge, as with colour preference, can be of assistance in selecting the required remedy.

Astrological star- and sun-sign archetypes

The twelve signs of the zodiac represent twelve archetypal modes of expression. The concept originated in Babylonian astrology and was later developed further by Hellenistic tradition. In the West, astrology is founded on the movements and relative positions of celestial bodies such as the Sun, Moon and planets. These are analysed by their movements through the twelve spatial divisions of the zodiac and their geometrical aspects relative to one another. The popular, simplified, sun-sign astrology that considers only the zodiac sign of the Sun at a person's date of birth has resulted in the twelve-well-known sun-sign archetypes. These archetypes are broad-based, whereas the atavistic and mythological archetypes are more specific. There is definite overlapping. Identifying a person's sun-sign and those aspects of its profile that accord with the emotional makeup of the patient, can enable the physician to home-in on a specific atavistic or mythological archetype. For example: a person born under the sun-sign of Leo may well present with a personality matching the profile of Lac leoninum (Lion) or Aurum (gold – Apollo). These observations also apply to the twelve animal signs of Chinese astrology and the totem animal signs of the Native Americans.

Reference

1   Tressider J. *The Hutchinson Dictionary of Symbols*. London: Duncan Baird Publishers, 1997. p155.

17

THE FOUR ARCHETYPAL TEMPERAMENTS

The Greek philosopher, Empedocles (492–432 B.C.E.), claimed that there *elements historical intro* are four basic forms of perceptible matter: earth, water, fire and air. Hippocrates (460–350 B.C.E.) coupled this concept to the theory that all illness could be attributed to four bodily fluids or humours: phlegm, black bile, yellow bile and blood. Health could only be maintained if these basic humours were in perfect balance and the presence of disease indicated that one or other was in excess or deficiency. The Hippocratic School of medicine adopted this theory as its fundamental axiom. The efforts of its physicians were therefore directed to either increasing or decreasing the volume of these humours in the patient's body. Medicines, especially emetics and laxatives, diet and often bloodletting were commonly employed.

Aelius Galenus or Claudius Galenus, better known as simply Galen (c130–c200), was a physician to four successive Roman emperors and also to Roman gladiators. He inherited the Hippocratic humours from the Greek tradition and from them elaborated his theory of the four fundamental types of human temperament and constitution: the phlegmatic (phlegm/earth), the melancholic (black-bile/water), the choleric (yellow-bile/fire) and the sanguine (blood/air). These categories slot comfortably into the four chronic miasmatic states: *Psora* – phlegmatic – earth; *Sycosis* – melancholic – water; *Syphilis* – choleric – fire; *Tuberculosis* – sanguine – air). *Carcinosis* encompasses all four elements, humours and temperaments.

Galen believed that these character traits were inherent, each springing from an excess of its corresponding humour. His conclusions and use of invasive methods to relieve internal pressure, accounted for the popularity of bloodletting in Europe, one thousand five hundred years later.

Setting aside the excess or lack of humours as causative, what seems antiquated and, therefore, worthy of being discounted, proves, in the light of miasmatic theory and clinical experience, not mere fanciful speculation, but grounded on valid premises. The association of the four fundamental elements with the four temperaments, links these concepts to both the chakra energy system, with its theory of ascending consciousness, and to miasmatic emotional progression.

The designations of the four temperaments have entered common idiom and literature and are of value in highlighting a dominant trait in an individual's disposition. Though mixed temperaments are common, one or other invariably comes to the fore when the individual is under stress. Acknowledgement of the four temperaments has always been intrinsic to homeopathy and common to homeopathic parlance. The temperaments sum up, in a tidy nutshell, the overall emotional disposition of a subject. When Calc-carb and the carbonates are termed phlegmatic (psoric) and when Nat-sulph is said to be melancholic (sycotic), Nux-vom choleric (syphilitic) and Phosphorus sanguine (tubercular), a simple designation carries a wealth of content – the temperaments are archetypal! This being so, it is of value to consider and differentiate their identifying features so that they may be better compared with the major archetypes of the materia medica. In doing so, I am assisted by a thoughtful lecture entitled, *The Physiognomy of the Temperaments,* delivered in June 1961 at the British Homeopathic Congress held in London, in June 1961. The speaker was Austrian born physician, Norbert Glas (1897–1986), who fled from the Nazis in the 1930s and settled in Britain.[1]

I differ from his perspective, however, in that I associate the phlegmatic temperament with earth, not water, and the melancholic with water, not earth.

The Phlegmatic Archetype – an aspect of the Calc-carb Archetype

The well-fed and healthy baby gives a very characteristic picture of the phlegmatic temperament. It usually appears content unless it is hungry or thirsty. In the baby, one can marvel at the eagerness with which it latches on and the satisfaction it derives from suckling. The phlegmatic temperament demonstrates that the human lives very strongly in the stream of their nutrition. They enjoy this more than those of another temperament.

The physiognomy of the phlegmatic tends to roundness and fullness, due to a constitutional inclination to accumulate fat (Calc-carb, Graphites). The face has a peasant-like broadness with a wide brow, round cheeks and chin, a nose that is short and broad and eyes that are round and beady and twinkle with humour. In the older phlegmatic, the lower third of the face becomes heavy with a fullness filling the angle between the jaw and the neck, producing a double chin. Likewise, the area between the eyebrow and the upper lid often becomes full and puffy (Kali-carb) and with the slackness of age may wrinkle over the lid. The body may be plump and solid from an early age; the danger of becoming overweight is soon apparent. From plump to fat, to corpulence, to obesity, is merely a matter of time, lack of discipline, lack of exercise and overindulgence. They are lazy, lethargic and slow moving. Their gait, though heavy due to their solid build, is not the hanging heaviness of the emotionally-burdened melancholic; it is more a cumbersomeness. Food and drink sustain their mood, which is generally cheerful and happy. To Norbert Glas, Shakespeare's Sir John Falstaff is the most famous example of the phlegmatic gourmet, delighting in the indulgences of the table, the wine bottle and mirth. The phlegmatic is an earthy, jovial, jocular, good-natured kind of person (Graphites).

The temperament of the phlegmatic is as grounded and stolid as their physical deportment. They are generally introverted and insular (Calc-carb), shy, withdrawn, quiet, reserved, unemotional, complacent, passive, unruffled, relaxed and easy-going. They prefer a quiet, routine and ordered life, free of the unexpected and the stressful. Their thinking is conventional, conservative, pragmatic and practical. They like to plan well ahead and are not spontaneous or adventurous; they dislike uncertainty and change and much prefer the known, the familiar and the tried. Their circle of friends is small, but intimate, and in their friendships, they are affectionate, sincere, warm, caring, devoted and very loyal. It takes a lot for them to break off a friendship, regardless of the other person's behaviour. They would rather have others visit them than bestir themselves; but friends are warmly received; they are attentive, and their home is a haven. While sharing little of themselves, they are sincerely interested in others' feelings and lives, are empathetic and caring, and build up intimate and enduring relationships, which they are at pains to preserve. They are always willing to compromise to preserve harmony.

Despite their warm, affectionate, sentimental nature, their feelings rarely surface, they keep them hidden. Behind a façade of stoic, carefree indifference, lie repressed, unresolved emotions. They can nurse a grievance and are passively aggressive, which they express by non-compliance or going slow. Confrontation is distressing to them. To avoid conflict they remain non-committal, do not take sides, compromise, and go along with the majority. They are not proactive and are reluctant to make a decision, especially when to do so will get them involved; they delay and procrastinate until reaction is forced upon them by a crisis (Graphites). Though reluctant to get drawn in and involved, once committed, they are deliberate, determined and persevering.

Known as '*the watcher*', they are observers rather than doers; listeners rather than talkers. They know the right questions to ask and are attentive to the answers. People confide in them and find them interested, empathetic and able to give good advice. They can evaluate situations objectively, in an unprejudiced way, and mediate between those who are at odds (Graphites, Mag-carb). People regard them as unhurried, calm, composed, cool-headed, steady, dependable, sympathetic and kind. Hidden from others is their reluctance, hesitancy, indecisiveness and fear of commitment.

Routine, structure, systems and protocol suit their ordered, undeviating, phlegmatic temperament and they excel at gathering, classifying, analysing and evaluating facts. But, they also have an eye for the bigger picture. The young are slow to learn, but once they have learned, retention is excellent and they can successfully apply what they have learned.

They are introspective and contemplative by nature and strive for greater self-knowledge. Many are religious by nature, very conservative, strictly observant and unquestioning of their faith. Their charitableness, selflessness, compassion and rectitude may be marred by self-righteousness. Their laziness, aversion to exercise and inactive, sedentary life may induce a sluggish torpor that can bring on depression.

In this picture, the carbonate archetypes are clearly discerned, particularly Graphites, Calc-carb Kali-carb, Nat-carb and Mag-carb.

The Melancholic Archetype – an aspect of the Aurum Archetype

The eyes are the windows of the melancholic soul. The melancholic, submerged in grief is indifferent to surroundings and the disinterest manifests in lowered eyelids, denoting limited and withdrawn focus. They are too lazy and lacklustre to lift their lids and extend their range of vision to embrace that which is now no longer of consequence. Consciousness turned inwards, removes brilliancy from the eyes, which take on a certain dullness, like one weary from mental fatigue at the end of an exhausting day. It is as if the individuality of the melancholic is less embodied. This, over years, devitalises and modifies the physical vehicle. The bones of the face seem unusually delicate as if depleted of mass. The limbs in contrast are heavy, especially the feet, which affects the gait and takes the spring out of the step, which is flat and shuffling, the soles scarcely lifting from the ground. The features are elongated, very much like those of Isaac Newton. The brow is deeply furrowed above the root of the nose and the eye brows are drawn up at their inner ends as if in anguish or pain. The nose is long, thin and angular. The nostrils narrow and more oval than round. The tip of the nose points down, as if weighted by gravity. This is exaggerated by the sagging stance of the introverted, self-occupied melancholic: shoulders stooped, head declined. Above all, the mouth reflects the misery of the melancholic state. The lips are thinned, the upper more than the lower and the compressed line of the mouth curves downwards at the corners, as if, never to be lifted again in a smile. Frédéric Chopin was Norbert Glas' example of the melancholic, and, to illustrate the typical features of the temperament, he provided a little-known portrait of the composer by a fellow Polish painter. In commenting on this very sad depiction of the great man, Glas wrote:

> The sadness of the eyes, the mouth, the bending of the head to the side – something very characteristic for many melancholics – the narrowed chest and the beautiful hands with the long fingers – all this can be considered as a sign of the pains with which the soul is affected by life. How much, too, do we feel the sorrow in Chopin's music! The climax of that heaviness is achieved in the wonderful Funeral March of his famous Sonata op. 35 in B flat minor.[1]

The melancholic is more introverted than the phlegmatic. They are very insular, private and reserved, keeping their thoughts and feelings to themselves. They are secretive and hold their cards close to their chest. They value time alone in their own space, dread crowds and social happenings, which they find trying and exhausting. They are not comfortable with 'small talk'.

Of an introspective nature, they are deep-thinkers and take life too seriously and suffer accordingly. The melancholic is known as '*the thinker*' and their thinking pains them. This accounts for their agonised eyebrows and furrowed brow. Being a water-temperament, they are highly emotional, very sensitive to what people think of them and how others will judge their work or what they have created. This leaves them very vulnerable to hurt.

They contemplate life and find it imperfect, unpredictable, out of control and hostile. They conclude that life cannot be trusted, and neither can people. To counter this, they take control, strive for perfection and close off their emotional world. They set unrealistically high standards for themselves and others. This can only result in disappointment, which mortifies them. They are self-deprecating, uncompromisingly critical of themselves and feel they have failed. They impose the same exacting demands on others and are harshly critical of their performance.

In keeping with their need to be perfect in a perfect environment, they may be meticulous, ordered and fastidious in every detail of their lives, or, their perfectionism may be expressed eccentrically. It may be idealism, a fantasy of perfection, never realised, always doomed to bring disappointment and disillusionment. Due to their sense of personal imperfection, they easily blame themselves for anything that goes wrong; similarly, they easily take on guilt.

Mistrusting life, they constantly worry about the future and the impact their decisions will have. This makes them exceedingly cautious and considered in weighing up their options. They do not look to others to help them decide; they are independent, self-reliant, purposeful, very focused and involved. As if life was a game of chess, they deliberate long and hard before making a move. To this end, they ask endless, exacting questions. Aiming for the perfect outcome, they need to know all the answers. They are never willing to take a risk and possibly make the wrong choice and be found incompetent. This 'anal attitude' leads to many arguments with those who are wanting to get a move on, but the melancholic cannot compromise with any issue. This is not a 'choleric' need to 'call the shots' or to be a dominant 'alpha'; it is about a logical approach, well thought out and promising the best result. It is about the issue in question, not about precedence or personality.

The mind of the melancholic is rational, logical and analytical and demands to know. They are too analytical, agonising over every detail, thus, impeding or halting forward-progress – 'paralysis through analysis!' They cannot be spontaneous and are never rash or impulsive. Being unable to plan in advance, is sure to put them into a panic. Once they have come to a conclusion and determined their course of action, nothing will sway them. They stubbornly and tenaciously follow their chosen path. To diverge, would be to question its perfection and doubt their judgement.

They gloss over, and forget, the good and positive things and home in on that which is negative. With any happening, they always assume the worst. The role of 'devil's advocate' is easy for them, since taking the critical, negative position is what they always do. Their inherent pessimism, stemming from their perception that life is intrinsically flawed, makes them cynical, sceptical, and paranoid. It is easier for them to dislike and reject someone, or something, than to love and embrace them. In dealing with people, they are very wary and suspicious. They expect concealed agendas and look for hidden meaning behind words, gestures and behaviour. They weigh people up very carefully before putting trust in them.

They choose their partner, friends, preferences and interests with their usual caution and care, but once committed, they hold them close and are attentive and loyal; never neglectful or remiss. To be the chosen friend of a melancholic is an honour; their friendship is not lightly given; the recipient has a friend for life. Fleeting fancies, fickleness and flavours of the month are sanguine traits, not melancholic.

Their fine-tuned, intense, nervous sensibility is also aesthetic, empathetic, intuitive and psychic. The hidden turbulence of their feelings and emotions may be sublimated through the creative and performing arts. What they avoid divulging or displaying in their personal lives, they express through literature, poetry, music, dance or drama. Often, they are unusually gifted, but their success and the acclaim they receive does not allay their innate self-effacing modesty. They have difficulty accepting compliments and will often deflect or deflate these by making some self-critical, derogatory observation. Their deeply caring nature and ability to read other people and pick up on their feelings, suits them for the caring and teaching professions.

Unfortunately, these varied traits exist against a background of melancholia that may haunt them throughout their lives. Their response to stress is more likely to be tears, anguish and despair than irritability or anger. They are very sensitive to hurt, misconstrue others' intentions and take offence easily, which can bring on depression.

The Choleric Archetype – an aspect of the Ferrum Archetype

El remedy

Roundness of cheek and twinkle of eye denote the phlegmatic; dullness of eye and down-turned mouth denote the melancholic, but it is the jutting jaw and steely gaze that announce the choleric. The jaw is commanding, its rectangular lines accentuated, prominent and often cleft. This bold, masculine statement is augmented by widely-flared nostrils, like those of an enraged stallion or fire-breathing dragon, and brilliant, riveting eyes, blue, grey or black, dart fire from beneath beetling brows when roused to anger. The body follows suit with muscular neck, broad shoulders, deep chest and powerful legs. Athleticism lost with age, the powerful physique thickens to corpulence, but the flashing eyes and craggy jaw lose nothing of their truculence. Though short of a dashing uniform and the trappings of war, here stands the warrior Ferrum, facing life and daring it to do its damndest.

The description may seem excessive, but the flamboyantly extrovert nature of the fiery, choleric invites hyperbole. His carriage is erect, and he propels himself forward with bold, purposeful strides, each step striking the ground fully on the heel. His is a heated temperament: fired by passion, ardour and a testy temperament. Leaders of armies, directors of companies and conductors of orchestras need to be choleric to marshal their forces. Whereas, the melancholic is partially disembodied, the choleric is fully and intensely embodied. Whereas, the will of the melancholic is caught in the dragging currents of turbulent emotions, the will of the choleric spirals in the heat and surge of the blood and the rapid-fire spontaneity of the amygdala and reptilian brain that clenches the fist, stamps the floor and bangs the door. But, just as the waters of grief can be sublimated, so can the fire of temper.

The choleric has the capacity to become fully aware of themselves as a human being and to express this intensely in their vocation. Just as he compares Chopin with the melancholic, so Norbert Glas compares the choleric with Beethoven. The tempestuous maestro evidenced to the full, how fire can be expressed positively and creatively. All the many paintings of Beethoven portray the strength and power of the choleric temperament: the fierce determined set of his features, the resolute mouth and incised chin, flared nostrils, beetling brow and the magnificent breadth and depth of his forehead. His body was sturdily built. When depicted walking, his hands are clasped behind his back, elbows jutting out to the sides and his body inclined forward, as if his head would lead his feet. It is recorded that 'he would go through a meadow or a wood like a storm, not looking to the left or the right – listening only to the inner music which sounded within him'.[2]

The converse of this sublimation is possible; the fire of the choleric can be degraded and put to ill-use, even gross wickedness. Many of the worst criminals of the world are of the choleric temperament.

The choleric is a strong-willed, forceful and assertively extrovert. Their energy is essentially masculine, regardless of their gender. At an early age, they display their innate alpha standing in the hierarchy of life, initiating games, taking charge and dominating other children. The bully of the playground is invariably a choleric, but so too are those who protect and defend the bully's victims. Their self-confidence, self-reliance and independent nature soon become evident. They can look after themselves and take responsibility; they show initiative and enterprise. Cholerics have an abundance of energy and drive; they can excel academically and shine in sport. Leadership comes naturally to them. They are good competitors, but very poor losers. Getting beaten, brings out the very worst in them.

Later in life these qualities can take them to the top, whatever their work or profession. They are ambitious and competitive and work towards being the best and attaining the top position. Though circumstances may prevent this, nonetheless, in all their dealings with people, they want to be dominant: the top dog, the one in charge and the one who makes decisions, for themselves and others. They are very confident and self-sufficient. Independence is an essential part of being a choleric, since, to be dependant is to be diminished to a beta standing. They are bold, courageous and, at times, audacious, thriving on intensity and high drama, especially in the pursuit of prestige and material success.

They are a mine of ideas, plans and objectives, which are not 'pie-in-the-sky', fanciful speculation, but practical and achievable. The choleric is the typical A-type personality: the *'doer'* or *'driver'*, orientated towards goals and successful outcomes. They need to be in control, exert authority and make snap decisions. They are often gifted, high-powered businessmen: highly-intelligent and with exceptional organisational and leadership skills. Their intellectual orientation is dominantly left-cerebral: analytical, logical and pragmatic. On the negative side, they are driven and dictatorial, impatient, intolerant, quick-tempered, unsympathetic and uncompromising. Even though they may thrive on challenges and opposition, incrementally, the pressure mounts and exacts its toll. They are tense and stressed. Although, at their peak, their energy seems limitless and they can function on minimum sleep, insomnia may become a problem and burn-out a constant threat. Alcohol relaxes them, but there is always the danger of abuse. It increases their irascibility, impatience, intolerance and outbursts of temper.

Being anti-authority and anti-establishment, they will enthusiastically fight with militant zeal for a cause, not out of compassion or empathy for the downtrodden – since, they are largely insensitive to the feelings of others – but for the opportunity to assert their own authority and challenge the alpha dominance of the regime. This false-altruism is so bound to their own deep need for alpha status that it can become fanatical.

Full of their own importance and self-esteem, they are arrogant, forceful, overbearing and unpleasantly condescending to those they deem inferior. People they are not on good terms with have usually in some way challenged or scorned them, or their alpha energy offends and threatens them. They take great pleasure and satisfaction from hearing of any discomfiture, humiliation or misfortune such a person may suffer.

They are controlling and assertive and see challenge, competition, contention and conflict as the normal dynamics of human interaction. They rise to any challenge, welcoming it as an opportunity to prove themselves, to show that they are tough, strong and courageous, even ruthless. Where the melancholic hides and represses grief; the choleric hides and represses fear.

Their thinking is sharp, quick and decisive. Always in a hurry, they are impatient and intolerant of delay and want people to jump at their command. Things must happen at the snap of their fingers. They demand efficiency and competence and are highly irritated by incompetence. Short-tempered and irascible, they are easily moved to anger, which can be explosive, even violent.

With friends, who pose no alpha threat, they form strong bonds. They are loyal and supportive and as a matter of honour will put themselves on the line in defence of those they deem 'blood-brothers'. The ties are often forged in military service or in sport. However, betrayal of such a friendship is never forgiven or forgotten.

Though ever eager to give advice and pressurise others into doing things their way, they resent being given advice. That someone should have the temerity to do so, affronts them and is perceived as presumptuous and intrusive. It is an old adage that what we dislike most in others is what we harbour within ourselves. The choleric's extrovert nature leads them to be intrusive and to meddle in others' affairs. Minding one's own business is not a choleric trait.

They take pride in their brand of honesty: telling the blunt truth regardless of sensibilities and social niceties. In speaking their mind, they are spontaneous and impulsive and may 'put their foot in their mouth'. To prove they are above decorum and to give emphasis to their words, they will lace their language with superlatives and expletives. When challenged, they assert their authority by drawing themselves up tall, inflating their chest, raising the pitch of their voice and fixing their adversary with a withering glare. Their easy access to adrenaline and cortisol comes to their aid, heightening their colour and causing fire to dart from their eyes. Primordial forces are brought to bear, designed to intimidate the foe and restore order – and the dominance of the choleric!

When obstacles bar the choleric's way, like Beethoven storming through the woods, they single-mindedly plough their way through to their determined goal.

Being hierarchical animals, they are defiant of authority and rebel against convention, which they unconsciously experience as the imposition of another's alpha will. Their boastful, self-opinionated attitude often gets them into arguments. They always have to be right; always have to have the last word. They are convinced that they are right and stubbornly resistant to evidence that they are wrong. Differences of opinion become heated and acrimonious. They need to gain the upper hand; others must submit or defer to them. They demand respect and bear a grudge against those who belittle them or trifle with them. Unfortunately, these hierarchical dynamics are carried over into their family life; they are arch-chauvinists and often misogynistic.

The Sanguine Archetype – an aspect of the Phosphorus Archetype

The element associated with the sanguine temperament is air, which by its very nature gives an impression of lightness and expansiveness – un-restrained, free and ungrounded – unfettered by consensus, convention and tradition. In terms of thought, air relates to the unbounded sphere of fancy, imagination and inspiration. The associated chakra is the 4th or heart chakra (Anahata) – known also as the love chakra; the associated colour is green and the associated miasm is *Tuberculosis*.

The phlegmatic and the melancholic temperaments may be termed passive or introverted emotional archetypes. They both give an impression of indolence, of not being fully participatory in the life experience. The phlegmatic temperament: earthbound, overcome by physical substance, like the oyster, tethered to a rock, sessile, waiting for life to come to it; reactive, not proactive – fearful and insular – wearing a shell to ensure survival. The melancholic temperament: water-bound; at the mercy of the counter-currents of duality: the attraction and repulsion of opposites, the push and pull of good and evil and the turbulence at the divide between the conscious and the unconscious, where Id and ego/superego contend over the expression or repression of emotions. Both temperaments are inad-equately and incompletely engaged in the 'Now.'

With the advent of the choleric, psychic energy swings into activity and is extraverted, but in primitive, hierarchical mode. The sanguine tempera-ment enhances the degree of activity and the degree of extraversion in a refined and creative way.

The sanguine person moves with alacrity and grace. Their eyes are lively and observant, taking in their surroundings with interest and curiosity, passing from one object to another. They are sparkling and luminous, and, as they gaze this way and that, their radiance is enhanced, like precious jewels capturing the brilliance of light from their many facets. It is, as if the eyes of the sanguine reach out to embrace their world and converse with it, lingering here, tarrying there, savouring all the colours, textures and shapes within their orbit. Consequently, the lids are open wide, and the eyes appear large and luminous. Just as the compelling eyes are ever-animated, so too, the face of the sanguine is seldom in repose, constantly changing expression in accord with their vibrant sensibilities. In comparison, when the melancholic is listening to someone, the face remains heavy and impassive, unless some tender chord is touched that may move them to tears. When their interest is captured, the sanguine is fully tuned in to the one speaking and their mind is already framing a question, comment or answer. Like a gundog on the alert, they are poised to speak, their lips vibrating slightly in their eagerness to spill the yet unspoken words that tremble on the cusp. Though the sanguine may become impatient and restless if they are at odds with what is being said, when the speaker has their full sympathy, they are a rapt audience, with a quick and ready understanding.

Air is the element associated with the sanguine temperament. This links the archetype to rhythm: the rhythm of breathing, and, on a deeper level, the rhythm of the heart, the circulation and the blood, conveying 'air' to every cell of the body. The rhythm of the breathing and the rhythm of the heart are intimately related to the prevailing emotions and feelings within the psyche: the tides of the soul/ego-self complex. This is the sphere of the sanguine, thus, the critical component of this temperament's physiognomy is the nose and the contour of the cheeks that frame it.

There are two types of nose that characterise the sanguine temperament.

The first, is a comparatively short nose that is tilted upwards – the upturned nose, described in French as: *les nez retroussé*. If we accept what Leonardo da Vinci postulated: that the soul fashions the features from within like a goldsmith embossing his material, then the unique delineation of a face gives insight into the inclinations and aptitudes of the one wearing it. This must be particularly true of the nose: the portal of our breathing, a function intimately related to our emotional life, and the seat of olfaction, the primal faculty essential for survival and emotional memory. Persons with a *retroussé* nose generally have a quicker, but more shallow breathing rhythm. In esoteric terms, the nose breaths in the life experience for inner reflection and breathes out the ego/soul-response. This leads one to conclude that such a sanguine individual can communicate easily with the holding environment, but the inner reflection on what they have taken in is shorter or more superficial, and the response rather more spontaneous and impulsive than considered. 'They can be people, who are quick in their reply, quick in their appraisal of the world, but quick also in their feelings, which may change from one moment to the other.'[1] They tend to be shallow and capricious!

The other characteristic nose, equally as common as the first, is a large nose, reminiscent of the melancholic, but without the heaviness and downward droop and more finely modelled or sculpted. The wearer of this kind of nose takes deeper and longer breaths, which provides more air-content in the lungs. 'The quality of their feelings is more deeply involved with the whole personality.'[3] They have an inclination for considered reflection, gravitas and measured response. If the larger nose of the sanguine is also aquiline, it indicates a capacity for great fortitude.

Musing once more on the physiognomy of great musicians, Glas proposes that such artists, being intensely immersed in rhythm and the soul's stream of feeling – singularly sanguine spheres – should have the 'most extravagant kind of noses' and that it would be interesting to 'show a collection of the noses of great musicians'. Glas recommends for study, the noses of Tartani, Purcell, Verdi, Wagner and Mahler. But, for his outstanding example, he chooses Mozart, who in his life, personality and genius exhibited all the qualities of the sanguine temperament to the highest degree, and also, in 'the overwhelming form of his nose, which can be traced back to boyhood.'[3]

Feeling, breathing, circulation and rhythm are ever-entwined: in life, a ceaseless unison of vibration. Music as an art form is similar: in constant flow and movement, like the air and the lungs and the heart and the blood; never still, always changing, unbroken undulations of rhythm and vibration from commencement to conclusion. Through understanding the mystery of the sanguine temperament, we can perceive the therapeutic power of music.

The sanguine-type lives strongly in the rhythm of the breath and this has a modelling effect on the features, especially the upper part of the cheeks extending outwards from the nose: a certain fullness of the upper-cheeks, giving an elfin-like high-cheekbone contour to the face, setting off to perfection their large, expressive eyes. Anyone gifted with a special warm and engaging smile, will, if only for a moment, capture at least some of this physiognomic magic. A magic that Norbert Glas recognises in Leonardo da Vinci's paintings of Saint Ann, Leda and John the Baptist – 'it gives the face the expression of lightness, something of the invisible wings of the soul.'

The profoundly phlegmatic has a ponderous, earthbound gait; the miserable melancholic a resigned and desultory shuffle; the forceful choleric a bold, military stride. In contrast, the exhilarated, buoyant sanguine has an elevated step: a light manner of walking, an ease of movement, the very surface beneath them seeming to waft them forward – a floating, weightlessness, as if skating. Their weight is carried mainly on the forefoot, and sometimes, particularly when eager and excited, on the toes. This is wonderfully exhibited by children and young people, particularly when their spirits are high. If forefoot-walking is exaggerated in adults, it reflects unfavourably on the underlying personality, hinting at an overstated sanguine state: a vivacious superficiality, combined with vanity and conceit.

Being archetypes, the temperaments are morphic fields, which have general as well as individual influence. When one of the archetypal temperaments becomes markedly prevalent as a personality theme in society, it can influence the fashion or trends of the time and direct the cultural development of the period. Typically, this influence occurs in waves, sometimes flowing and dominant, sometimes ebbing and recessive. The Sanguine stiletto-heel and the Choleric padded-shoulders are prime examples of this phenomenon.

The Sanguine is an extroverted, active, energetic, fun-loving, gregarious, talkative, vivacious optimist.

They are sociable, friendly, outgoing and enjoy company. It is easy for them to start up a conversation and establish a new friendship; they are open and engaging; make eye contact, smile readily, talk freely and easily; and are at ease with physical contact, openly showing affection and empathy by a hug, a touch of the hand, an arm around the shoulders. They are not prejudiced or complexed about social standing, education, race or religion and can mix comfortably with a wide range of people, adapting and accommodating as need arises. Parties and get-togethers are their delight; the more people, the better; they are pleasure-seekers, always in the mood for fun and a goodtime. They love to circulate, like a butterfly going from flower to flower; they enjoy seeing and being seen. Everyone is their friend and because they do most of the talking and little listening, all they may ever know about the other person is their face and name. The Sanguine is familiarly known as 'the talker.' This said, they do have an ear for juicy gossip and if you want the world to know your affairs, tell them to a Sanguine. By nature, they are lively, effervescent and charismatic and attract a deal of attention, enjoying centre-stage, showing off and being the life of the party. They are their own best audience. The young Sanguine while having an emotional melt-down or temper tantrum will have one bright eye on the mirror, fascinated by their own performance. In like manner, the grown-up Sanguine will employ melodramatic histrionics to capture the attention and sympathy of their audience. They are adept at playing the 'drama queen'.

They thrive on compliments and flattery and being popular. Their lively sense of humour, sparkle, enthusiasm and light-hearted cheerfulness are contagious and add to everyone's fun. They are sure to be invited back. They invariably arrive late. Unreliability and lack of punctuality are serious shortcomings, and these are compounded by the amount of time taken in making sure they look their very best and their desire to make a grand entrance. Their dress may be trendy, eccentric or revealing; all the better to shock, create a stir or attract compliments.

There is a certain child-like quality to their personality; they appear much younger than they are, and retain a refreshing, often cultivated, naiveté well into later life. This is part of their charm. Even their conceit, vanity and self-indulgence are captivating and easily forgiven, being part of such an irresistible package. They are very much in the moment, but not on a deep level – not in the real 'Now'. Just as they seem to skim over the ground, so they skim over life, keeping it shallow and superficial, avoiding the rocks and hard places, or making light of them. They are spontaneous and very impulsive and will often leap before they look. Always with an eye for good looks and charm, they are easily infatuated and soon imagine themselves in love. They are sensual, passionate and uninhibited, but fickle by nature and soon become bored: always the butterfly in search of nectar. Escapism is a pervasive influence. In the blur of activity, distraction, entertainment, bright lights, chatter and revelry, they do not have to focus on serious and upsetting matters. In relationships and friendships, the same holds true. They avoid deep issues and grave matters, and, thus, escape hurt and involvement. Nursing grudges and grievances is foreign to them; they are far more likely to forgive or forget – and they naively expect others to do the same. Likewise, their own behaviour, wild, wanton and reckless as it may be, does not burden them with remorse or guilt.

Though they seldom pause long enough to hear another person's story, when misfortune strikes someone close to them, they are very empathetic and in their intensely-emotional way give help and support, but the frenetic nature of their life soon distracts them and draws them away to matters less distressing. Out of sight, out of mind, is a Sanguine truism.

They love the good things in life; money is like sand between their fingers, spent on luxury and pleasure. Fine possessions add to their glitter and their glamour. Money enables them to keep their carousel spinning fast, so that life will always be in soft focus. Due to their hectic, non-stop lifestyle they tend to be very disorganised; surrounded by disorder in which only they could possibly know where anything is.

Their fickle, superficial, butterfly nature that never comes to rest, can, however, be caught in an aesthetic net and brought to intense focus. They are very creative and artistic, gifts that can be expressed in many different ways: the arts, poetry, literature, drama, music, dance, fashion, cuisine, photography, etc. They are imaginative, talented, innovative and adventurous and often Bohemian and avant-garde. They bring to their chosen artistic expression, energy, enthusiasm, passion and unique flare, and yet, still have time and energy to enjoy the social whirl their much-admired work invites.

Boredom is their anathema; they have little tolerance for the mundane and routine and boring company soon drives them away. They are high-energy, emotionally-charged people, who must be always on the go; entertaining and being entertained. Despite the intensity and drama of their emotions, they are generally superficial and ephemeral.

The greatest risk for the Sanguine is that their need for escapism may result in alcohol and substance abuse, addiction to gambling, or the craving for the adrenaline high of dangerous pursuits.

These sketches of the four archetypal temperaments give valuable insights into the nature of the four atavistic archetypes that best exemplify their profiles: Calc-carb – the phlegmatic; Aurum – the melancholic; Ferrum – the choleric; and Phosphorus – the sanguine.

References

1 Glas N. The Physiognomy of the Temperaments. *British Homoeopathic Journal* 1961. 50(4). p258.
2 *Ibid.*, p176.
3 *Ibid.*, pp185–187.

18

EVOLVING THE HOMEOPATHIC ARCHETYPE

Proving sensitivity

When a substance undergoes a proving (pathogenetic trial), the comprehensiveness of the remedy picture will vary according to the quality of the proving, the efficiency of the collating protocols, the number of trialists and the age and gender differences within the trial group. But, most critical of all is the number of provers that are highly sensitive to the substance. The more hierarchically fundamental the trial substance is (e.g. *Sulphur, Calc-carb, Lycopodium*), the more sensitives there will be in any given group and the wider the range of symptoms will be.

Since all constitutions are complex and multi-layered, it is possible for a prover to respond, with varying degree of sensitivity to a wide range of potentised substances. With most, sensitivity will be insufficient to produce a florid picture of the remedy. However, a small percentage of trialists and patients prove markedly sensitive to a wide range of substances. They are a boon to proving programmes and a bane to treatment regimes. Fortunately, most of these hyper-sensitives have relatively strong constitutions, possessing a vital force that is always on its toes and quick to react to dynamic stimuli. This type of constitution must be differentiated from one that reacts to a wide variety of material things e.g. chemicals, allergens, foods, etc., denoting morbid susceptibility and weakness of the vital force.

The novice homeopath can take comfort from the knowledge that the average trialist is able to respond to a variety of substances in potentised form – a truth well documented in the early days of homeopathy, when Hahnemann's small group of provers were personally involved in many different trials. What is true of trialists is also true of patients. Each patient has a range of sensitivity, enabling them to respond to a range of different substances lying within their sensitivity band.

The task of selecting the similar remedy from homeopathy's extensive materia medica can be very daunting for the young in experience, especially for those who have been taught that a mythical *exact* simillimum selected for an equally mythical *totality* of symptoms is essential to bring about cure. Fortunately, the varied sensitivity of most patients provides welcome latitude. Providing the physician prescribes as similarly as possible on the basis of the recorded symptoms, a reaction will be initiated, bringing further symptoms to the surface, possibly in the form of significant dreams. The initial remedy, even when not striking the bull's eye, metaphorically shakes the constitutional apple tree, causing apples to fall. These may be confidently added to the patient's picture to provide the next prescribing template.

The complexity of the human psyche presents a labyrinth that has more than one entry point.

Evolving the homeopathic archetypal image

A successful proving produces a spectrum of emotional, intellectual and physical symptoms, which through careful analysis can be confidently ascribed to the specific action of the particular substance. These provide an initial archetypal profile. The emotional content is of first importance, particularly uncharacteristic moods and feelings; *fears*; *dreams*; a changed sense of reality, comprising altered outlook, prejudices and preferences; and peculiar *fancies and imaginings* regarding environment, circumstances, things, people and themselves. These fancies are referred to as *delusions*. The more out of character, out of context and out of proportion symptoms are, the more significant they are in building up the profile of the archetype.

All substances must be considered archetypal. Through potentisation and serial dilution, the unique archetypal energy of the substance is progressively released into the carrier medium, captured, and preserved.

Proving dynamic

When a homeopathic potency is administered to a sensitive prover, the frequency pattern of the archetype permeates the constitution of the prover and becomes a centrally based influence upon the vital force, extending via the personal into the collective unconscious. Here, a reciprocal response is elicited, and the archetype energised by the specific frequency of the potency rises from the deep unconscious to assert its presence in the mental, emotional and physical spheres. The response is from within outwards and from the centre to the periphery. For the period of the trial, the prover is in the grip of the aroused archetype, to a degree consonant with their sensitivity to its influence.

Healing dynamic

In the patient, the process is identical, but here, the selection of the potentised substance is based on the closest similarity possible and its effect is strategically monitored and sustained. The centrifugal dynamic of the energised archetype releases contained energy of repressed emotions, unresolved issues, forgotten suffering, rejected and unrealised aspects of the self that are responsible for the archetypal similarity and sensitivity to the potency. The mobilised, previously repressed energy moves outwards, weakening and progressively erasing its own morbid external image.

It is the reaction of the vital force that produces the emotional and physical symptoms of the proving and it is the reaction of the vital force that facilitates healing. Proving phenomena and healing phenomena are due to one and the same process. Hahnemann's injunction to participate in provings because of their beneficial effect is so valid.

Most provings are not conducted with a view to healing, therefore the curative process of the proving is only partial, but the successful production of symptoms, due to resonance with the proving substance, indicates susceptibility to its healing influence, and if marked, further formalised treatment with the substance should be pursued.

From the earliest pathogenetic trials conducted by Hahnemann and his colleagues, the variability in provers' sensitivity to a given substance was noted.

> Amongst any group of provers there would be those who produced either no symptoms at all, or few of any value; those who showed a definite sensitivity and experienced significant symptoms; and a small number, often a single person, who evidenced exceptional susceptibility to the remedy's influence, yielding an entire spectrum of symptoms, many of them 'strange, rare and peculiar'. Likewise, in treating cases with a particular remedy, it became apparent that, as with provers, a certain type of patient or constitution proved to be particularly vulnerable to the healing power of the specific remedy. The exceptional prover and the successfully treated patient often showed common, shared characteristics of build, complexion, features, demeanour, character, beliefs, mannerisms, habits and behaviour, which added together produced a remedy and patient profile that became recognisable – *a homeopathic archetype*.[1]

The remedy portrait gathered from accumulated experience, fleshes out the framework created by provings and cured cases, creating an archetypal presence. The skill of intuiting a patient's remedy by recognising the key features of the archetype they resemble, is born of long experience. It gives the physician a 'gut-feel' about a case. Often, the attendant symptomatic picture simply provides confirmation of the patient's constitutional remedy.

Fundamental homeopathic archetypes

Three of the most fundamental remedies of the materia medica are *Sulphur, Calc-carb* and *Lycopodium*. Each possesses a strongly developed archetypal profile, reflected in their external appearance, their physical features, their behaviour, their emotions and their self-image.

Sulphur

Sulphur, a substance associated with volcanic activity has a fiery, explosive temperament, puffed with self-conceit and confidence, loud-mouthed, full of ideas, theories and advice for others, blissfully unaware of their own shortcomings. Sulphur is an archetype redolent with masculine character-istics. Lazy by nature, he is often a couch potato, or an armchair philoso-pher, large on opinion and small on effort. However, their ability for speculative thought may give rise to innovation and invention. *Sulphur* has a masculine energy, whether male or female, which is bold, brash, bom-bastic, belligerent and in keeping with the B's that so aptly describe him, he is a pushy, overbearing bully. Hot, like a volcano, he is a sweaty indi-vidual with a ruddy, flushed complexion; red, fleshy lips and ears, unruly hair, a generally unkempt, dishevelled appearance and could not care less what others think of him. In build, he is either thin or heavily built. The thin type is sallow complexioned with red cheeks; bony and stooped with a round-shouldered, sway-backed posture and a penchant for slouching, leaning and reclining, rather than standing. The robust type is ruddy, muscular and corpulent though firmly fleshed, and loves the high-life and good food. Both types may have a craving for alcohol.

Calc-carb

Calc-carb, is impure calcium carbonate derived from the middle layer of the oyster shell and shares the archetypal profile of this shell-bound, rock-anchored mollusc, indicating a nature as introvert as Sulphur is extravert. It is feminine in its presentation. The need for a protective shell reveals a fearful, apprehensive disposition that considers life hostile and views it with trepidation. They are shy, self-conscious, timid, easily embarrassed, and, unlike Sulphur, are not venturesome, fearing anything new, different and unfamiliar. Their fears are legion: heights, claustrophobia, dogs, insects (especially spiders), infections and cancer; and they suffer from social phobia, fear speaking in public and dread ridicule. The shell is built slowly, in layers, over years, a process that requires patience, dedication, stubborn perseverance and an ordered, structured approach, all of which are characteristics of this water-dwelling archetype. Fire: Sulphur, is volatile, aggressive and masculine. Water: Calc-carb, is deeply emotional, internally turbulent, yielding and feminine. Open the shell: the creature inside is soft, pale, cold, clammy and terribly vulnerable. From an early age, the Calc-carb archetype is inclined to gain weight easily even to the point of obesity, their flesh is soft and flabby, their muscles lack tone and their ligaments are lax, disposing them to sprains and strains. Their handshake is limp, their hands cold and clammy. They have a pallid complexion, but the least exertion, particularly ascending, leaves them breathless, flushed and exhausted.

Lycopodium

Lycopodium is prepared from the yellow spores of a creeping plant, the common club moss, *Lycopodium clavatum,* which is descended from the Lycopsids: tall, tree-like ancestors that flourished some 350 million years ago and towered dominantly over their peers. This decline in size and stature has left the Lycopodium archetype with an inferiority complex, a sense of inadequacy and lack of self-esteem, which is paradoxically often in conflict with a high degree of ability and competence. Unlike Calc-carb, their remedy for this weakness and vulnerability is not a shell, but an over-compensating drive to excel and achieve success, wealth and influence. They hide their sense of inferiority, inadequacy and insecurity behind a veneer of confidence, bravado, arrogance, hardness and irritable-intolerance. Their focused dedication towards reinstating their stature and status, makes them selfish, egotistical, aggressive, ruthlessly competitive, dictatorial and highly sensitive to criticism, contradiction and comparison. The yellow spore has a hard capsule and a soft oily centre, which emulates the profile of the archetype: externally hard and tough; internally soft and vulnerable; and an oily ability to obsequiously flatter and butter-up those in a position to help them up the ladder to success. The energy displayed is unadulteratedly masculine; so much so that most symptoms are right-sided. They are sallow-complexioned, often prematurely bald and grey, wear a perpetual frown, startle easily and are full of male mannerisms, affectations and vanities designed to make them look confident, nonchalant and in control. When nervous and intimidated, they may whistle tunelessly to themselves. While their upper bodies are thin and underdeveloped, from the waist down they tend to present a fuller figure, with well-developed buttocks, thighs and calves.

Archetypal profiling

These brief sketches of three very prominent archetypes often met in society and often seen in practice, show how good profiling can provide easy access to the constitutional type. They reveal how imaginative and intuitive appraisal of the source and substance of a remedy, be it the volcano, the oyster or the spore of the club moss, can provide invaluable information about the archetype, even without recourse to provings. The universe has been 'proving' substances for millions of years and their archetypal profiles are symbolically realised in the wonders of the Creation. Knowing that the loving, caring Cosmic Intelligence is responsible for the phenomena of the physical universe and that survival of the fittest and natural selection are not merely the result of random mutations in genetic material, but the result of Divine Intent, we are entitled to view all manifestations of this higher purpose in anthropomorphic and archetypal terms.

It is evident that the remedy picture that emerges from provings alone is just a starting point. To this we must add the generic picture of the sensitive, constitutional type and also the characteristics that can be intuited from a thorough knowledge of the source material e.g. the volcanic associations of Sulphur and its role in human physiology; the natural history, morphology and habits of the oyster; the ancestral history of the club moss and the properties of its spores. To do this effectively, requires an anthropomorphic perspective, enabling us to recognise human qualities in the volcano; human behaviour in the sessile, reclusive community life of the oyster; and human frailty in the regressive evolution of the Lycopsids.

Ralph Twentyman, with whom I shared a keen interest in mythology, drew attention to the importance of this archetypal vision in his essay on *Argentum* in *The Science and Art of Healing*, when, with characteristic eloquence, he stated:

> The human soul responds to the processes and substances of our world through myth, legend and poetic imagery, and these may be considered the revelation of a higher reality lying latent, like a sleeping princess, within the natural phenomena. They constitute, one might also say, a homeopathic proving in a very clear and heightened form. In contemplating these images and symbols, we may be led deeper into the hidden genius of the substance and its remedial

actions than by confining our attention strictly to the realm of material effects and the statutory rubrics of official provings.[2]

This way of looking at nature has largely been lost due to the persuasive and erosive influence of science and its insistence on empirical evidence as the basis of truth; limiting consciousness to a three-dimensional universe, measured by time and space; presenting the material world as the only reality, despite its inconstant, ever-changing nature. This left-brained, masculine perspective disdainfully views feminine intuition and imagination as the province of art, not science. Yet, science owes much to the workings of speculation and fantasy, witnessed in its debt to the alchemists, who possessed a reverence for the Creation that eludes the modern scientist.

The Doctrine of Signatures

The shaman and medicine men of old regarded everything about them as being an outward expression of the Divine; all things were sacred: the mountains, the streams, the forests, the grasslands, the ocean and all that dwelt there; everything, no matter how great or how small, was created, sustained and blessed by a hidden godlike force, which was powerfully visible in all the manifestations and phenomena of nature. To identify this sacred force in a star, a rock, a tree or an animal, or in the wind, the storm, the lightening or the earthquake, as a particular god or goddess is dismissed today as primitive and pagan. In doing so, we lose contact with an arcane truth, which we otherwise only experience when deeply moved and entranced by a work of art, the splendour of our world or the majesty of the night sky. Northrop Frye, the influential and highly-respected, Canadian literary critic and theorist, captured this dichotomy in these profound words:

> Man lives, not directly or nakedly in nature like the animals, but within a mythical universe, a body of assumptions and beliefs developed from his existential concerns. Most of this is held unconsciously, which means that our imaginations may recognise elements of it, when presented in art or literature, without consciously understanding what it is that we recognise.[3]

What the shaman recognised and honoured was the differentiation of a universal, wise and loving, divine power into the various forms and forces of the manifest world. Thereby, the Absolute Godhead assumed the guise of individual divinities, which according to the attributes of the particular form or force were understood to possess either masculine or feminine energy. At first glance, this would appear to represent a pagan pantheism, which although intrinsic to the vision of Paracelsus, is foreign to minds programmed by the three religions of the Middle East. However, on earnest contemplation, this vision reveals the greatest truth. A truth that imbues the creation with the immanence and imminence of the Divine, and when embraced sustains this sacred awareness in the fibre of the being, even in times of grave duress. Monotheism by contrast, although stating that all is God, and God is all, fails to perpetuate the same sense of constant, divine immediacy and participation that shamanic vision inspires.

Though childlike, this vision is not childish. It pushes away the stifling prejudices of *logos* (reason and intellect) which lacks the means to see the higher Reality behind the façade of the material world. It permits us to retain our consciousness of the mythical universe referred to by Northrop Fry; a consciousness that we touch when someone walks over our grave, when our hair stands on end and our blood runs cold, when we cross our fingers, and when we are transported out of this world on the wings of poetry, music, dance or fantasy into a realm where gods and goddesses, heroes and dragons truly abide.

Belonging to shamanic wisdom, handed down from ages past in the medical traditions of many cultures, is the *Doctrine of Signatures*, a postulate first formulated in the Middle Ages and espoused by Paracelsus, who included it in his writings. The understanding of this doctrine is that all substances, mineral, plant or animal, bear a therapeutic signature implicit in their external appearance and characteristics, which informs regarding their specific ability to cure certain illnesses. By this, it is understood that every substance demonstrates its healing potential in symbolic form. What Hahnemann truly thought of this postulate is uncertain, because he was at great pains to distance himself from Paracelsus, the alchemists and any doctrine that might seem tainted by mysticism. This reserve stemmed not so much from disbelief – he showed himself to be strongly influenced by alchemical thinking and methodology in his passionate pursuit of chemistry – but rather from his conviction that homeopathy could stand on its own feet without addition from other sources. Furthermore, desiring to bring homeopathy to the attention of his allopathic peers, he could not risk jeopardising his arguments with any concepts that might be construed as Paracelsian or mystic. Professionally, he discounted the doctrine as '*the folly of the ancients.*' These words, coming from the Master, created contention among his followers. To this day, some still echo his scepticism.

Whatever Hahnemann's deepest feelings may have been, the shamans of old had no doubt. Psychically tuned to a deeper Reality and sensible to the omnipresence of Divinity and the pantheon of powers pervading the physical realm, their world was sentient, enfolding and beneficent. They knew that the Great Earth Mother would not only have blessed her earth-children with remedies for their ailments, she would have designated each a therapeutic signature, whereby, its healing virtue might be recognised: an encoded token accessible to human insight and intuition. Over gener-ations, through implementing such clues, the shamans assembled an enduring legacy of herbal knowledge, which they bequeathed to posterity.

Therapeutic signatures repose in all qualities, properties and features of a medicinal substance. In the instance of herbs and trees, all characteristics of appearance, preferred habitat, vigour of growth, abundance, propagation and seasonal changes are indicative – also the colour of bark, leaves, blossoms and sap; the number of petals; the fragrance of leaves and flowers; the colour, taste and configuration of fruit; and a plant's value or danger to insect, animal or human life.

The shamans soon realised that among the greatest poisons, the greatest remedies are to be found. Hence, the poisonous effects of a plant became a key part of its therapeutic signature. From this consideration, the *Doctrine of Signatures* naturally evolved into the *Doctrine of Similars*: what a plant (or substance) can cause in a poisonous dose, it can cure in a therapeutic dose.

Later this doctrine extended to minerals and animal remedies. The art of recognising and understanding archetypal forms and matching these to the sick in mind and body was established.

In modern times, this art has been expanded considerably; the advance of science adding much more information to our knowledge of the medicinal substances used in homeopathy: the chemical properties of the mineral remedies, isolation of plant glycosides and alkaloids and their physiological effects, plant classification, the natural history of animals and the analysis of animal poisons and secretions.

The art of homeopathy is the art of deciphering metaphors: the metaphor of the substance and the metaphor of the subject and matching the one to the other. The process of acquiring an understanding of the characteristics of a substance and of a subject is the same. In Frans Vermeulen's words, both need to be 'consulted' or 'interviewed'. In the case of a substance, the consultation involves the gathering of information about that substance from every possible source and viewpoint, gleaning the essence and totality of its signature. The picture compiled from this accumulated evidence provides a profile equivalent to that achieved in the case history of a subject. Remarkable parallels and similarities between the essence of substance and subject are revealed. Such clear correspondences should convince even the most sceptical of the validity of the doctrine of signatures. The 'consultation with the substance' provides a wealth of valuable detail to supplement the remedy information contained in the materia medica.[4]

The toxicology (poisonous effects) of a substance adds important details to its remedy picture. It demonstrates the organ and system affinities of the substance and the pathological states it can cause and therefore cure. This supplies critical information since provings with potentised remedies reveal the subtler, functional effects of the substance and not its capacity to provoke structural change or damage. When the substance is psychoactive (psychotropic), causing alteration in perception, mood, consciousness, understanding and behaviour, as do Stramonium, Opium and Cannabis, mental symptoms and conditions brought about by ingestion of the non-potentised substance prove a rich source of information regarding the emotional states that the substance will benefit when prescribed homeo-pathically.

References

1 Lilley DJ. The Homeopathic Materia Medica. In: Kayne SB (editor). *Homeopathic Practice*. London: Pharmaceutical Press. 2008. p80.

2 Twentyman R. *The Science and Art of Healing*. Edinburgh: Floris Books, 1989. p151.

3 Frye N. Introduction. *The Great Code: The Bible and Literature*. New York NY: Houghton Mifflin, 2002.

4 Lilley DJ. The Homeopathic Materia Medica. In: Kayne SB (editor). *Homeopathic Practice*. London: Pharmaceutical Press. 2008. p87.

Part two

THE PSYCHE

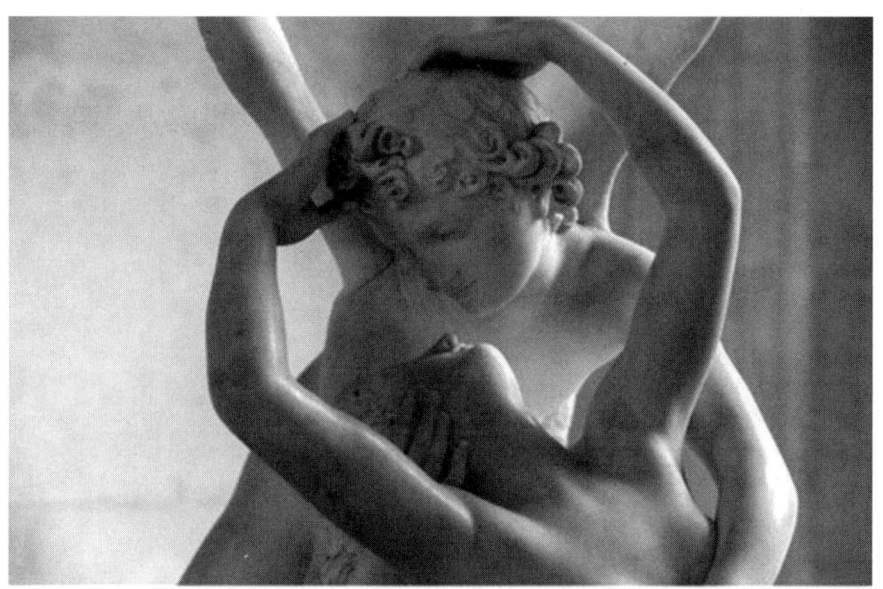

19

JUNG'S RITE OF PASSAGE

The theories of Sigmund Freud (1856–1939), the Austrian neurologist who founded psychoanalysis, have always been given more credence by medical orthodoxy than those of Jung. The empirical nature of Freudian psycho-analysis and its patriarchal-based psychology are more in keeping with scientific, Western medicine than the maternal emphasis of Jung's analyti-cal psychology in which the pre-eminent archetype is the Great Mother Goddess, incorporating all her varied facets: devouring, destructive, nurtur-ing, protective and creative.

The concepts of analytical psychology developed by Carl Gustav Jung (1875–1961), the Swiss psychiatrist and psychologist, are complementary to the philosophy and principles of homeopathy. His theories regarding the topography of the psyche are invaluable in the interpretation of psycho-logical material derived from homeopathic provings. They give meaningful structure to the painstaking methodology of homeopathic case taking and

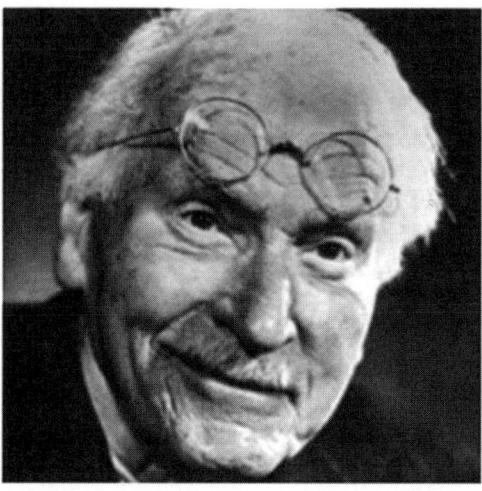

Figure 19.1 *Carl Gustav Jung (1875–1961)*

(Image: Almay)

the subsequent analysis of the emotions, feelings, compensations, projections, prejudices, values, perceptions, drives and behaviour that come to light during the unfolding of a case; particularly the evaluation of fears, delusions (imaginings) and the interpretation of dreams. Reciprocally, homeopathy is the therapeutic arm of analytical psychology and provides, through its pathogenetic trials and process of cure, clear proof of the theoretical conclusions that Jung propounded.

The disparity between the Freudian and Jungian systems of analysis was strongly influenced by the different upbringing of their founders. Jung experienced his father, Paul Achilles Jung, a poor, rural pastor in the Swiss Reformed Church, as a conservative, predictable and dependable but weak man, and his mother Emilie, who came from a wealthy well-known Swiss family, as dominant and powerful, but eccentric, neurotic and highly unpredictable. She was a source of great stress to him; a woman of contradictory and fanciful emotions, so extreme that he was convinced she had two personalities. She was given to bouts of depression, and, when he was about three-years-old, 'deserted' him to receive several months of hospital treatment for a vague illness that Jung later attributed to the difficulties and tensions that existed between his parents. The effect of this prolonged separation from his mother, and her continuing periods of absence, was a widespread, eczematous skin eruption, presumably brought about by a combination of emotional stress and constitutional vulnerability. On a deeper level, the experience germinated into the conviction that *separation* and *fear of abandonment*, especially from the all-important mother figure was far more central to psychopathology than all the sexual reasons, such as 'fear of castration' or 'penis-envy,' that Freud favoured. The insecurity and unpredictability engendered by his mother's swings between ecstasy, during which she experienced visitations from spirit beings, and depression, during which she could not cope with life, left Jung with a very ambivalent attitude towards her and a general mistrust of women, whom he judged to be innately unreliable. These were subjective, patriarchal prejudices that he would analyse with objective candour during the psychic catharsis that afflicted him many years later.

For the first nine years of his life, until the birth of his sister, Jung was an only child. This, together with an exceptional intellect, which placed him far above the mental capacity of his companions at the country school he attended, provided a childhood characterised by solitude. This fostered a naturally introspective disposition much inclined to self-analysis: a process that would come to serve him well in understanding the complexities of the human psyche.

In contrast, Freud's childhood in Vienna was blessed by having a warmly-expressive, protective and loving mother who adored him. His father Jacob Freud, a Jewish wool merchant, had been married twice before when he met Sigmund's mother Amalia Nathansohn, and already had two children. Jacob was a strong patriarchal figure: a strict disciplinarian and the voice of authority in his home. Sigmund was born with a caul nine months after their marriage and Amalia interpreted this as a very positive omen for the boy's future. Apparently, his parents favoured him over his siblings and despite their difficult circumstances strove to give him a good education. They were rewarded for their sacrifices through the excellence of his academic achievements. He had a deep love for literature and shared with Hahnemann a mastery of languages, becoming proficient in seven. His great joy was reading Shakespeare in English. Coming from this background, Freud's elaboration of the concept of the typically masculine, moralistic superego with its emphasis on conventional norms and consensus opinion, driven by conscience, responsibility and fear of retribution is understandable. Possibly foreshadowing his fixation on the sexual influences affecting the development of the psyche was the four weeks of exhaustive and inconclusive zoological research he participated in as a medical student, dissecting hundreds of eels in search of their elusive male reproductive organs.

Critical to the different bias these two brilliant minds developed was the religious background from which they emerged. Jung came from a Christian family. His father Paul was a 'kindly but undistinguished' pastor, and his mother Emilie was the youngest daughter of Samuel Preiswerk, a distinguished theologian, president of the pastors of Basel and professor of Hebrew, whose devotion to the language stemmed from his conviction that it must be the language spoken in Heaven. He was also a convinced spiritualist, who held regular conversations with his deceased first wife and was certain that when he composed his sermons she protected him against evil spirits.[1] His second wife, Jung's grandmother, who like other members of her family was apparently clairvoyant, shared Samuel's belief in the immediacy of the spirit world. Her daughter Emilie, Jung's unstable mother, inherited this feyness, which at night offset her depressions with enthralling spirit visitations. Her son, equally sensitive to otherworldly influences, picked up on the mysterious transformation she often manifested at nightfall and shared some of her psychic feelings and images, which must have been frightening. Far from scaring him off, however, this early introduction to dimensions beyond the physical keened a lifelong interest in the occult and the unfathomable. Growing up in the country brought him into contact with the local peasant community and the rural interest and belief in occult phenomena. This natural, comfortable relationship with a spirit realm, that was seen as constantly interacting with the material world, did much to reinforce his own predilection for the arcane.

Although Jung was brought up in the Christian faith, its tenets did not satisfy or persuade him.

> A good deal of Jungian psychology can be seen as part of Jung's attempt to find a substitute for the orthodox faith in which he was reared, but against which he started to rebel at a very early age.[2]

He would thoroughly investigate philosophy, mythology, alchemy and the traditions of Christianity, Hinduism Buddhism, Gnosticism and Taoism, but the conclusions enshrined in his remarkable psychological theories are highly original and mostly derived from personal inner experience, his work with patients and particularly from tortuous self-analysis arising from the mental upheaval that he experienced in 1913, at the age of 38. He was convinced that life had meaning beyond material goals and that its true purpose was spiritual attainment. He likened it to a journey of transformation, which he called *individuation*, through which the impure soul achieves its innate spiritual perfection and the divinity of the Self is realised. In his autobiography, Jung writes of an imperishable world, as opposed to this transitory one.[2]

Freud's upbringing was far more stable and solidly grounded in his allegiance to his secular Jewish origins and identity, which would prove of significant influence in the development of his intellectual and moral outlook. Although regarded by some as essentially conservative and by others as a controversial non-conformist, the content of his psychoanalytical ideas always remained committed to rationalistic values.

Anthony Storr, a psychiatrist and trained Jungian analyst, comments on this difference between the two:

> Jung cannot be explained unless it is remembered that, for him, unlike Freud, natural science was not enough. There had always to be a background of something supernatural, which could not be explained away by the rationalism that took hold upon men's minds at the end of the nineteenth century, and which appealed so strongly to the hard-headed and somewhat pessimistic Freud.[3]

Jung's perspective derived particularly from his subjective experiences and pertained to the evolution of the soul through the realisation of its innate potential; it produced a philosophy that was uplifting, positive and optimistic. Freud's perspective was primarily objective and empirical and failed to recognise the spiritual nature and purpose of life, the existence of the human soul and Spirit and the existence of an afterlife; it produced a philosophy which was not inspiring, gave no higher purpose to life and was, therefore, essentially pessimistic. Freud remained a sceptical agnostic throughout his life and regarded metaphysical investigations as pseudo-science and distraction for immature minds.

Jung acquired nine years of clinical experience working with psychotic patients while practising first as assistant to the eminent psychiatrist Eugen Bleuler and then as senior staff physician at the Burghölzli Mental Hospital, the renowned Psychiatric Clinic of the University of Zurich, where he was appointed lecturer in psychiatry in 1905.

He gained a reputation for himself in the psychiatric world through his research on word-association testing. This resulted in the publication of a formal text on the subject: '*Studies in Word Association*' in 1906. Knowing of Freud's ideas about the unconscious through his '*The Interpretation of Dreams*' (1900) and his promotion of a new method of therapy, '*psychoanalysis*', Jung made contact with Freud and sent him a copy of his published work. The following year, in March 1907, Jung went to visit Freud in Vienna.

Jung, who was then 30-years-old, remembered the discussion between himself and the 50-year-old Freud that took place as being interminable, lasting fully thirteen hours without a break; an indication of the esteem in which they held each other and of their shared interest in the dynamics of the unconscious mind. Six months later, Freud showed his respect for his younger colleague by sending a collection of his published essays to Jung. This was the beginning of an intense period of correspondence and collaboration between them, which lasted six years, ending traumatically for them both in 1914.

To Jung, Freud appeared the archetypal image of an august, wise father-figure; a strong, influential being contrasting markedly with his own insipid father; a man free of the superstitious limitations of conservative Christian philosophy; boldly prepared to brave the criticism of his peers with novel and contentious concepts. Freud recognised in Jung, a young man with a remarkable intellect, equal to his own, and a potential disciple eminently capable of furthering the spread of his psychoanalytical theories. It was a time when his concepts were causing much controversy and Freud needed advocacy from psychiatric collaborators and colleagues outside his Vienna circle to validate and disseminate his ideas. Jung's research had brought him international recognition and he was resident physician and lecturer at one of the most respected psychiatric clinics in Europe. His word would carry weight. Freud also valued Jung because unlike the majority of Freud's closest associates he was not a Jew, which made him even more of an external, unbiased opinion.

Given their widely different philosophical paradigms, the initial intensity of their professional and psychological infatuation and hopes of a collaborative future could not be sustained. Despite Jung's deep respect, admiration and need for Freud, he was soon aware of serious areas of disagreement between their perspectives.

Central to this divergence was Freud's scepticism regarding religion. Without a spiritual foundation, without the essential insight that the patient is a spiritual being fraught with the conflict of opposites inherent in the duality that reigns in the physical realm, Freud's explanations of the causes of psychopathology fell far short of the mark. Lacking an esoteric base, these focused on the libido as pivotal to the formation of the core personality; its repression being key to disturbances of psychological health. While Jung did not discount the role of the libido in the development of individuality, he did not regard it as the crux, but as a vital part of the great panoply of opposites supporting the symbolic structure of the Universe; a numinous force whose contrasexual elements, the masculine and the feminine, the supreme pair of opposites, seek to be reconciled through sacred union to become a symbol of wholeness. Since duality, the manifestation of opposites, is the inevitable consequence of descent from the infinite to the finite, from the Real to the relative: the return to our Source, to our innate Divinity, our Oneness, must require the reconciliation of opposites. This unification of the contradictory, the incongruous and the paradoxical became critical to the healing method of Jung's analytical psychology and is fundamental to the homeopathic method of cure through similars.

Another primary difference between Freud and Jung was their understanding of the nature of the unconscious. To Freud, the unconscious was the repository of repressed feelings and thoughts, which distorted the patient's emotional life, and the goal of psychoanalysis was to bring these repressed images into the light of consciousness. This was achieved through encouraging a patient to talk about dreams and engage in free association: speaking openly for and about themselves and working through their difficulties and problems through a free flow of thoughts and ideas, without judgement or interpretation. Jung concurred with this conception of what he termed the 'personal unconscious, but he also perceived the existence of a far deeper and universal level of the unconscious: the collective unconscious, the realm of archetypal forms developed over the millennia. These symbolic images drawn from the myriad manifestations of the Universe and life's collective experience form an unconscious field of archetypally charged energy, which, when stimulated by specific patterns impinging upon it from the personal unconscious, causes an archetype of corresponding character to emerge and seek expression through the psyche, often in the form of dreams, intuition, inspiration or emotional expression. The energy flow is concordant and centrifugal, hence harmonious and healing. The action of the most similar potentised homeopathic remedy selected on the basis of dominant emotions, feelings and significant dreams acts in unison with this natural phenomenon, bringing cure by working from within outwards.

At first, Jung remained silent about his misgivings and put aside his judgement and criticism in favour of continuing to corroborate with Freud's work and enjoy the emotional comfort he derived from their relationship. Freud's paternalism nourished a part of his psyche that had previously been starved of a father figure: a role-model to esteem. However, much as he wished to avoid contention with Freud, this suppression of his professional opinion was unnatural and eventually had to yield to his own development and his desire to share his findings with others. To this end, he decided to embark on authorship and in the process of writing his book in 1911–12 entitled, *The Psychology of the Unconscious*,[i] he was brought face to face with the radical degree of difference existing between his conceptions and those of Freud and the realisation that if he was to honour his own integrity, he would have to express the criticisms, which he had never voiced publicly. Knowing the pride of the man and the great store he set by Jung's support and approval, Jung feared that what he had to say would damage or end their friendship.

Anthony Storr writes of this critical point in Jung's life:

> This idea disturbed Jung to such an extent that he was unable to proceed with writing for two months; a fact which attests the emotional importance to him of his relationship with Freud.[3]

In fact, as early as 1909, Freud had seen reason to gently admonish and chide Jung by letter about his preoccupation with the occult, in this instance, the possibility of poltergeist phenomena, which Jung had discussed one important evening, despite knowing of Freud's pragmatic scepticism. In doing so, Freud, although he was only 53 at the time, draws about him the mantle of the wise-old-man, who knows better and is not given to the mental dalliances of youth. His comments reveal a sense of betrayal, pique, entitlement and condescension, which did not bode well for their future relationship and must have warned Jung of the inevitability of a future rift, should he step out of line. The letter also clearly indicates that he expected, indeed, insisted that Jung should follow in his footsteps.

---

[i] This book was revised and republished ten years later, with the title, *Symbols of Transformation*.

> Dear Friend . . . it is remarkable that on the same evening that I formally adopted you as an eldest son, anointing you as my successor and crown prince . . . that then and there, you should have divested me of any paternal dignity, and that the divesting seems to have given you as much pleasure as investing your person gave me. Now I am afraid that I must fall back again to the role of father towards you in giving you my views on poltergeist phenomena . . . I therefore don once more my horn-rimmed, paternal spectacles and warn my dear son to keep a cool head and rather not understand something than make such great sacrifices for the sake of understanding . . . I also shake my wise grey locks . . . etc.

After giving an example of the limited 'specifically Jewish character of my mysticism', he closes the letter thus:

> I therefore look forward to hearing more about your investigations of the ghost-complex, my interest being the interest one has in a lovely delusion, which one does not share oneself.[4]

Two years later, in May 1911, Freud was clearly aware of a growing distance between them and wrote a gentler letter to Jung with a careful warning that if he continued with his occult investigations it would ultimately damage his reputation.

> Dear Friend . . . I know that your deepest inclinations are impelling you towards a study of the occult. . . . There is no stopping that, and it is always right for a person to follow the biddings of his own impulses. The reputation you have won with your *Dementia* will stand against the charge of 'mystic' for quite a while. With cordial greetings and the hope you will write me again after a shorter interval this time.[4]

Scarcely a month later, Freud wrote again, but in conciliatory tone, prompted by the discovery that his close associate in the psychoanalytical school, the Jewish Hungarian analyst Sándor Ferenczi, was also investigating the paranormal.

> Dear Friend . . . In matters of occultism, I have become humble ever since the great lesson I received from Ferenczi's experiences. I promise to believe everything that can be made to seem the least bit reasonable. As you know, I do not do so gladly. But my hubris has been shattered.[4]

There can be no doubt that the great man was acutely concerned about the activities of his 'prodigal son' and feared a schism between them; a fear that encompassed both his deep affection and his professional interests.

The breakup that was forewarned in 1911 became final in 1913, following an increasingly acrimonious conflict between them as the 'son' tested the strength of the 'father' and the validity of his psychoanalytical concepts and the 'father' repudiated those of the aspiring 'son', who sought to usurp him. Eventually, it was a clash between two large egos and emotions ran high. At their last meeting at a congress in Munich, 7–8 September 1913, the atmosphere between them was most disagreeable. Lou Andreas-Salomé, a Freud sympathiser, who was present, wrote:

> It is not so much that Jung diverges from Freud as that he does so as if he could rescue Freud and his cause *through* these divergences. . . . A single glance at these two shows which of them is more dogmatic and power-hungry. Two years ago, there was robust gaiety and exuberant vitality in Jung's booming laughter, but his seriousness now is made up of pure aggression, ambition and intellectual brutality.[5]

It was an attempt at switching father-son roles, perpetrated with all the savagery seen in the wild when some younger male challenges the dominance of the alpha male; and it came at great cost to both. The final rupture caused Freud great distress and was experienced as a 'great loss'; Jung, however, now aged 38, succumbed to huge emotions welling up from repressed regions of the unconscious where the unresolved conflicts of the supreme opposites, the masculine and feminine within him, born of the ineffectual, imageless father and the unpredictable, forsaking mother, were in ferment. With the overthrow of the substitute father, the unadulterated hubris of the masculine, threw off the vestiges of maternal dominance, and, assuming unbridled authority, cast him into a cauldron of delusion and emotional torment: a horrible 'confrontation with the unconscious.'

For a time, he balanced precariously on the brink of insanity, feeling 'menaced by a psychosis.' Apocalyptic visions beset him, hinting at incipient schizophrenia, but in 1913 also presaging a very real-world catastrophe of disastrous proportions that lay ahead. In the throes of these disturbing delusions, visions, imaginary conversations and visitations, Jung held onto his sanity by invoking the feminine within him through writing, drawing and painting, 'activities that helped him to regain a degree of control over turbulent fantasies,'[6] and by training himself to dream in a new way:

> What I did . . . was to make at night an exact reversal of the mental machinery I had used in the day. . . . By assuming a passive attitude at night while at the same time pouring the same stream of libido into the unconscious that one has put into daytime work, the dreams can be caught, and the performance of the unconscious observed.[7]

Although he suspected that he had 'some psychic disturbance' and feared he might lapse into insanity, he also continued to see himself as a receiver of revelations and a channel for inspiration. This gave him the trust that his mental condition was an essential learning experience for the work that lay ahead. This conviction strengthened him and forced him to subject himself to intense and continuous self-analysis during 1914–1918, certain that he would gain vital insights into the working of the unconscious mind. During this period, apart from learning to capture his dreams, he developed the therapeutic, meditative technique of inducing hallucinations that he termed *'active imagination'*, by which visualisations and fantasies are permitted to well up from the unconscious unhindered by judgement or analysis, while the conscious mind responds imaginatively as if the drama being enacted were real. Dreams can also be worked with in this way. The process provides a bridge between the unconscious and the ego-consciousness, and, if taken deeper, between the collective unconscious (the 'Spirit in the Depths') and the personal unconscious. It invites the unconscious to freely act-out, through symbolic imagery, repressed, unrealised and unresolved material held within the depths of the psyche. Active imagination may also be achieved through automatic writing or through creative work and activities such as painting, sculpture, music, dance, arts and crafts – all of which are essentially feminine – as is homeopathy!

Herings Law

The method is in keeping with Hering's Law of Cure: healing taking place from within outwards, from the unconscious to the conscious and from the mind to the body. Homeopathic treatment acts in the same manner as active imagination, taking the rich material of dream, fantasy (delusion) and fears (negative imagery) and through the action of a remedy capable of eliciting and energising similar images within the unconscious, releasing and dispersing their pent-up energy in a healing process. Active imagination used on its own is not without danger, because, for the ungrounded and unstable, the method may leave the subject in a transitional state in which fantasy becomes reality; also traits and characteristics realised through imagination and dream may become ingrained rather than being worked through and dissipated. Homeopathy obviates this risk; the healing process of release from within is taken to its natural conclusion while unburdening the unconscious and restoring the integrity of the conscious mind.

The process swamped Jung:

> An incessant stream of fantasies had been released, and I did my best not to lose my head but to find some way to understand these strange things. I stood helpless before an alien world; everything in it seemed difficult and incomprehensible. I was living in a constant state of tension; often I felt as if gigantic blocks of stone were tumbling down upon me. One thunderstorm followed another. My enduring these storms was a question of brute strength.[8]

Jung painstakingly documented everything he experienced in numerous small journals, which he later transcribed to a large, red leather-bound book, which has become iconically known as the Red Book. Throughout, the text is meticulously illustrated by reproductions of the paintings and drawings executed during the period of his breakdown. For JC Andrijeski, in his *'Journey into Jung's Red Book: Liber Primus'*, the book chronicles the 'deconstruction of a mind . . . the beginnings of this process for Jung, and all its requisite fear, ranting and expounding both for and against its need, are documented in detail in *Liber Primus.'*[9] The rampant masculine is everywhere apparent, self-absorbed, inflated with self-esteem, filled with narcissism, bombast and excess, yet threaded through with humility and fear; a mind searching and struggling to find order in chaos and thereby synthesise a logical psychological edifice, which would prove of help to himself and possibly for others.

> I had to try to understand what had happened and to what extent my own experience coincided with that of mankind in general. Therefore, my first obligation was to probe the depths of my own psyche.[10]

During this dark period in his life, he continued seeing patients, but due to the flux of emotions and conflicting energies that threatened to unhinge his mind, he often did so in an erratic and harsh manner. The errant masculine held him in its sway, usurping kindness and empathy with the heel of a tyrant. He, who had always maintained that an analyst should never bully, manipulate or even influence patients, began to transgress these rules even reducing a patient to tearful submission.[11]

Then one day, out of the kaleidoscope of previously male-dominated fantasy images, emerged the presence of a woman. He was methodically writing down his fantasies and inwardly questioning himself about the value of what he was doing and whether it was truly scientific.

His inner dialogue ran:

> What am I really doing? Certainly, this has nothing to do with science. But then what is it?' Whereupon, he heard the voice of a woman within him say: 'It is art.'

His reaction was denial:

> I said very emphatically to this voice that my fantasies had nothing to do with art, and I felt a great inner resistance. No voice came through, however, and I kept on writing.

Then came the next assault, and again the same assertion:

> That is art.'[12]

He attempted to draw her into further discussion, but there was only silence. He significantly concluded that 'the woman within me' had no voice of her own. He had inadvertently touched the very quick of his torment: the stilling and subjugation of his feminine aspect. From early childhood, in resentful reaction to desertion (rejection) by his mother and compensation for the inadequate masculinity (castration) of his father, he had choked 'her' off and wilfully asserted his manhood. His primordial struggle for supremacy with Freud had exaggerated this conflict of opposites to a pathological degree.

The initial refusal to accept the assertion of his feminine voice was symptomatic of the heedless authority imposed by the masculine side of his psyche, but he had heard her voice speaking out of the desolation of his wilderness and there was no way back. in his autobiography, *Memories, Dreams, and Reflections*, written in his eighties, he says (my italics).

> I was greatly intrigued that a woman should *interfere* with me from within . . . Later I came to see that this inner feminine figure plays a typical, or archetypal, role in the unconsciousness of a man, and I called her the "anima." The corresponding figure in the unconscious of woman I called the "animus".[12]

She was essential to his cure! He described the process clearly in his autobiography:

> I felt awed by her. It was like the feeling of an invisible presence in the room. Then a new idea came to me: in putting down all this material for analysis, I was in effect writing letters to the anima, that is, to a part of myself with a different viewpoint from my conscious one. I got remarks of an unusual and unexpected character. I was like a patient in analysis with a ghost and a woman![12]

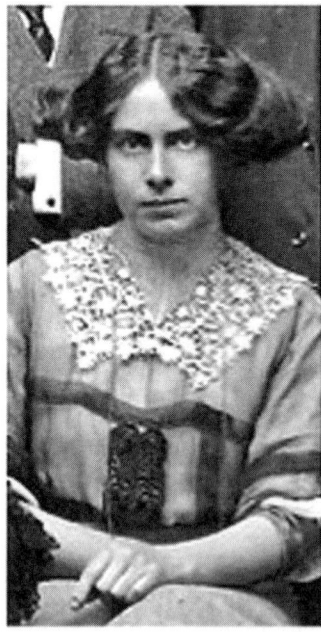

Figure 19.2 Antonia (Toni) Anna Wolff (1888–1953) pictured in 1911 aged 23
(Wikipedia)

Our inner reality creates our outer reality, and the conscious advent of Jung's anima from his unconscious was soon reflected in the presence of her physical counterpart projected in the person of Antonia (Toni) Anna Wolff (1888–1953), a young Swiss woman who had been under his analysis. During the worst period of his confrontation with madness, he had found himself unable to continue with her treatment. Toni had incredible, wild and cosmic fantasies, but he was too preoccupied with his own to cope with hers. Though he felt involved with her, he broke off her analysis, and did not then know what to do.[13]

He was irresistibly attracted to her. She had beautiful, soulful, large, brown eyes and dark hair, and like other loves of his life, she matched the memory he had of the attractive dark-complexioned maid who had looked after him during his mother's absences in hospital. As he acknowledged, unlike his wife Emma, she represented the type of girl who had come to represent an aspect of his anima. The attraction was mutual, intensified by his having been her therapist and mentor. Considering his mental state and her need for him, it is probable that it was she who took the initiative and instigated their intimate relationship. Inevitably, she was drawn into his suffering and shared the severe storms that beset him. It was a time of extreme stress for them both, but her presence and love saved him. As a patient commented: '. . . she acted on him like a brake, saving him from going over the edge. Without her he wouldn't have made it. She brought him back to reality.'[13]

Ronald Hayman who wrote *A Life of Jung* explains the dynamics of the intense relationship that developed between them:

> His love for Toni . . . was born out of transference, counter-transference and a discovery that their fantasies coincided, overlapped, interlocked.[14]

With these words, he inadvertently describes the relationship between a patient and the well-selected homeopathic remedy: the delusions, dreams and fears of both must *coincide, overlap and interlock* for healing to take place. Toni and Carl provide a grand example of how the relationship of similars heals. She was like a homeopathic remedy to him, and, therefore, able to do for Jung what his wife Emma, whom he loved in a different way, was unable to achieve. She saved his mind.

She was also essential for the formulation of his theories of the structure of the psyche. She acted like a psychic antenna for him, capturing and bringing order to the disparate images, fantasies and voices that assailed him. Later, she too would become an analyst. One of her patients who experienced her abilities gives us this insight:

(I felt) as if I were even nearer Jung's inner wisdom when I was with her than when I was with him in the flesh. She was in some way the inner side of his work. . . . She mediated Jung's mind and intuitive ideas directly, for she had been part of their creation from the unconscious.[14]

Jung wrote positively of this cataclysmic time:

The years when I was pursuing my inner images were the most important in my life – in them everything essential was decided. It all began then; the later details are only supplements and clarifications of the material that burst forth from the unconscious, and at first swamped it. It was the *prima materia* for a life's work.[15]

References

1   Stevens A. *On Jung*. London: Penguin Books. 1999. p5.

2   Storr A. *Jung*. London: Fontana Press 1995. p9.

3   *Ibid*., p9.

4   Jung CG. *Memories, Dreams, Reflections* Appendix 1. Letter: Freud to Jung, April 16, 1909. London: Fontana Press. 1995. pp397–399.

5   Hayman R. *A Life of Jung*. Bloomsbury. London 2002. p169.

6   *Ibid*., p175.

7   *Ibid*., p176.

8   Jung CG. *Memories, Dreams, Reflections* Appendix 1. Letter: Freud to Jung, June 15, 1911. London: Fontana Press. 1995. p201.

9   Andijeski JC. *Journey into Jung's Red Book: Liber Primus*. White Sun Press 2010. Kindle Edition.

10 Jung CJ. *Memories, Dreams, Reflections*. London: Fontana Press 1967. p225.

11 Hayman R. *A Life of Jung*. Bloomsbury. London 2002. p182.

12 Jung CG. *Memories, Dreams, Reflections*. Fontana Press. London 1995. p210.

13 Hayman R. *A Life of Jung*. Bloomsbury. London 2002. p185.

14 *Ibid*., p186.

15 Jung CJ. *Memories, Dreams, Reflections*. London: Fontana Press. 1967. p200.

20

PSYCHE – SPIRIT – SOUL

From these rites of passage, Jung was able to conceive a map of what he termed the *psyche*, in which its various structures and functions could be defined. These structures must not be perceived as anatomically delineated or as discrete energies; they are dynamic and therefore represent fields of energy, which are charged with specific qualities and potentials; they are interactive and in constant flux. In physical terms, they are metaphorical and abstract, but they provide a body of assumptions that provides a working model, which can be visualised and utilised. These structures are the most fundamental of all the archetypal forms and provide the key to understanding the functions of the psyche. Their presence and effects may be recognised in ourselves, in others and in the remedy pictures of the homeopathic materia medica.

The terms spirit, soul, psyche and self are often used loosely and interchangeably, their real meaning blurred by casual semantics. Our purpose, which is the linking of the sciences of spirit, archetype and homeopathy, necessitates working definitions of these terms to avoid ambiguity. Since the concepts they identify are open to contrasting opinions and beliefs, my perspective may differ from that of other philosophies and systems, including those conceived by Freud and Jung, but will provide a reliable foundation for what needs to be discussed and compared in this work.

The Psyche

In strictly psychological terms, the *psyche* represents the totality of the human mind, incorporating both the conscious and the unconscious elements. This is a practical definition devoid of esoteric meaning, but limits its application, for the psyche encompasses far more. To the ancient Greeks, the word *psyche* was numinous; it had spiritual and mystical significance. The basic meaning of the Greek word was '*breath of life*' and from this '*spirit, soul, ghost*' and ultimately '*self*' were derived.

The etymology of the word indicates a basic meaning embracing concepts far wider than just the mind and its various levels of consciousness. In his allegory, *Metamorphoses* or *The Golden Ass*, Apuleius, the Roman author of the second century A.D., relates the classic love story of the beautiful princess Psyche and Cupid [Eros], the God of Love. Fittingly, the story brims over with universal motifs common to myth, folktale and romance, including: the mysterious divine lover, Eros, and the innocent, ingenuous, enraptured heroine, Psyche – the earnest injunction to keep the liaison secret – the violation of this pledge – the malicious mother and jealous sisters – the box that must not be opened – the irresistible curiosity that ensured that it would be – punishment, for the transgression, by the imposition of impossible tasks, among them descent into the fearful depths of Hades – all accomplished with divine assistance and crowned by reunion, the triumph of romantic love and the immortalisation of Psyche. A story as rich in psychological metaphor as the psyche is in its ambit and content. To classical Greek philosophy, Psyche, having transcended her human origins, became the very embodiment of the soul: mortal, yet immortal; confined yet unhindered by the body; capable of crossing the boundaries between heaven, earth and the underworld and surviving death.

Freud, lacking the notion of spirit, soul, eternity and immortality, restricted his concept of the psyche to a psychological structure made up of three components, the largely unconscious *Id*, which drives the basic instincts; the partially conscious *Super-ego*, which acts as an internal critic, exacting behaviour based upon the internalised values and norms of consensus morality; and the conscious *Ego*, which mediates between the urges of the Id and the prohibitions of the super-ego – a balancing act that necessitates artifice and repression – ingredients for psychological dysfunction and disease. These components of the psyche will be considered later.

Jung did not always make a clear distinction between *psyche* and *soul*. On balance, he favoured the term psyche over soul and regarded it as '*the totality of all psychic processes*'. He used the term *spirit* to simply define the non-material aspect of a living person (thoughts, intentions, ideals), e.g. a spirit of endeavour; or to describe an incorporeal being detached from a human body (ghost, wraith, shade, ancestral soul). At times, he would use soul instead of spirit when referring to the core, heart or centre of the human psyche. In general, his image of soul was a functional complex, or innate *personality*, rather than the Christian concept of a transcendental essence. Much of what are generally considered to be qualities of spirit and/or soul, he ascribed to the *Self*.

These various shades of meaning and usage, which developed over time as new theories were being developed, make clear-cut definitions of such intangible concepts imperative!

In *Healing the Soul*, the psyche will be given the widest delineation possible, used as a term to define a complex, individualised energy field and all its non-physical phenomena: an objective, transpersonal appellation pertaining, as Jung envisioned, to the totality of all psychic processes, but also to the entire Spirit – soul – ego-self – emotion – mind complex, which gives rise to these processes. Unlike the soul, the psyche is transpersonal; it has no face, destiny or existence of its own; it is not synonymous with either the Spirit or the soul; it is an all-embracing definition for psychological processes and psychic structures, not an entity. *It is also a domain, the field of contention between the sovereign-elect: the soul, and the usurper: the ego-self.*

In this work, the soul is not equated with the personality, which it far transcends, or the Spirit, which is its goal. The soul is the hero we are, the immortal traveller on a mystic journey in search of the 'Holy Grail' of Self-enlightenment: the realisation of our Divinity. Through many life times, the hero-soul is destined to confront and contend with the villain-ego-self: a pseudo-self, which, through the fear and doubts of the soul, has usurped its position and identity, shrouding its pristine purity with layers of compensatory personality, denying it expression. The arduous journey of the soul is an inward one towards its own radiance; a goal achieved by casting off the obscuring structures of the ego-self to reveal the effulgent glory of Spirit.

Homeopathy, is soul-medicine; its immaterial dynamis reaching the divide between soul and ego-self, enabling the dismantling and expulsion of the ego-self from the domain of the psyche.

Self or Spirit

[handwritten marginal note: Jungs Self as unus / individuation]

Jung perceived the Self as being the goal of individuation: the process by which the various archetypes and complexes of the psyche become integrated and unified into a coherent whole. The path of individuation culminates in the realisation of the Self by the soul: it merges with the peerless qualities of Spirit. Taking this concept to its ultimate, the Self is synonymous with the individualised Spirit: the eternal, omnipotent Divinity at the core of every soul: its True Nature, Essence or Being. The Self may also be termed the 'true or higher-self' of the soul – the 'false or lower-self' being the ego-self: the psychological structure unconsciously erected by the immature soul in defence of its perceived isolation, inferiority and vulnerability, and with which it misguidedly comes to identify itself.

In Eastern philosophy, the Self is known as the *Atman*. It is the immortal *Essence* of the individual and is in a constant state of *Being*, while the soul is ever in a state of *becoming* that *Being*: a state it achieves when it finally merges with the Atman or Spirit. Jung referred to the Self as *the archetype of archetypes* and this concept is truly in keeping with its ineffable majesty.

The more aligned the soul becomes with the Self, the better able it is to adapt to its environment and to changes within that environment. The better the soul adapts to life, the better able it is to express the qualities of Self and deny the promptings, prejudices and preferences of the ego-self.

Qualities denoting a life lived through the Self

Virtues of the Godly

- Basic trust.
- Wisdom: uninterrupted adherence to spiritual knowledge and values.
- Purity of being, thought and action.
- Unconditional love.
- Truthfulness.
- Empathy.
- Service.
- Surrender (adaptation) to what is unfolding.
- Being centred in the "Now".
- Groundedness.
- Fearlessness – fortitude.
- Optimism – non-conceptual (unconditional) positivity.
- Joyousness.
- Ardour – enthusiasm, energy, intensity.
- Dispassion.
- Creativity.
- Self-restraint and self-discipline.
- Renunciation of ego-desires.
- Freedom from attachment, need or dependency.
- Generosity.
- Selflessness.
- Studiousness.
- Kind forthrightness.
- Harmlessness.

- Peacefulness.
- Tolerance.
- Forgiveness.
- Freedom from anger.
- Freedom from fear.
- Freedom from hatred and malice.
- Freedom from jealousy and envy.
- Freedom from criticism and comparison.
- Freedom from purposeless activity.
- Freedom from gossip.
- Cleanliness and orderliness.
- Refinement.
- Modesty.
- Humility: freedom from ego-pride.

These virtues, in any philosophy, denote goodness or godliness. In glancing down this list, even perfunctorily, *'unless things mortal move us not at all'*, we are aware of an inner resonance, an echo within ourselves that indicates that a sensitive and responsive chord of truth has been struck. We intuitively know that this is how we should be, not occasionally, not under certain circumstances, not only in relation to certain people, but as our constant on-going state. If we should do more than just glance and study each virtue carefully, we sense beyond and deep to the echo, a longing for that serenity of being that can engender such perfect poise amid the turbulence of life's events. Dwell on the longing and the urge to achieve it arises. Whether we can hold this urge and respond to it consistently or not, we need to know that it comes to us from the Self; from the Spirit within, calling us to return from whence we came; in truth, it comes from ourselves. The paradox lies in the fact that we need to attain what we already are. The perfection, power and eternal nature of the Self are already ours waiting to be realised. So often in my moments of frailty, Dr Letari said to me: "My son, if you but knew the infinite power residing within you, you would have no fear."

The Self is not remote, it is pervasive; it is not static, it radiates and influences our lives; it is not silent, it speaks through the voice of the conscience; it is not unfamiliar, it is our very Essence. The Spirit or Self has no goal other than drawing us to itself, since it already is all that it needs to be.

The symbolic representation of the Self is the *mandala*, a Sanskrit word meaning *'circle'*. This complex, intricate, circular design is also a powerful symbol for the Godhead and the Cosmos. When the energy system that pervades us and radiates from us is visualised, it is perceived as a complex, patterned, multi-coloured, rhythmically-pulsating mandala positioned in an ordered field of energy comprising an infinity of similar points of focussed density. This indicates a profound truth: that at any given moment, each one of us is placed precisely where we need to be!

Representing the goal of self-realisation, mandalas are employed in many spiritual traditions for the purpose of assisting the devotee or aspirant to create a sacred space, to focus the consciousness and to meditate on at onement with the Divine.

The Soul

The soul is the hero on a quest to find the Holy Grail of Self-realisation. The hero's journey is the path of individuation, through which the soul attains wholeness or perfection. The way is arduous and cannot be accomplished in a single lifetime, for the soul is multifaceted and complex. It takes many lifetimes and the surmounting of many different challenges before the soul has the required maturity, vision and self-reflective awareness to assume the role of hero and begin its spiritual odyssey. The soul is the immortal *'becoming'*, that travels through cycles of life in the spirit realm, its natural domain, and shorter periods of physical incarnation, during which the soul is afforded the invaluable opportunity of putting into practice spiritual lessons learnt upon its journey towards transcendence.

As in hero myths down the ages, only the one with purity of heart has the power to draw the sacred sword from its scabbard of stone. Each incarnation is perfectly tailored to give the soul the opportunity to unfold and advance towards its sacred goal. Nothing in the soul's life is ever arbitrary or coincidental from the moment of conception to the moment of transition to the afterlife. Everything that transpires does so with reason, and, regardless of how traumatic, the purpose is always beneficent. Even when terrible tragedy strikes, it must be witnessed against the backdrop of imperishable immortality: the soul cannot die; the body is a temporary vehicle; there is more than one lifetime; the physical domain though actual is not Reality.

The soul is the repository of lifetimes of experience, a complex endowment with aspects that need to be fulfilled or overcome. Accordingly, when the time is right, the soul is drawn once more into the cycle of life and given the opportunity for further unfolding. The stage is set, the constellation of characters essential to the life experience of the developing soul is arrayed; some of the significant personages are present as the curtain rises, others will appear on cue when their roles dovetail with the destiny of the soul.

Some are not of this world, they are spirit beings appointed to protect, assist, inspire and direct the soul through the experiences and creative opportunities that life affords. They are themselves souls on the path of individuation, tasked, because of their standing, experience, learning and desire to serve, with the role of guides and inspirers. These *'elders'* are catalysts in the process of the soul's spiritual evolution. Personal to the individual soul are the *'gatekeeper'*, the personage specifically assigned to protect the psychic boundaries of the soul from impingement by unwanted and undesirable influences in the psychic environment, and the *'personal guide'* or appointed mentor, the *'guardian angel'*, who throughout life attends and supports the soul at every step of its physical adventure: through thick and thin, through joys and heartaches and through triumph and tragedy. In addition, there are gifted, like-minded souls, who are drawn to assist and inspire any creative or altruistic work the incarnated soul embarks upon. No matter the field of service or creativity pursued by the soul, there will always be adepts in the world of spirit able and eager to lend their talents to its endeavours. At birth, we enter this world seemingly naked and alone, and, at our passing, we depart, seemingly naked and alone, but in truth, we are never alone, there are always those about us, who love and cherish us unconditionally, working tirelessly in subtle, but persuasive ways, to aid our spiritual advancement.

The life of the soul is orchestrated to provide opportunities for its spiritual growth. But, to make things happen, the soul must be convinced that life has a spiritual rather than a materialistic purpose and bring its focus, curiosity, enthusiasm, commitment and perseverance to the task of developing spirituality and attaining the 'virtues of the godly'. 'Knock and it will be opened, ask and it will be given, seek and ye shall find' are injunctions oft repeated and of vital importance. The Cosmos is always doing its part, but the soul must initiate the start of the journey.

The soul creates its own reality through the assemblage of focus, energy, optimism, initiative, participation, adaptation, determination and virtues. Without these, it is merely treading water, waiting for the oceanic drift of the Cosmos to provide progress and enlightenment: a state of psychic torpor in which the soul is oblivious or indifferent to the jolts sent to waken it and the cues to direct it. Taxing events are experienced as cruel twists of fate – undeserved, purposeless suffering – rather than opportunities for learning and progress. This misconception (delusion) fosters disillusionment and despair (*Psora*), scepticism and cynicism (*Sycosis*) and paranoia (*Syphilis*), which become engrained in the nature of the lower-self.

The body, with all its genetic, racial, familial and miasmatic advantages and disadvantages, provides the perfect vehicle for the soul's journey. Soul endowment, physical make-up and the demands of destiny are synchronised.

From the marriage of soul and body, the ego-self (ego-personality or ego) is conceived: an errant, compensatory pseudo-self, born from the soul's *lack of basic trust*: the perfect adversary for the soul on its journey towards Self-realisation.

The ego-self is the disease from which the soul suffers. It possesses traits not yet mastered by the soul, unresolved challenges from the soul's past. Dominating and controlling the psyche, the ego-self, according to its inherent nature, transmits a frequency pattern that attracts a corresponding external reality that appropriately tests the soul. To neutralise the discord of the ego-self is to change the holding reality positively

The acquisition of basic trust is pivotal to gaining mastery of the ego-self. Trust in the Cosmos and in the higher-self must be sustained and unwavering for the compensatory structures of the ego-self to be dismantled.

The ego-self, born of mistrust, fear and delusion, dreads annihilation (the loss of its individuality); it resists the development of trust, which will bring its downfall, clinging, tooth and nail, to its identity, its fears, its prejudices, its preferences and its pleasures. Through doubt, fear and rationalisation, the ego-self undermines the soul, negating its influence.

Resolutely deployed, the strengths of the soul are equal to mastering the ego-self and overcoming the lack of trust on which it is founded. But, the ego-self is a wily and tenacious opponent. It deludes the soul into thinking that its identity is one with the soul.

Incorporating negative aspects of the evolving soul, the ego-self possesses the means to impose its fears, beliefs and prejudices on the soul. The soul that largely identifies with the ego-self, takes on its reprobate ways and accepts the distorted reality perceived through the subjective filters of ego-vision. Rather than the soul nullifying the ego-self, the ego-self drags the soul down to its level of perception. In identifying with the ego-self and its vision of reality, the soul abdicates dominion over the psyche and submits to the dictates and devices of a self-serving despot.

Subsumed in the quicksand of the ego-self, the loss of soul-identity constitutes the source of emotional suffering that lies at the heart of mental and physical disease. Life's events seen through the warped filters of the ego-self, loom large and are fraught with difficulties, devoid of meaning, and culminate in decline and death. Fear, loss and grief are erosive ingredients that overthrow the homeostasis of the body.

Disease is essentially a departure from the spiritual virtues of the Self through the soul colluding with the delinquency of the ego-self. As must be repeatedly emphasised, the ego-self represents the essence of the illness from which the soul suffers; it is the part of the psyche that needs healing. Disease is not primarily emotional, mental or physical; it lies in the nature of the ego-self. This spotlights the serious limitations of conventional medicine, whose therapeutic parameters do not extend beyond the chemical and the structural. The high potency of the homeopathic remedy, matched to the profile of the ego-self, directly addresses the cause of disease at soul level.

The challenges that the ego-self presents for the soul are the consequence of all that has transpired during the soul's previous life experiences. The past confronts the soul in the character of the ego-self – in circumstances and events – and through individuals sharing its stage – all orchestrated to lead the soul forwards. This is spoken of as *karma*, the law of cause and effect: 'as you sow, so shall ye reap'. This law is always operative, not in a punitive sense, exacting atonement for past misdemeanours, but as opportunity for reparation, building and progress. Love and forgiveness are the watchwords of the Self and of the Cosmos. Reward or punishment, eat or be eaten, are the values of the feral ego-self born into a hostile dog-eat-dog, eye-for-an-eye, tooth-for-a-tooth dimension – imbedded assumptions and Shadow energy that the ego-self projects onto the Cosmos – thus, alienating the soul from Reality.

Contrary to the negative view of the ego-self, the travails of life are not exacted as punishment for past misdeeds. Fashioned from weaknesses still to be overcome, propensities not curbed, and strengths not yet realised, the challenges of life, even the most painful, are stepping stones on the ascent of the soul. With progress, the trials that face the soul become ever less traumatic and far more subtle.

Although there are individuals who retain some fragmentary memories derived from previous lives, generally, the incarnating soul loses *conscious* memory of its former existence. This is essential to progress. Constant recall of memories from the soul's past would prove a heavy burden, since the soul is constantly evolving from a less enlightened existence to one more refined and advanced. Deeds perpetrated without thought or moral consideration in the soul's spiritual adolescence, or sufferings inflicted upon the soul by others during the course of previous incarnations, if remembered and revisited, would afflict the soul with fear, grief, guilt, shame, resentment, prejudice and hate and sully the freshness of a new life. The detail and content of past-lives is of no consequence to the evolving soul, but it is the essence of those lives that quickens the conscience.

On an *unconscious* level, the continuity of memory is retained, and the accumulated influence of past incarnations is written in the nature of the ego-self, the qualities of the soul and the dynamics existing between the two. From early childhood, innate patterns of behaviour and the absence or presence of morality, point to characteristics reflecting the soul's long history of contention with the ego-self, the road it has travelled and the progress it has made. The innate nature of these characteristics indicates their source; they are not inherited, learnt or conditioned, they are intrinsic to the soul/ego structure. *'Nature' is always more fundamental and formative than 'nurture'*.

Regression through therapy and hypnosis is a means by which forgotten events may be accessed and recalled, not only from present life, but also from past life experience. When we know that reincarnation is an essential element in the evolutionary cycle of the developing soul and not just a philosophical or religious concept, such evidence is not surprising. Indeed, it would be strange if it were not so. The memory and influence of past lives is indelibly written in the essence of the soul. Just as the experiences of our current life impinge on our nature and influence the direction our lives take; the soul's karmic history subliminally affects both the innate tendencies of the soul and its present-day environment. Cause and effect extend in unbroken continuity from the distant past into the remote future. *We are what we are because of what we have been, and what we will be in the future is profoundly affected by what we are now.*

But, here, a warning needs to be given, regression into past life experience through hypnosis and suggestive questioning is fraught with danger, apart from the risk of imparting false memories based upon suggestion, imagination and wishful thinking. As explained, the natural erasure of past-life memory during incarnation is not without good reason. Intrusion into this unconscious domain, even when ostensibly for therapeutic reasons, e.g. seeking explanation for present life fears and emotions, may trigger recollections better forgotten, which are usually revisited with all the vivid, raw intensity of the original event without full access to the context in which they occurred. These undiluted emotions can be extremely traumatic and lasting in their effect, commensurate with actual, present-life experiences. Originating from unresolved shocks to the ego-self, they feed into its current structure, reinforcing its fundamental lack of trust and further disempowering the soul. Fascination with previous life experience is characteristic of the fickle ego-self; it is diagnostic of its inability to focus positively on the present, its need to vindicate its inadequacies in the light of past suffering, or its wish to escape its mundane lot through fantasies of an infamous or inflated past.

At infrequent intervals throughout his life, my father experienced flash-backs into his own past-lives, during which he was involved in historic events unrelated to anything he had ever experienced vicariously through literature or films. During these spontaneous episodes of recall in which he felt himself projected into distant times, he was either an observer or a central figure in the events that appeared before his mind's eye. These were not always pleasant. During one such occurrence, I saw him break out in a sweat and become distraught, anxious and pale. Although, he did not supply me with details, the images and sensations he experienced were obviously harrowing. He never sought these distant recollections; they occurred without his bidding. He accepted them as part of his heightened psychic awareness and their occurrence as a sign of having weakened his boundaries through fatigue. He assured me that by no means were all such flashbacks distressing; some were joyous and uplifting.

It is apt to repeat here the stirring poem of Joseph Campbell, the master of myth, that captures the mystery of the Hero's Journey:

> We have not even to journey alone
> The heroes of all time have gone before us
> The labyrinth is thoroughly known; we have
> Only to follow the thread of the Hero Path.
> And where we had thought to find an abomination
> We shall find a God
> And where we had thought to slay another
> We shall slay ourselves
> Where we had thought to travel outward
> We shall come to the centre of our own existence
> And where we had thought to be alone
> We shall be with all the world.[1]

The God discovered at the centre of the labyrinth is the Self: the divine Essence of the soul, its source and goal. The Self is the treasure guarded by the mythical dragon that must be metaphorically slain before the treasure can be attained. The dreaded dragon is the ego-self; the soul's own ego-personality, built up over the ages through lack of basic trust; a dragon that will only yield the treasure it mantles through mortal combat. The centre of the labyrinth lies at the core of the soul's being, not external to it; it is the inner sanctum of the soul, the battleground where the struggle for supremacy between soul-self and ego-self must be fought. A ruse the ego-self employs in its fight for self-preservation is to convince the soul that through achieving the Self, the individuality of the soul will be lost forever, with all it holds dear, subsumed in the awesome, maw of the Infinite's, absolute solitude. In the event, the triumphant Hero, instead of being alone, through fully *becoming* the Self achieves the blessed state of *Being* in which he or she becomes one with all that is – omnipotent, omniscient and omnipresent – a state of transcendent bliss and perfect at Onement.

* * * * *

In the light of the above several vital, fundamental tenets need to be laid down before proceeding further. These are themes that will be returned to repeatedly on the journey forward into the mystery of the psyche.

- A Supreme Cosmic Power (Universal Intelligence/Divinity) created the manifest and un-manifest universe – the physical and spirit dimensions.
- The Creative Power is omnipotent, omniscient and omnipresent.
- The Power embodies truth (unity), law, wisdom, perfection and love.
- The Creation is an eternal process emanating from and governed by the Universal Intelligence acting with infinite love and wisdom.
- The Creation is perfect; it has no imperfection.
- The Creation is permeated by and inseparable from the Power that created it.
- The Spirit or Essence of each individual (the Self) is perfect, one with the Universal Intelligence and therefore one with the Creation; it is the Divinity within us.
- Differentiation from the perfect unity of the Universal Intelligence gives birth to the soul.
- The soul is the immortal individuality carried from life to life: it cloaks the perfection of the Self.
- Through differentiation from the Self, the soul loses the realisation of its divine, essential nature and experiences loss of basic trust.
- Loss of basic trust creates the ego-personality or ego-self: the greater the loss of trust the more powerful the ego-self becomes.
- The ego-self is a psychological structure created by the soul to compensate for its loss of basic trust; it is primarily fear-based; it is in all ways inferior to the soul.
- The characteristic traits of the ego-self are determined by innate nature rather than external circumstances and are expressed archetypally.
- The ego-self displaces the soul as the executive agent of the psyche and persuades the soul that it is the soul's true identity.
- The ego-self is the source of all miasmatically based disease!

The ego-self perceives the Creation and the circumstances of life through filters distorted by lack of basic trust and persuades the soul that the Creation is not holding, perfect and loving.

Reference

1   Campbell J. *The Hero with a Thousand Faces*. Noveto CA: New World Library. 2008. Chapter One.

21

THE BIRTH OF THE EGO-SELF

Ego-self

In absolute terms, the Self – the Being, Essence or Divinity at the heart of the psyche – is the *archetype of archetypes*. On the platform of the relative plane, the ego-self, the usurper false-self, is the *architect of archetypes*, for its presence and influence in the life of every soul gives rise to the diversity of archetypes playing out the destiny of the world. Whereas, the Self or Spirit is eternal, numinous and one with the Universal Consciousness, the ego-self is transient, protean and discrete: a creature of duality. It is the ego-dragon that mantles the Divinity of the psyche and calls the hero-soul forth to do battle for this treasure of all treasures.

It is true to say that there is nothing that exists, nor anything that we can sense or in any way apprehend, visible or invisible, that is not the Universal Consciousness, the Absolute, the Cause without a cause. This includes ourselves. Yet, here, a profound paradox exists, for the relative dimension is ever a sphere of paradox. The ego-self that challenges the soul for dominion over the psyche is for that soul the only aspect of the entire creation that *is not Divinity*. The paradox is fully perceived, when it is understood that that self-same ego-self that is not Divinity to the soul it challenges, *is Divinity* to all other souls, even when in the guise of a Hitler or a Harold Shipman. This is a profound concept, difficult to comprehend, but when understood, makes the soul aware of its most pressing responsibility: the disempowering of the ego-self and its elimination as a force within the psyche, for the soul can only merge with its Essence or Divinity when the ego-self ceases to stand between the two. And, the soul is made conscious of being immersed in an ocean of Divinity – *an ocean of love* – no matter what is transpiring in the 'Now'!

Every substance is permeated by Universal Consciousness; every living form is animated by soul, possesses a level of sentience and is subject to the basic instincts of the Id. As evolution produces higher forms, so the soul force animating them expands its influence, gains greater expression and independence. Within all life an evolutionary drive exists, blueprinted by the Universal Consciousness, mediated by the Id, catalysed by the evolving soul principle, executed by genetic mutation and screened by natural selection and survival of the fittest. From the interplay of these creative forces, the resplendent beauty and infinite artistry of our living planet come into being. Contrary to the conclusions of materialistic science, nothing is random, everything is designed with intent, aesthetic awareness, an eye for excellence and fashioned with love!

In the beginning, cosmology informs us that there was only the singularity, an infinitely dense, infinitely small, infinitely powerful point of absolute potential. From the moment this point suddenly expanded in an immense explosion of energy – creating space, time, cause and effect – the One created the many – Unity created duality. Archetypally, the cardinal duality of the relative plane arises through separation of the Cosmic or Sacred Feminine (*Yin*) and the Cosmic or Sacred Masculine (*Yang*); a division that occurs at the very moment of creation. From the brooding blackness of the Void, the Womb of the Cosmic Feminine (the Great Mother Goddess) emerges the dynamic red of the Cosmic Masculine, giving form, substance, structure and motion to the Creation. In this sequence, the Cosmic Feminine is the primary creative force.

The divergence of the two fundamental archetypal forces of the Cosmos is momentous for it sets the stage for the hero's journey through 'the shadow of the valley of death', laying down a primordial dichotomy within the psyche: a schism that underlies the contention between age-old adversaries: the hero soul (*Yin*) and the trickster ego-self (*Yang*): a struggle that will initiate the psychic discord that leads to disease. The 'hero path' is the soul's arduous journey towards individuation and the attainment of the Sacred Emerald, the gem of love – the mythical Holy Grail: a quest that necessitates the psychic merging of the feminine and masculine principles: a conclusion that heals through unseating the imposter (the ego-self) and restoring the rightful heir (the soul) to the throne of the psyche.

Genesis is an archetypal event of stupendous proportions. The vast scale of its physical phenomena is tangible evidence of the action, direction and intent of invisible, sentient forces. This design is played out not only cosmically, but also archetypally, for the universe, in all its majesty and magnificence, is expressly created for the ascent of the individual soul from innocence to omniscience. At the birth of a baby, the entire Cosmos is focussed on the event; an empathetic attention that never abates throughout life on earth and life in the hereafter. As in the expanding universe, where galaxies are hurtling apart towards infinity and the elements in stellar alchemy increase progressively in atomic weight, so the separation of *Yin* and *Yang* archetypally is dynamic, and, while continuous, increasingly perturbs the homeostasis of the psyche. The separation *is born on the wings of consciousness and intellect. Yang* intellect/logic parts from *Yin* instinct/intuition and the two will only merge again through *wisdom*.

As the primitive, aboriginal mind advances from the uncluttered simplicity of a life close to nature – primed with psychic faculties alert to the unseen world beyond the physical and conscious of the guidance of ancestors – towards intellectual and technological complexity, the soul forsakes the warm, nurturing feminine embrace of *Yin* (mythos, nature, instinct, intuition) and is drawn into the cold, harsh, masculine world of *Yang* (logos, science, civilisation, intellect). At the extreme point of divergence between the feminine and the masculine stand the godless, the amoral, the fanatical, the implacable, the cruel and the totally materialistic; those in whom the feminine is utterly stilled and the masculine ego-self is rampant. This state parallels the remote reaches of the cosmos and the archetypal qualities of the heaviest elements.

One day, the expansion of the universe will reach the critical point when energy needed for further expansion is expended; the force of gravity will become supreme and contraction of the universe begins. As in the cosmos, so in the psyche: as the soul gains ascendency over the ego-self, the power of the ego-self wanes; *Yin* and *Yang* will converge and finally unite as the soul achieves individuation (Self-realisation). Consciousness is the catalyst that promotes both divergence and convergence of the feminine and masculine within the psyche: *intellect separates the two forces, wisdom unites them*. In the divergent dynamic, intellect and the elaboration of the ego-self are entangled. Conversely, wisdom, the demise of the ego-self and the convergence of the feminine and masculine principles are entangled.

As the soul evolves from animal innocence towards intellectual sophistication, the polarities of duality and the elaboration of the ego-self put the soul to the test. The advent of the ego-self is an inevitable consequence of burgeoning intellect and essential for the spiritual progress and transcendence of the soul. *The hero-soul must have an opponent.*

The presence of the ego-self is heralded in animal life, evidenced in the differing 'personality traits' displayed by members of the same species when responding to a common challenge in the wild, even when difference in gender, age and experience is discounted. Varied behavioural response, based on innate 'personality', increases as creatures ascend the hierarchical pyramid of life and is distinct among carnivores, reaching greatest disparity among apex predators. The presence of individual personality is clearly manifest among primates, most developed in the great apes and very marked in our closest relative, the chimpanzee. In the higher primates, the defining of personality comes with expanding *animal consciousness*, emotional capacity and the development of social and hierarchical relationships. Jane Goodall, the English primatologist, ethologist and anthropologist, who for more than 50 years studied the behaviour of wild chimpanzees in Gombe Stream National Park, Tanzania, was at first impressed by the harmony of life within chimpanzee troops. She was touched by their gentleness and their capacity for altruism and found them, 'for the most part, nicer than human beings'. Only later did she discover that chimpanzees can be brutal – that they, like us, have a darker side to their nature[1] – that bullying, jealousy, hatred, selfishness, infanticide, kidnapping, gang-warfare, cruelty and murder are all part and parcel of chimpanzee behaviour: sure signs of the presence of the invidious ego-self.

Despite these warning signs, *animal consciousness* is generally ruled by the innate wisdom of instinct. Duality in the animal world remains a harmonious interplay between the masculine and feminine principles. *Yang* gives the alpha male or female aggressiveness, boldness and assertiveness, while relative lack of *Yang* causes the beta male or female to show less of these traits and display submissive behaviour. The earliest signs of increased intelligence, emotional capacity and ego-personality usually remain wholesome and balanced, governed by hierarchical dynamics and the ritualistic enactment of domination and submission, in which all conflicts are resolved without hurt and the homeostasis of the troop or pack is preserved. The strongest and most assertive alpha male exercises sexual precedence, which ensures the propagation of the most positive emotional and physical characteristics.

The departure from homeostasis must have progressively occurred as *hominid-human emotional and intellectual consciousness* passed a critical transition point that released our pre-human or early human ancestors from the innate wisdom and restraints of instinct. A momentous change, impossible to capture anthropologically, but frozen forever in the myth of Adam and Eve and the Garden of Eden when, at the instigation of the serpent (the embodiment of the duplicitous ego-self), the innocent primal pair ate of the apple of the Tree of Knowledge of Good and Evil – the tree of intellect and duality – and were banished from Paradise (instinctive wisdom). Although, later manipulated by the patriarchy to place the blame for man's downfall firmly on the shoulders of 'woman', this myth exemplifies how a simple parable can encapsulate concepts of great import.

Judging from chimpanzee behaviour, this transition could have come about remarkably early in hominid evolution and over a relatively brief period. It was primed to happen! As much as we may conjecture that the early-hominids, Australopithicus and Paranthropus, were more prone to ego-based social unrest than modern-day chimpanzees, we cannot determine how severe this might have been. Nor can anthropology define when the ego-self first began to seriously disturb homeostasis. But, there are certain anatomical and cultural signs, which, taken together, provide us with a time period in human evolution when the ego-self was definitely well established. There are important indicators: the advent of a sophisticated tool technology; anatomical changes in the human skull indicating the potential for complex speech; death awareness and an after-life philosophy, evidenced in burial rites and respect for the dead; and engagement in cave painting. These were definitely all in evidence around 50,000 years ago, at the start of the Upper Palaeolithic, when the evolution of human culture quite suddenly accelerated.

The symbolic Eden scenario must, therefore, have taken place far earlier and we can justifiably surmise that the ego-self began to interfere in 'human' welfare possibly as early as *Homo erectus* (1.9 million to 70,000 years ago) and certainly amongst *archaic humans*: a broad category of pre-modern humans that includes *Homo heidelbergensis* and the Neanderthals (*Homo neanderthalensis*). The latter, appeared some 200,000 years ago and died out in Europe more or less 40,000 years ago. The Neanderthal genome differs from modern humans by only 0.12%. This small difference produced a far more robust, powerful frame and markedly coarser features, characterised by a very long, large, wide nose, a low brow and a receding chin. However, the Neanderthals were by no means unintelligent; they made advanced tools, buried their dead and probably communicated by speech. Their extinction was in all likelihood due to more than one factor. About 55,000 years ago, the weather in Europe began to fluctuate wildly between extreme cold and more temperate conditions. The heavily built Neanderthals, although well suited to survival in severe cold, could not adapt to these extreme swings, which impacted on their preferred habitat and made subsistence difficult. However, of more importance than climate change must have been the increasing movement of modern humans into the Neanderthal range. History always tends to repeat itself and if we reflect on the fate of the Native Americans, the Incas, the Arctic Inuits, the Aboriginal Australians and other indigenous peoples round the world; it takes little imagination to conjure a scenario of discrimination, displacement, abuse, violent conflict and genocide. All signs of a well-established aggressive, rapacious ego-self.

Given that *Homo heidelbergensis*, the common ancestor of the Neanderthals and modern humans, evolved from *Homo erectus* at least 600,000 years ago, it is safe to presume that the mythical confrontation between Adam and Eve and the snake was prior to this. Though speculative, these reflexions give a rough estimate of how long ago the ego-self began to emerge as a disruptive force in the human psyche and kindled the evolution of the chronic miasms.

Once the human mind became independent of instinct and attained freedom of choice (ate of the fruit of the Tree of Knowledge), humanity inevitably began to step out of harmony with Nature's laws. As the ego-self assumed dominance over the soul, the duality within the human psyche became exaggerated and the divergence of the feminine and masculine principles increased to subversive proportions. Hierarchical precedence and ritualistic dominance and submission were superseded by the self-serving imperatives of the ego-self.

The ancient texts chronicle the dire consequences of this transition from instinctive (primarily *Yin*) to intellectual life (primarily *Yang*) in the biblical myth of Cain and Abel, the sons of Adam and Eve. Coming so early in Genesis, the myth reflects age-old wisdom regarding the nature of the ego-self and its duplicitous, destructive nature. Cain, the elder brother, became a farmer and tilled the land, whereas his younger brother, Abel, became a shepherd tending his flocks. When the time came for the brothers to give offerings to the 'Lord' (Mother Nature), Cain presented produce he had grown on the land and Abel presented some newly born lambs with their fat. Mother Nature acknowledged the younger son's offering with pleasure and gratitude but disregarded and rejected the elder son's offering. Cain was 'furious and downcast'. Mother Nature asked Cain why he was so angry and when Cain remained silent, Mother Nature explained that if he had given unconditionally, out of the goodness of his heart, without desire for reward (as Abel had done), his offering would have been accepted. As he had given only out of desire for praise and recognition, 'sin crouches at the door'. For his gift to be acceptable, he had to first master his self-serving desires and learn to give out of love and generosity. Filled with resentment, indignation, anger, envy and hate (emotions characteristic of the ego-self), Cain defiantly turned his back on Mother Nature and invited Abel to accompany him into the fields. There, once out of sight, 'he rose up against Abel, his brother, and killed him!'

Yet again, a well-known myth sums up, in a few telling images, the difference between functioning through the scheming, egotistical desires of the ego-self and the effortless, bountiful flow of unqualified goodness celebrated by living through the soul. Though simple, the parable encapsulates extreme complexity. It does not equivocate, it exposes the worst villainy of the ego-self: the primal sin – fratricide – the murder of a sibling soul! The murder portrayed is symbolic; it does not have to be physical; far worse, is the slow, insidious, emotional murder perpetrated in so many homes and in so many of society's institutions. The story highlights core, negative emotions that are primed within the structure of the ego-self. All are based on fear: the original emotion forming the foundation of the ego-self due to the young soul's lack of basic trust as it moves out of the warm embrace of instinctual life (*Yin*) into the glare of life lived through the intellect (*Yang*). Unconsciously, the soul feels severed from Mother Nature (*Yin*), exposed, naked and impotent. The ego-self, the *Yang* warrior, takes shape as a compensation for these deficiencies and built into its armour forged from doubt, fear and suspicion are resentment, anger, defiance and rebelliousness. Envy, pride and hatred are ever on call; disillusionment, depression and despair will be their legacy.

The myth highlights the sense of entitlement and expectation of reward that are so characteristic of ego-self motivation and behaviour. If thwarted, this presumption arouses grievance and anger against Mother Nature – Providence (*Yin*) – 'God'; jealousy and hatred towards those whom Mother Nature has blessed (the pure and innocent of spirit [*Yin*]); and the repudiation of guidance (intuitive wisdom [*Yin*]). A fatal step follows: defiance and a vindictive, retaliatory act against Mother Nature (*Yin*) – against the 'Lord' they *consciously disown and deny, but unconsciously resent and hate*. The victim against whom this arrogant, masculine pique is directed is the helpless, innocent child of Mother Nature, the very embodiment of *Yin* – Abel – the wolf – the rhino – the environment! The interplay of forces denotes the divergence of the masculine principle from the feminine: a separation that fosters tension and conflict and leads to the abuse of the feminine: the tragedy of human life and the root of disease. *The primal eldest sin: a brother's murder, was an act of misogyny!*

Cain's reaction to the rejection of his offering and Mother Nature's reprimand, demonstrates his unmitigated hubris, his recalcitrance, his rejection of Divinity, his contempt for spiritual values and his willingness to sacrifice others to salvage his pride and display his rebellious independence. These are brazen attributes of the ego-self.

And Mother Nature asked of Cain,
"Where is Abel, thy brother?"
Sullenly, Cane lied,
"I know not!"

And then, with incomparable insolence, he petulantly blurted out,
"Am I my brother's keeper?"
Mother nature asked again,
"What hast thou done?"

When Cain made no reply, Mother nature, showing that nothing is ever hidden, declared:

"The voice of thy brother crieth unto me from the ground."[2]

In succinct terms, Mother Nature reveals to Cain what life transgressed by the ego-self entails:

> And now art thou cursed from the earth, which hath opened her mouth to receive thy brother's blood from thy hand. When thou tillest the ground, it shall not henceforth yield unto thee her strength; a fugitive and a vagabond shalt thou be in the earth.[3]

The ego-self creates its own reality, visioned through warped perspective and convoluted by delinquent behaviour. Life's events faithfully reflect the distortion, which is evidenced in the strife and despair that beset humanity. Out of touch with Divinity and Mother Nature, the vagrant ego-self is a fearful fugitive on planet Earth.

At last, Cain responds from a deeper level of his psyche: "My punishment is greater than I can bear." There is a trace of soul in his acknowledgement of punishment for misdoing and in his expression of hopelessness. In his lament, he concedes the existence of a Supreme Being and his need for its influence and protection in his life:

> Behold thou hast driven me out this day from the face of the earth; *and from thy face shall I be hid* ... everyone that findeth me shall slay me.[4]

The answer of Mother Nature was for all souls, not only Cain:

> "Therefore, whosoever slayeth Cain (soul), vengeance shall be taken on him sevenfold."

And Mother Nature set a mark on Cain (ego-self) lest any finding him (soul) should slay him.[5]

The mark of Cain is branded upon the ego-self, distinguishing it from the soul. To perceive the *mark of Cain* in others is to recognise the actions of the ego-self and not to judge or 'slay' (condemn) the soul it masks, whether it be a Caligula or a Jeffrey Dahmer. No matter the vilest deeds perpetrated by others, the enlightened observer knows that paradoxically everything that transpires through such deeds is perfect and necessary. Those who are implicated are souls in transit, living out their archetypal destiny, providing others with challenges vital to their unfolding.

When a myth or parable is deciphered in this way, the method used is the same as for the analysis of dreams, since, as Joseph Campbell stated, myths are universal dreams and a dream is a personal myth. Dream analysis is invaluable to the practice of homeopathy. The indicated remedy will often call forth directive wisdom from the patient's higher-self in dream form. As thematic dreams change their content, they become a means of measuring progress. When initial layers of disease have been peeled away, *a significant dream may announce the need for a change of remedy and provide clues for its selection.*

In interpreting the meaning of ancient texts, allowance must be made for symbolic terminology, which if taken literally would at times seem excessive, e.g. the 'Lord's' words: vengeance, slaying and sevenfold – depicting an extremely wrathful, vengeful, autocratic divinity: a warped projection from the human ego-self unfortunately impressed upon the Abrahamic religions down the ages; subtly contributing to miasmatic disease through indoctrination and religious fear. A key rubric that stands out in this regard is *doubt of soul's welfare*, containing: *Arsenicum; *Aurum; *Lachesis; *Pulsatilla; *Lil-tig*; *Sulphur*; *Veratrum*; Belladonna; Calc-carb; Crocus; Cyclamen; Digitalis; Hyoscyamus; Kola; Lycopodium; Nux-vom; Selenium; Stramonium. Note the presence of the three members of the toxic *Solanaceae*: Belladonna, Stramonium and Hyoscyamus: key archetypes in the conflict between the soul and the 'beast principle' of the psyche.

Applied to the individual, '*vengeance*' pertains to the dire consequence of 'bad' action and '*slaying*' to the prejudiced judgment and condemnation of others, but applied to the propensities of humanity at large, the immediate meaning of the words remains apt, for vengeance and slaying abound on planet Earth.

With this myth in hand, it is possible to return to the evolutionary setting, and provide a human narrative. With expanding intellect and increasing freedom of choice (eating of the Tree of Knowledge of Good and Evil) ominous changes took place in the dynamics of hominid life. The villain of the piece strides onto centre stage: the *ego-self Cain, the perpetrator*, the dominant alpha figure charged with the aggressive aspect of the Id (*Yang*). The submissive beta figure, embodying the libido aspect of the Id (*Yin*), is the *victimised ego-self Abel*. Released from instinctive control, the hierarchical and ritualistic behaviour essential to the harmony and security of troop or tribe becomes unstable and subject to the tyranny of the ego-self. The abuse of Abel by Cain commences and the psoric miasm takes root, born of deficiency, fear and grief. Overtime, domination becomes oppression, oppression becomes persecution and persecution becomes genocide. Aggression, no longer simply a display of strength to express and exert dominance, is acted out in cruel, malicious, murderous ways and submission becomes deprivation, subjugation and enslavement. The 'haves' and 'have-nots' are soon established in early human society: the broad-based Cane and Abel psoric archetypes, represented by Sulphur (alpha) and Psorinum (beta), respectively, and their infantile forms: the aggressive, angry, high-stool tyrant, Chamomilla (alpha) and its counter-part, the timid, weeping, nursery pushover Pulsatilla (beta).

In all this, we find ethology, psychology, miasmatic theory, materia medica, mythology and symbolism coming together seamlessly.

The Cain and Abel dynamic within the psyche is inevitable and integral to the contention between soul (*Yin*) and ego-self (*Yang*); a conflict that catalyses the attainment of Self. The implicit nature of abuse of the feminine by the masculine indicates that it is inherent to duality; it is primordial and archetypal and does not owe its origin to secondary factors such as cultural-era, social mores or religious doctrines. These merely exaggerate or mitigate its expression. The mastering of this phenomenon is personal to each one of us; like Mother Nature, we too, regardless of our gender, must put the mark of Cain on our ego-self, know *him* well and never ingenuously take *his* hand and be led into the fields.

The primordial nature of the split between the feminine and masculine principles is graphically and aptly demonstrated in the evolutionary path taken by our closest living relatives: the bonobo (*Pan paniscus*) and the common chimpanzee (*Pan troglodytes*) of Central Africa, which share 98% of our genome.

Re-enacting, the divergence of *Yin* and *Yang*, some 1.5 to 2 million years ago, the formation of the Congo River divided the common ancestor of the two *Pan species* into two geographical groups: one north of the river and the other south of the river. Because of the expanse of water and the indif-ferent swimming ability of these primates, the two groups remained perma-nently separated, and, over time, speciation took place.

Symbolically, the manner of the rift is significant. Water is the metaphor for the unconscious, personal and collective; it is also the symbol for intuitive and received wisdom and for the flow of destiny. The river itself possesses an added connotation. Swollen with waters from many sources, the great river flows inexorably towards the ocean with which it merges, allegorically portraying the return of all diversity and differentiation to its boundless origin: the primal, undifferentiated state of Unity. Implicit to the Cosmic return is the conjugation of the supreme opposites, *Yin* and *Yang*, a blessed union, which, lived out in the dynamics of the psyche, denotes the demise of the ego-self.

In Hinduism, the Ganges, is personified as Ganga, the supreme river goddess [*Yin*], who is depicted in myth as cascading from heaven, cush-ioned and channelled by Shiva [*Yang*], cleansing the earth [conscious mind] and penetrating to the underworld [unconscious mind]. Similarly, in Middle Eastern philosophy, the image of a heavenly stream flowing down vertically through the World Axis or Tree of Life in Paradise, and then flowing horizontally to the four points of the compass, was a similar metaphor for divine energy and spiritual nourishment coursing through the whole universe. Each of the four cardinal quadrants of Gaia is permeated by one of the four emanations of the Tree of Life, bestowing upon each their unique symbolic and archetypal attributes.

Viewed metaphorically, the cleaving of western-equatorial Africa by the Congo, dividing the ancestral *Pan* ape's domain into North and South, is powerfully archetypal and has deep esoteric meaning. Like a dream, the event and its consequences unfold before intuition's eye, disclosing the wisdom of a deeper reality revealed by the apotheosis of the river.

Each of the four compass points possesses specific archetypal attributes. This was well known to the various tribes of Native Americans. Not unexpectedly, North and South bear opposite symbolism and whereas North is perceived to be predominantly masculine (*Yang*), South is understood to be predominantly feminine (*Yin*).

The North encompasses the energy and environment of the far Northern hemisphere: the lands of ice and snow; soaring, ice-capped, mountain ranges; temperate forests; the mighty belt of iron ore and coal-deposits that provided the tools for human, technological acumen. This is the quadrant dominated by the masculine, *Yang*, attributes of intellectual knowledge, logical understanding and deductive reason – the zone of invention, discovery and reductionist science – the world of the Sulphur and Ferrum archetypes. It is the source of the explorer, the adventurer, the conqueror and the warrior, and, set loose upon the South: of the Visigoth, the Viking, the Hun, the Tartar and the Conquistador, whose bloodthirsty warmongering and rapacious aggression are proverbial. The North encompasses both ice and fire – intellect and war.

Though typified by life far north of the tropics, this Northern archetypal force pervades the planet. No matter where one stands, north remains archetypally North, and for the south-placed observer bears the Northern stamp. In present times, this dynamic is starkly displayed by the opposing ideologies of North and South Korea.

North is always associated with West; both are dominantly *Yang*. The West and East quadrants are not defined symbolically by longitude in the way North and South are defined by latitude. West symbolises the culture and materialistic philosophy of the Western World and East symbolises the culture and spiritual philosophy of the Eastern World.

North of the Congo, the *Yang* influence upon the ancestral *Pan* ape was derived from both North and West, whereas, south of the Congo it stemmed from South and East. While North's orientation is intellectual,

West is pragmatic, materialistic, grounded and goal-focussed, all predominantly masculine perspectives. Its primal element is earth. In concert, on the material plane, North and West, masculine fire and earth, overpower and subordinate, South and East, feminine water and air.

South, like North, holds sway over the entire expanse of Gaia. South is always archetypally South, no matter how far north one's position may be. This may best be understood by comparing the intellectually controlled Scandinavian or Swiss temperament with the emotionally expressive Spanish or Italian temperament. Though both stereotypes evolved north of the equator, their obvious differences exemplify the archetypal effect of their position relative to each other.

The focus of South is far more emotional than intellectual, and the quadrant evinces the *Yin* attributes of empathy, caring, nurturing, inclusiveness, artistic expression, aesthetic sensitivity, trust and adherence to faith. It fosters sensitivity, imagination, fantasy, creativity and devotional fervour and favours music over the clash of arms, romance over ambition, leisure before industry and making love rather than waging war. Softness prevails in the south and hardness rules in the north (Hitler would have done well to heed this when he relied so heavily on his southern-allies). Water is the element associated with this quadrant and fittingly it was water that delineated the southern and northern ancestral *Pan* territories in Central Africa millions of years ago.

South is always associated with East; both are dominantly *Yin*. East is the beginning, the awakening, the dawn of realisation and the ascent towards the light of spiritual wisdom. East heralds the advent of the hero and the beginning of the hero's journey on the spiritual path towards Self-realisation (individuation). Its primal element is air. Air levitates earth and water quenches fire; when dominant and in concert, South and East sublimate the attributes of North and West and bring transcendence.

These four quadrants represent *morphogenetic fields* (for convenience and ease of expression, termed: *morphic fields*): fields that can determine the pattern, structure or form of things; hold and transmit collective memory and instinctual behaviour in species; and influence the emotions, thinking, behaviour and creativity of individuals and even nations. In theory, if animals learn a new skill in one place, similar animals raised under similar conditions should subsequently tend to learn the same thing more readily all over the world.[6] At a deeper level, morphic fields hold all archetypal memory: a spectrum of frequencies bearing the image of all that has been, is and will be: a repository of archetypal forms, which can be formatively and creatively activated through resonance: a vibratory accord that is keened and amplified by intent, focus and repetition.

This hypothesis is termed *formative causation*, which affirms that all plants and animals draw upon and contribute to the collective memory of their species. The memory held within the field of nature is known as *morphic resonance*. Rupert Sheldrake, an English biological scientist and researcher in parapsychology, elucidated these controversial concepts in his books: *A New Science of Life*[7] and *The Presence of the Past*.[8] Of the latter work, Professor Paul Davies of Arizona State University, an eminent English physicist, cosmologist and astrobiologist wrote,

> Bold, clear and incisive . . . a sweeping challenge to the very fundamentals of established science.[9]

These words, written by the best science writer either side of the Atlantic, recognised the gauntlet thrown down by Sheldrake in the face of accepted scientific opinion. The response highlighted the hidebound inflexibility and severely limiting, materialistic fundamentalism inherent in scientific thinking. After some favourable reviews in scientific journals, the community woke to the very real challenge posed by this erudite 'heretic' within its midst and closed its ranks. His theories were repudiated as an exercise in pseudoscience and he was discounted as a misguided eccentric. His genuineness, concern for truth, persuasive eloquence, clarity of thought and public appeal only add to the quite heated rebuttals he evokes; a sure sign that his ideas expose weaknesses in the scientific paradigm, just as homeopathy has always done.

Sheldrake's theories complement homeopathic science and accord with the concept that water and rectified spirits (medicinal alcohol) can be imprinted with the memory of an archetype and 'downloaded' into the constitution of an individual with whom the image resonates to bring about a healing response. Formative causation and morphic resonance may be compared with Jung's theory of the collective unconscious, in which all individuals draw from and contribute to the collective memory of humanity and repeated patterns of thinking, perceiving and behaving coalesce and shape archetypal profiles. In accordance with the hypothesis of formative causation, the four quadrants of the compass are morphic fields of formative energy, each resonating with its respective archetypal image and capable of exerting a corresponding affect upon organisms evolving within its sway.

In the Congo, the permanent division of the territory of the common chimpanzee ancestor into a northern and southern zone, separated by a great river, had a remarkable effect on the evolutionary path taken by the two groups of apes, despite their common origin and the close similarity of their habitat. The genetic starting point for each was identical. The only variable was the respective morphic field within which each of the two species would evolve. Over a period of less than a million years these patterned fields inexorably persuaded remarkable emotional and physical differences to emerge between the species and these changes were consonant with the archetypal power of the cardinal points of the compass as intuited by the Amerindians.

North of the river, the common chimpanzee, *Pan troglodytes*, evolved from the ancestral form, as it did in other areas of West and Central Africa and also in Gombe where Jane Goodall made her studies of chimpanzee behaviour. This northern species, the 'chimp' most familiar to humans, is powerful and robust and lives in strictly male-dominated hierarchies in which disputes are generally settled without resort to violence. However, top-ranking males tend to be highly aggressive even during dominance stability, though ritualistic display is generally preferred over violence. It takes little provocation to make a chimp raise its hair, pick up a branch and challenge and intimidate anyone perceived as weaker than themselves: they are very much into status.[10] Dominant males are often in dispute, backed by lower ranking males, who are characteristically fickle in their support, regularly changing sides and ever alert to sexual opportunities that arise when dominant males are preoccupied with each other. Social hierarchies among adult females are much weaker. Common chimpanzees are highly territorial and far more likely to be violently aggressive over land-rights than over mates. As Jane Goodall reported, chimps patrolling borders are extraordinarily hostile to males from outside the community and may brutally attack intruders, often killing single males.

South of the river, lives the bonobo, *Pan paniscus*, the endangered and 'forgotten ape', some 30- to 50-thousand individuals clinging to a dwindling habitat; poached and hunted for bushmeat by the heavily armed militias in the area. Due to the war-ravaged state of the central Congo, and the animal's timidity, very little fieldwork has been done.

Previously called the pygmy chimpanzee, this gentle, peace-loving ape is more refined, gracile and less robust than the common chimpanzee. It has relatively long legs, pink lips, a dark face, a tail-tuft through adulthood and long parted hair on its head. While large male chimpanzees far exceed any bonobo male in bulk and weight, there is little difference in their height. The bonobo's posture when walking bipedally, gives it an appearance more like a human than a common chimpanzee and its appreciably longer legs enhance this impression. Like humans, bonobo facial features are clearly different one from another and very mobile, indicating that facial recognition and expression are important when socialising and communicating. Their society, in contrast to the chimpanzee, is entirely

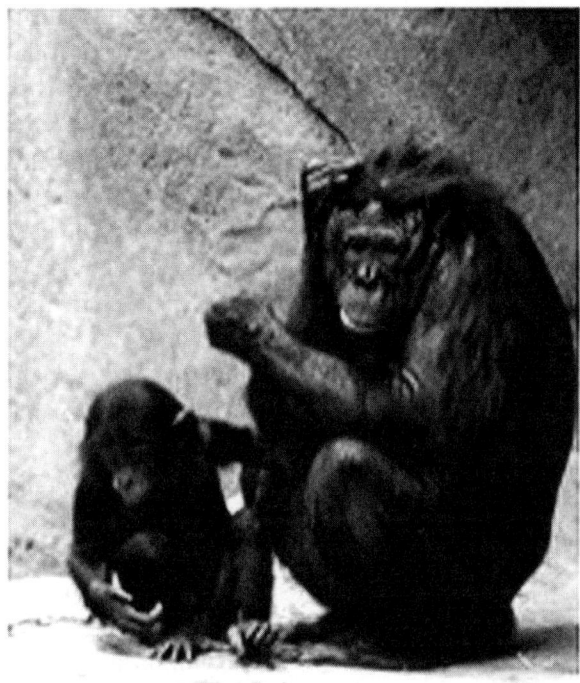

Figure 21.1 Bonobo mother Lana, age 25, and daughter Kesi, 2, at the San Diego Zoo in 2006

Credit: WH Calvin: Ape Bonobo San Diego Zoo

matriarchal; females are dominant and enjoy higher status than males. Males derive their standing in the ape community not from their own alpha qualities, but from the status enjoyed by their mothers. The mother-son bond is very strong and remains so throughout life; any attempt to sever this alliance leads to protective, female aggression. In accord with this feminine domination, Bonobos are more inclined to express altruism, compassion, empathy, kindness, tolerance, patience and sensitivity than the common chimpanzee and they are considerably less aggressive.[7]

Sexual activity plays an important and diverse role in bonobo society, being used as a greeting, for bonding, and as a means to decrease tension, avoid conflict and seek reconciliation. Significantly, the bonobo is the only non-human animal known to engage in face-to-face sexual activity, tongue kissing and oral sex. Bonobos engage in sex in virtually every possible partner combination, putting paid to Freud's persuasion that homosexuality is pathological and a perversion of the normal sex drive. Their eroticism is so varied it borders on the imaginative rather than being merely instinctive, but it is always relaxed, non-aggressive, casual and affectionate.

Although their sexual appetite is high, reproduction rate is low. As with humans, the libido has been released from its purely procreative role and is motivated by affection, bonding and pleasure, aspects that are ignored by ideologies that condemn non-reproductive sex. From the example set by these closest cousins of ours, it is clear that very few human sexual practices can be regarded as unwholesome and unnatural.[7] This is of great import given how often moralistic imprinting blights human sexuality with the belief that sex is somehow intrinsically dirty and sinful.

Unlike chimpanzees, Bonobo males and females prefer sexual contact with outsiders to aggressive display and violence. When members of different communities meet, they may mingle socially, have sex and groom one another; behaviour never observed among common chimpanzees. It is clear that Bonobos would much rather make love than war!

Research has revealed distinct differences between the brains of bonobos and chimps. The bonobo brain is more developed than that of the chimpanzee in those regions thought to be vital for sensitivity to the distress of others and for feelings of anxiety. There is also a more extensive neuronal connection between the amygdala, the repository of emotional memory, and the anterior cortex, the keyboard of the will, indicating better impulse control, more forethought and caution.[11]

Inexplicably, the bonobo is not vulnerable to infection with the simian immunodeficiency virus (SIV), which is found in at least 45 species of African primates, including the common chimpanzee. The SIV retrovirus is believed to have crossed the species barrier from the common chimpanzee and the sooty mangabey monkey into humans, resulting in HIV-1 and HIV-2, respectively. Infected, wild chimpanzees would seem to suffer from an AIDS-like sickness similar to human HIV-1 patients. Since it is estimated that SIV has been present in monkeys and chimpanzees for over 30,000 years and probably much longer,[12] its failure to infect the bonobo, so closely related to the chimpanzee, is startling and demands explanation.

Unless one is a mainstream scientist, the natural history of the two *Pan* species of ape, one north of the Congo and one to the south, provides a clear instance of the role morphic fields and formative causation play in the evolution of life forms and the development of behavioural characteristics. Projected onto the human stage, it is apparent that given resonance these fields exert a modelling effect on constitution, disposition and behaviour. The diversifying influence of the primordial feminine and masculine principles on form, features, feelings and functions is clear to see, as is their distinct channelling of the basic instincts of the Id; the masculine North favouring aggression and the feminine South favouring the libido aspect. The masculine principle encourages the selfish, aggressive traits of the ego-self, while the feminine principle brings out traits that are caring, inviting and embracing – qualities pertaining to the soul. Both extremes are coupled to physical characteristics that reflect these qualities – coarse, muscular and robust north of the river – refined, gentle and gracile to the south.

A presiding ego-self with a dominant masculine and recessive feminine energy is the most potent cause of miasmatic disease. When life is lived through the soul rather than the ego, the feminine is dominant, but fortified by an empowering, recessive masculine energy: a combination that gives emotional and physical resilience and resistance to disease. These configurations explain the vulnerability to SIV of the masculine orientated chimpanzees in the north and the innate resistance to SIV of the feminine bonobo to the south. As always, the universality of Cosmic law is apparent. Sublimation towards soul-values and distancing from ego-self-desires constitutes a healing process, even in incurable and terminal disease.

As early as 1927, Ernst Schwartz (1889–1962), the German born anatomist who first stumbled on the bonobo and recognised it as a distinct species, compared life on the Parisian Left Bank of the Seine with the life of the bonobo living on the left bank of the Congo. Both rivers flow to the west, therefore, their left banks are to the south. His comparison was valid for the Left Bank of Paris has always been traditionally home to the Bohemian world of artists and writers, a world in which more feminine energy is to be found. It is less frenetic, less sophisticated, less materialistic and more laid-back than the north: a haven for the creative mind. This equates with the peaceful, relaxed, sexually orientated life of the bonobo and their unconventional ape society. The Parisian Right Bank, with its banks, business corporations and affluent tradition may be compared to the aggressive, competitive, masculine society of the chimpanzees north of the Congo.

Situated at the heart of Gaia, in the equatorial rain forests of Central Africa, close to the cradle of humanity, the tiny, threatened enclave of the gentle bonobo, surrounded and infiltrated by the male madness of internecine war and genocide, provides a poignant commentary on the present state of the planet and a stark profile of miasmatic disease. Knowing the infinite scope of formative causation and morphic resonance and the constant, powerful influence exerted by morphic fields that hold all images of life, the need to conserve these precious, innocent beings, who exemplify the way life should be lived, becomes doubly urgent.

Influences determining the development and nature of the ego-self

The influences contributing to the development of the ego-self are manifold. Their very number emphasises the inevitability of the ego-self's appearance in the life of the soul and its essential role as the soul's antagonist on the path to individuation.

- *Lack of basic trust – the prime influence, stemming from the soul itself* due to loss, into the Shadow of the psyche, of the nine Cosmic Concepts, Divine Aspects or soul Virtues that are the soul's spiritual heritage (perception of, surrender to and attunement with: universal Love, Wisdom, Truth [Oneness], Perfection, Harmony, Law, etc.). Although all nine Cosmic Concepts are lost to consciousness early in life, the individual soul is always most attuned to one of the nine, and, hence, most susceptible to its loss. The ego-self, or personality-type, that confronts the soul is a psychic structure unconsciously fashioned by the soul to compensate for the loss to consciousness of the specific Cosmic Concept with which the soul is especially attuned: *Ennea-type influences.*
- The incarnating soul departs the spirit world, descends onto the physical plane and is beset by a world of polarity (pain or pleasure) and paradox (soul- or ego-perception). The soul feels abandoned, alone and separate; it may feel that it has been banished from paradise and thus morally blighted, unworthy, un-loveable – a sinner. Having lost all sense of its immortal, spirit nature, the soul believes itself limited, vulnerable and mortal – a body, mind, ego-self complex – hence, it suffers: *incarnation influences.*
- The destined archetype: *archetypal influences.*
- Unresolved ego-characteristics carried over from previous lives: *karmic influences.*
- The morphogenetic field: *formative causation influences.*
- Holding environment: the degree of consistency, dependability and adequacy of the holding environment of the child: *nurturing influences.*
- Conditioning from parents, role models, culture, convention and religion: *imprinted influences.*
- Circumstances the individual is born into and the events of life: *situational influences.*
- Habits of thought, emotion and behaviour: *habitual influences.*
- Physiological and physical propensities: *genetic influences.*
- Chronic miasmatic disease: *miasmatic, constitutional influences.*
- Emotional and behavioural traits within the family: *familial influences.*

- Characteristics common to a particular race or nation: *racial influences.*

These influences, working together, build the psychological structure of the false- or ego-self: an influential, compensatory being able to compete with the soul, usurp its sovereignty of the psyche and impose its version of reality. This is evidenced in the millions of people gripped by emotions and feelings contrary to life lived from the perspective of Spirit. The combined weight of influences contributing to the emergence of the ego-self would seem insuperable, but what is intrinsically false, inferior and transient, cannot prevail over that which is true, perfect and eternal and the soul does not stand alone or unaided.

As complex and diverse as the ego-generative energies may seem, they are not arbitrary or at odds. They are drawn together to perfectly match the development and needs of the soul; a template created during the soul's long journey through lifetimes and constituted of the soul's spiritual strengths and weaknesses and particularly it's spiritually unresolved aspects and destined role in life. The disparate influences that combine to precisely correspond with the soul's level of unfoldment and needs, furnish an incarnation perfectly designed for the growth of the soul.

The trials, pitfalls and tragedies of life are opportunities for the evolving soul to hearken to the subtle, but insistent, call of the Self rather than the incessant clamour of the self-seeking ego-self. Whatever the challenge – the death of a loved one, the dashing of dearest hopes, the rupture of a relationship, the maiming of the body, a dread disease – life at its longest is short-lived and the soul and those it loves and loses are immortal; they cannot die! The vulnerability and suffering of the soul lies in its fealty to the ego-self, which has limited vision, is self-serving and fickle. The ego-self identifies with the body and the mind, and, regardless of the persuasiveness of imprinted faith, lacks trust and doubts immortality. The longest life is a mere blink of an eyelid in eternity, but to the ego-self, time is tedious during pain and fleeting during pleasure. The values of the ego-self are materialistic, and its sentiments are highly conditional. Child-like, it has a sense of entitlement and demands instant gratification. Like the serpent in the Garden of Eden, the ego-self persistently tempts the soul away from a life founded on spiritual values and attempts to impose its preferences, prejudices and perceptions on the soul. Even when in religious guise, protesting its faith with fervour, its belief system is the product of birth and conditioning; unquestioning, inflexible, often bigoted, yet wavering in the face of temptation and tragedy and liable to fanaticism.

Because of its eccentricities, faithfully forged from unwanted, unresolved and unrealised aspects of the soul, the ego-self is the ideal opponent for the hero-soul on its path towards Self-realisation.

The distorted perspectives of the ego-self draw the soul out of absolute Reality into relative reality: a 'delusion' of incorrect assumptions. These ego-based misconceptions create difficulties for the soul and elicit compensatory reactions. Emanating from the ego-self, the delusion, the difficulty and the reaction are out of tune with the spiritual path of the soul, impede its progress and challenge its integrity. The ego-induced trials and tribulations of the soul impinge on the emotional and physical health of the body, creating a disease patterned on the pernicious nature of the ego-self.

Deduced from this:

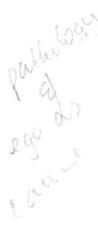

- *The ego-self is the disease that afflicts the soul.*
- *Being a permission of the soul, the ego-self is that part of the soul that requires healing.*
- *Being the disease of the soul, the ego-self is the disease of the body.*
- *The delusions of the ego-self and the difficulties and reactions they initiate, represent the very essence of disease.*

These concepts are crucial to understanding the fundamental nature of disease and to devising a curative healing regime. Despite whatever initiatory cause, chemical imbalance or structural change represents the perceptible aspects of disease, behind the scene stands the true culprit, the invidious, treacherous ego-self: the imposter who consummately slips into the role of the soul, lulling it into spiritual indolence and inertia; an imponderable adversary, proof against the weapons of conventional medicine, no matter how sophisticated. The body, mind and emotions are merely the playthings of the ego-self and therapy devised to counter its activities at these levels must fail. Only remedies sufficiently subtle to address the ego-self in the domain of the psyche and matched to its peculiar nature can unseat it. The most similar remedy in immaterial, potentised form has the necessary subtlety and accuracy to achieve success.

In the vanguard of the soul's defences stands the infinite power of the Id. Intolerant of ego-repression and chemical-suppression, the vital force, working ceaselessly and powerfully on behalf the soul, seeks to externalise and release negative forces generated by the ego-self in the *least harmful way possible*. This process must be recognised even in the worst clinical conditions, when the action of the vital force seems utterly self-destructive. Oft-times, because of grave constitutional disease and severe emotional trauma, soul-healing may even require a malignancy. The vital force, in directing the destructive energy of disease away from the mind and the emotions, may well threaten the life of the body; it would rather produce malignancy than permit insanity. A psychosis eclipses the soul and impedes its unfolding, while a malignancy, to a degree greater than most other diseases, weakens and erodes the ego-self. The refined sensitivity, deep compassion and altruism expressed in the profile of the cancer nosode, *Carcinosin*, are proof of this.

For all its power to subvert the soul, the ego-self structure is founded on weakness not strength. It takes shape as a compensation for the immaturity of the soul and its lack of basic trust in life. This lack of trust derives from identification with the body and the intellect; the perception that the processes of life are random, unthinking, pitiless and devoid of higher purpose; and from fear that the soul is beyond redemption or that death is the end of existence. The result is existential fear, which the ego-self attempts to seal-off from consciousness. It is a state of *primal terror*: a state encapsulated in what can be considered the primal remedy of the materia medica: Aconitum, commonly known as monk's hood or wolf's bane, a herb, which in myth, fittingly sprang from the saliva of Kerberos, the three-headed dog guarding the gates of the Underworld: the portal to the deep unconscious, to which such insupportable fear is relegated.

Primal fear is a combination of feeling disconnected, alienated, solitary and isolated; being expelled or rejected; being lost, abandoned, forsaken, threatened and in peril; and of being weak, defenceless and puny. This fear and these accompanying feelings and emotions – along with prolonged grief – provide the delusional foundation for the development of the psoric miasm upon which all other miasms are based. In volume three of *Healing the Soul*, we will pursue the evolution of the ego-self in the light of the five classic chronic miasms: *Psora –> Sycosis –> Syphilis –> Tuberculosis –> Carcinosis*.

Overcoming Cane

Healing the soul is an evolving spiritual process in accordance with Cosmic Intent. It is inseparable from individuation: the path of unconditional love and service that leads to Self-realisation. This being true, in addition to the primal power of the Id, there are many influences acting ceaselessly on behalf of the incarnated soul.

- Inspiration and guidance from the Self: the spark of Divinity at the heart of the soul.
- Inner dialogue with the higher-self (true-self) sensed intuitively and experienced through revelation and dreams.

Synchronicity

- Synchronicity: Cosmic cues, prompts and opportunities (significant coincidences).
- The support, guidance and inspiration of spirit helpers and guides attending and protecting the soul during its life journey.
- The circumstances of life – ever-orchestrated to the needs of the soul – life happens *for* the soul, not *to* the soul!
- The constellation of people the soul meets along the hero path from physical birth to physical death.
- Homeopathy and other forms of energy healing.
- Wise counselling from fellow-travellers.

In addition:

- Discerning the presence, influence and motives of the ego-self and recognising its cunning, self-seeking strategies (the "mark of Cane").
- Foiling the ego-self by:
  - Re-incorporation of the 'lost' Cosmic Concepts and Divine Aspects.
  - Alignment with the virtues of the Self – the Virtues of the Godly!
  - Positive surrender and adaptation to life's unfolding drama.
  - Passionate, creative, positive participation in the 'Now'.

Although the incarnated soul lacks awareness of the constant help, guidance and support of the Cosmos on its spiritual journey, they are ever-present. The soul's entire holding environment: situations and circumstances, significant people that constellate about it and its physical vehicle are a perfect prescription for the healing of the soul and the dismantling of the ego-self. Often the push that the soul needs to begin its spiritual odyssey comes in the form of a shock or loss, but gentler means can prove as persuasive for the sensitive soul already searching for spiritual truth: a remarkable blessing, a loving act, another's word or a passage from a book may be all that is needed for the journey to begin. Synchronicity is always operative, catalysing soul-healing by drawing the essential role-players and events together, seemingly by coincidence, but with purposeful intent.

Sometimes, the meaningful happening is the homeopathic consultation. The dynamic potencies of homeopathy specifically selected for the idiosyncrasies of the ego-self have the penetrative power and subtlety of action to touch the soul/ego level of experience, strengthening the soul's resolve, weakening the dominance of the ego-self and reducing inherited influences. The result is twofold: in the shorter term, improved emotional and physical health, and, in the longer term, *healing the soul of its ego-based disease.*

The encounter of homeopathic physician and patient is synchronistically timed, as are all events, but the meaningfulness of the exchange varies from patient to patient, even with a competent and experienced physician. Sometimes, the exchange is brief and inconclusive, often because the would-be patient is merely *'trying out'* homeopathy and being ignorant of the way homeopathy works and impatient for *'press-button'* results, fails to permit time for the healing process to unfold. Others are not ready for deep changes at the soul/ego level and are satisfied when the complaint for which they sought help has cleared. Fortunately, there are those whose time for healing at the deepest level has arrived; a time when physician, patient, spiritual need, circumstances, disease and homeopathic therapy come together in a sacred act of initiation, which ushers the patient into a new phase of life. Paracelsus considered healing at its deepest level to be healing of the soul, a process that requires the readiness (knowledge and skill) of the physician and the readiness (spiritual receptivity and preparedness) of the patient. Repeating his profound words noted in the first volume of this series:

> God has created remedies against diseases, and he has also created the physician; but He holds them back until the hour predestined for the patient. Only when the time has been fulfilled, and not before, does the course of nature and art set in.[13]

Important points to consider in overcoming ego-based disease:

- The patient's commitment and participation in the healing process.
- Emotional and physical symptoms and signs of illness are evidence that healing is required at a deeper level.
- The deepest level is the interface between the ego-self and the soul.
- The personality of the ego-self and its distorted perception of life (wrong assumptions, imaginings, misconceptions, delusions) the attendant difficulty and the compensatory reaction to the difficulty, lie at the core of ego-disease.
- The profile of the ego-self (the mark of Cane) is the most accurate guide to the selection of the correct remedy.
- The path to Self-realisation is a path of healing during which the soul overcomes the ego-self, replacing its values and perspectives with those of the Self (Abel must overcome and replace Cane).
- Healing at this level takes time, patience and perseverance.

- The healing work should ideally begin at the earliest opportunity, preferably prenatal, when the choice of homeopathic remedy is influenced by family history, outstanding characteristics of close family members, especially siblings, and by the mother's emotional and physical state: 'It is easier to build a child than repair an adult! (Greg Laurie).
- Early healing can avoid the fixations of the psychosexual development stages (see Chapters 23 and 24).

Levels of soul/ego attainment

From the influences previously enumerated, it is evident that even before birth important elements are already in place to bring about the elaboration of the soul/ego-self complex. To the endowed characteristics of the soul, derived from the experience of many previous incarnations, there are added inherited, constitutional and emotional characteristics built into the emotional/physical vehicle from various sources, all of which indicate marked disparity between individuals rather than the equality extolled by the idealist.

Reincarnation postulates the recurrent return of the soul to the physical realm for the purpose of development and unfoldment (individuation) through learning the art and practice of spiritual and creative living in circumstances that put such abilities to the test. This can be likened to the return each academic year of the pupil, scholar or student as they move through ascending grades of learning towards final graduation. However, whereas earth students may progress to the next grade on a minimum pass, in the school of the soul each lesson must be thoroughly learned and become part of the soul's moral fibre. Until this is achieved, the soul finds itself repeatedly faced by similar situations that test its spiritual response. During every incarnation, even those in which the soul may have evinced great evil, certain lessons are learned; even the most depraved, hateful and destructive individual may experience a moment of tenderness, a pang of conscience or a twinge of regret which plants a seed that someday will germinate. The soul comes into life with a history, a mixture of strengths to be realised, problems to be to be resolved and weaknesses to be overcome, and the life that unfolds for the soul is immaculately fashioned to bring these to fruition. After conception, the karmic history of the soul interacting with perceived or actual inadequacies in the holding environment contributes to the development of a unique ego-self.

The familiar cliché 'all men are born equal' holds true only at the deepest level. Equality is an absolute value, belonging to Spirit alone. The unrealised soul is ever in a process of transformation from ignorance to illumination and the ego-self, for all its strength and tenacity, is a compensatory structure within the psyche. While every soul is equal by virtue of its divine Essence, each is unique and enters life with its own level of spiritual attainment and ego encumbrance. This is infinitely diverse, ranging from the wicked to the wise, providing the stage of life with all the characters and situations necessary for testing and evolving the individual soul. One can only 'love one's enemy' if there is an enemy; one can only learn to 'forgive' if there is someone to forgive; and one can only 'turn the other cheek' after having been struck.

The level of spiritual attainment determining the standing of a soul is reflected in the afterlife where there are various levels of consciousness, ranging from those close to the physical dimension, which are more dense and peopled by souls still clinging to the material life and all its attractions, to the very highest, the exquisitely refined domain of radiant beings whose souls stand on the very cusp of the Divine.

Jung's Ego

Finally, in the light of what has gone before, it is of value for us to consider the functions of the ego as visualised by Jung. In his book, *On Jung*, Anthony Stevens, an experienced psychiatrist and Jungian analyst, gives a very clear exposition of Jung's evaluation of the ego.

[margin note: Jungs defn of ego]

- The ego is the centre of the conscious mind, therefore, the focal point of consciousness.
- The ego is what we refer to when we use the words "I" or "me" (hence, the ego-self).
- The ego carries our conscious awareness of existing.
- It also carries our continuing sense of personal identity.
- It is the conscious organiser of our thoughts and intuitions, our feelings and sensations (hence, the disease of the soul).
- The ego has access to those memories that are unrepressed and readily available.
- The ego is the bearer of personality (hence, the ego-personality).
- The ego mediates between the subjective and objective realms of experience (hence, the imposter).
- It stands at the junction between our inner and outer worlds.[14]

Jung also postulated that the way people relate to their inner and outer worlds is determined by which of two fundamental *attitudes-types* they belong to: the extraverted-type, primarily orientated to the outer world, or, the introverted-type, primarily orientated towards the inner world. Jung also noted that people differ in how they consciously make use of four basic *functions*, which he termed: *thinking, feeling, sensation* and *intuition*. He considered that in any individual one of these functions will be dominant, more highly developed through use and therefore superior. By conjoining each fundamental attitude-type with one of the superior functions, he was able to define eight major ego-types, e.g. the extraverted intuitive, the introverted thinker, etc.

Although the ego possesses all the qualities enumerated above, in essence they do not belong to the ego, they have been partially or entirely appropriated at the expense of the soul, the degree being dependent on the soul's ability to resist the intrusion of the ego and retain its authority. The ego is the usurper or pretender, who has wrested the cognitive throne from its rightful heir, the soul. This is a story often related in hero myths in which the evil, unprincipled, grasping younger brother, through unscrupulous plotting and betrayal, unseats the virtuous elder brother and banishes him from his birth right. The ego-self is an intruder and an imposter and not a fit executive to handle the affairs of the soul. This is the plight of the soul; it must regain its lost throne; a process that can be expedited by *depth homeopathy*!

References

1   Goodall J. *Reason for Hope: A Spiritual Journey*. New York: Warner Books, 1999.
2   Genesis 4:9.
3   Genesis 4:11.
4   Genesis 4:14.
5   Genesis 4:15.
6   Sheldrake R. An experimental test of the hypothesis of formative causation. *Revista di Biologia – Biology Forum* 1992. 86(3/4): 431–444.
7   Sheldrake R. *A New Science of Life*. 3rd edn. London: Icon Books Limited, 2009.
8   Sheldrake R. *The Presence of the Past. Morphic Resonance and the Habits of Nature*.London: Icon Books Limited, 2011.
9   Davies P. Book Review. Available online https://www.sheldrake.org/books-by-rupert-sheldrake/the-presence-of-the-past-morphic-resonance-and-the-habits-of-nature (Retrieved 09.03.2018.)
10 de Waal FBM, Lanting F. *Bonobo: The Forgotten Ape*. Berkeley CA: University of California Press, 1998.
11 Wikipedia. *Bonobo 66. Brain differences may explain varying behaviour of bonobos and chimpanzees*. Washington Post.com (12.04.2011). Retrieved 26.12.2012

12 McNeil DG, Jr. Precursor to HIV was in Monkeys for Millenia. *New York Times.* September 16, 2010.

13 Lilley D. *Healing the Soul* volume 1: Glasgow: Saltire Books, 2014. p56.

14 Stevens A. *On Jung.* London: Penguin Books (second edition), 1999. p30.

22

FREUD'S ARCHETYPES
OF THE PSYCHE

The Id, The Ego and the Super-ego

Although the analytical psychology of Jung more naturally dovetails with homeopathic philosophy and the psychoanalytical paradigm of Freud has found greater acceptance with conventional medicine, Freud's topography of the psyche and his concept of the sexual development phases of the psyche, provide invaluable insight into the workings of the human mind and the development of emotional dysfunction and disease.

Freud's secular perspective perceived neither the existence of spirit nor soul. Therefore, the structural model of the psyche he envisaged is devoid of an incorporeal essence imbued with spiritual yearning. *He proposed that the drives of instinct, the reason of intellect and the dictates of conscience rule*

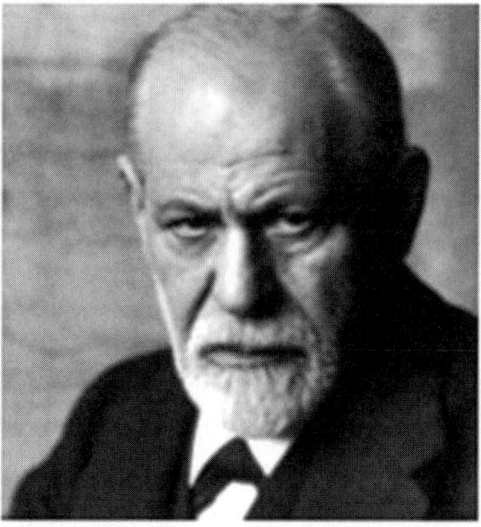

Figure 22.1 *Sigmund Freud (1856–1939)*
(Wikipedia)

the dynamics of the psyche. These dynamics reflect the interaction between three psychic agencies:

- The Id.
- The Ego.
- The Super-ego.

This topography, though devoid of the main character, the soul, still provides a useful working basis for understanding important elements of human psychology and behaviour. The mind tends to personify these three aspects of the psyche, but they must not be thought discreet; they are different aspects of consciousness, which are in constant and energetic interaction.

Freud 4

The Id

Representing the primitive, biological urges, the Id (*das Es*) is the most archaic component of the psyche: an *unconscious, patterned field of energy* that contains the instincts and provides all the drive and focus required to have them satisfied. The Id is operative in all instinctive animal behaviour; and is active from the moment of birth, ensuring the harmonious operation of body functions and eliciting behaviour essential to survival. In equal measure, the protective and propagating vigour of the Id is present in plants, witnessed in flowers, colour, perfume, fruit, resins, ethereal oils, alkaloids and glycosides.

When Freud introduced the concept of the Id, he wrote:

> To the oldest of the mental provinces or agencies, we give the name of *Id*. It contains everything that is inherited, that is present at birth, that is fixed in the constitution – above all, therefore, the instincts, which originate in the somatic organisation and which find their first mental expression in the Id in forms unknown to us.[1]

During infancy, before the other components of the psyche come into play, the influence of the Id is supreme. It is ruled by the *pleasure principle*, demanding instant satisfaction, with no sense of propriety, consideration for the appropriateness of time, place or circumstance, or concern about consequences. Its intent is always positive: movement away from pain or want towards pleasure and satisfaction. With development, awareness and self-consciousness, the demand for instant gratification of instinctive urges, needs and desires is gradually brought under control by the reason of the ego and the inhibitions of the superego. When this is poorly achieved, the subject will lack disciplined desire and impulse control, leading to thoughtless, reckless, selfish and impetuous behaviour, hurtful to themselves and others. When this is overly achieved, the subject is inhibited, held in check by a conservative straightjacket of convention and custom that represses emotions, feelings and behaviour.

The prime objective of the Id is survival, not only of the individual, but also of the species. It incorporates the basic instincts vital to self-preservation and the continuation of the species: *sex* and *aggression*. The former encompasses all the urges focused on sex and reproduction; the latter comprises the instincts that ensure survival through either attack or defence: the classic *flight, fight, or freeze* options that an animal has when faced by an aggressor. These drives and instincts operate through the functions of the reptilian brain, the limbic system, the adrenal glands and the autonomic nervous system, and they are intrinsic to the energy and functions of the first or root chakra.

With characteristic pessimism, Freud had a rather jaundiced view of the Id and in *New Introductory Lectures on Psychoanalysis* (1933), he described it as follows:

> It is the obscure, inaccessible part of our personality; the little we know of it we have learned from our study of dream-work and the formation of neurotic symptoms, and most of that is of a negative character and can be described only as being all that the ego is not. We come nearer to an understanding of the Id with images, and call it a chaos, a cauldron of seething excitement.... The instincts fill it with energy, but it has no organisation, produces no unified will, only an impulsion to obtain satisfaction for the instinctual needs, in accordance with the pleasure principle. The Id has no recognition of the passage of time ... knows no values, no good or evil, no morality.... Instinctual (drives) seeking discharge – that in our view, is all that the Id contains.[2]

Considering Freud's concept of the Id in the light of homeopathic philosophy, it is apparent that it can be equated with the instinctive functions of the *vital force*; functions that are intrinsic to its universal homeostatic and evolutionary role. However, contrary to Freud's vision, there is never chaos in the Id, only order – chaos is the province of the ego – and there is only a cauldron of seething excitement, *when repression has occurred*; then discord arises, creating dysfunction, which, if persistent, provokes morbid change. One with the universal vital force, the Id operates ineluctably according to cosmic law, and may be described in the words of Hahnemann as an *instinctively perceiving and regulating dynamis* acting constantly throughout nature as a harmonising, balancing, regulatory force, maintaining the homeostasis of the universe, our planet and all life. The instincts do not fill it with energy – it is the energy of the instincts; it is not devoid of organisation – its very function is organisation; it is not wanting of unified will – it is the inexorable will of the Creation: the mediator between the Supreme Consciousness and the material universe. The Id is, indeed, beyond time, beyond morality, beyond good and evil, beyond all duality; it is objective, impersonal and Cosmic. Like the seasons, like the tides, like the migration of birds and like the beating of the heart and the drawing of breath; it is autonomous and adamant. It is inherent in the maternal instinct, the suckling reflex, the rapture of infatuation, the ecstasy of orgasm, the drive to achieve, the desire to create and the longing for the Self; it is unadulterated positivity and unbounded potential. The Id is certainly all that the ego is not; it is authentic, obdurate and beneficent; never wavering or destructive. The basic instincts are innate, wholesome and in the animal state always ordered. It is only humans who step outside the parameters of natural law, display delinquency and become bestial: a deviation that is always the consequence of ego-choice (free-will), never evidence of a rampant Id.

The Id is immensely powerful. Like all force fields, it is imbued with momentum and rhythm. The unconscious tides of the Id must find expression; they must 'discharge' biologically and psychologically or be sublimated. Its power is such that any repression must lead to grave emotional and physical consequences. Homeopathically, this is well understood: the action of the vital force within a living form is always from within outwards, from above downwards and from organs critical to survival to organs of less importance. This is always the direction of balance, health and cure. Repression or inhibition of the Id opposes this and must impact on the health.

From these deliberations, it becomes clear that in homeopathic terms *the Id should be identified with the vital force*.

Freud defined the instinctive, reproductive force of the Id as the *libido*, which he limited to a dynamic manifestation of sexuality. Based on this theory, he conceived a sequence of psychosexual developmental phases during which the libido fixates on different erogenous zones. Jung, however, discerned the libido's wider significance, describing it as a neutral, psychic energy manifest in all physiological and emotional processes of life and subjectively perceived as the undefined '*striving and desire*', which drives each and every process. This broader understanding identifies, in addition to the sexual aspect, a powerful creative element in the force of the libido and recognises a dynamic connection between the two. The sexual and the creative drives are seen to be intimately related: they run parallel, feed and fire one another, and, most importantly, *the sexual drive can be converted or sublimated, not only through creative expression, but also through spiritual aspiration and endeavour*. The sublimation of libido energy is of central importance to the health of the psyche, to the soul's creativity and its progress towards Self-realisation. This observation is in line with ancient Tantric texts, which specify that sex has three distinct purposes: *procreation, pleasure and liberation.*

From time immemorial, the ego-self has had a curious relationship with the libido, as reflected in one the oldest myths of the Abrahamic religions: the story of Adam and Eve in the Garden of Eden, replete with a Tree of Good and Evil, harbouring the perfidious snake, a seductive creature of Satan, and bearing apples of temptation, poisoned with the overweening pride of intellect and the addictive power of sensual pleasure. Eating of the apple brought humanity's downfall and banishment from Paradise. The sexual connotation of this fall from virtue is witnessed in Adam and Eve's sudden awareness of their nakedness and their haste to conceal their genitals. Written into the myth is the warped perspective of the masculine principle of the ego-self that cloaks the glory of the libido with shame and makes the 'inferior' feminine principle culpable of luring the masculine into the mire of lust. The subliminal message infers that the sexual act, other than for procreation, is intrinsically base, animalistic and shameful. Thus, the immaculate, creative, libido energy of the Id becomes a force to be repudiated, suppressed and hidden beneath a veil of religious rectitude and hypocrisy. Heightened religiosity is often coupled to unhealthy sexual scruples: a pseudo-sublimation of the libido through puritanical prudery that sees virtue in celibacy. Religion and the libido are ever entangled in bitter contention. Repression, as distinct from sublimation, always spells corruption; beneath the cassock may fret a prurient, irresistible desire. The contention between libido and faith is exemplified in the Lachesis, Lilium tigrinum (tiger lily), Platina, Thuja, Origanum, Aurum and Anacardium archetypes. Religion is the tortuous path of the ego-self; spirituality is the sublime path of the soul.

The vast power of the Id highlights the necessity for sublimation. When a natural force is inhibited or repressed it is corrupted and projected onto the world and society with destructive consequences for the psyche, the community and the world (e.g. radical Islam). By sublimation, the libido energy of the Id is channelled constructively and creatively, and the danger of repression and corruption is avoided. This knowledge emphasises the special role of healthy activity, creative expression and spiritual development as the natural involution of the sexual drive takes place in middle age. *The libido aspect of the Id must flow* and this necessity is intrinsic to the Lachesis (serpent) archetype, which possibly more than any other remedy exemplifies the struggle between the libido and the ego.

Freud was conscious of the danger inherent in the repression of the instinctive drives and demands of the Id by the ego and identified this as pivotal to the development of what he termed *neurosis*, a word first coined in 1769 by the very same William Cullen, whose opinions, regarding the curative action of Peruvian bark (China or quinine) in the treatment of malaria, inspired Hahnemann to conduct the first homeopathic remedy proving. Although the term neurosis has largely fallen into disuse, it encompasses a wide range of emotional disorders from anxieties and phobias to obsessive, compulsive states, inappropriate behaviours and depression. More important than the psychological scope of the term, is Freud's awareness that if the ego-self foregoes an instinctual demand for satisfaction made by the Id, the demand may pass from consciousness, but remains primed, and appropriate triggers will arouse it again. If the Id's importunities continue to be thwarted, they will seek substitutive satisfaction and produce emotional and/or physical symptoms, which the ego-self will fail to recognise as being linked to the earlier repression. Freud went so far as to say that all symptom-forming phenomena could be justly described as being "the return of the repressed".

> If we survey the whole situation, it becomes clear that there is a simple formula for the arising of a neurosis; the Ego has made an attempt to suppress certain parts of the Id by an *inappropriate method* (repression) and this has miscarried, and the Id has taken revenge. Neurosis is thus the consequence of a conflict between Ego and Id ... (in which) the Ego, insists throughout on retaining its adaptability to the outer world. The opposition lies between the outer world and the Id, and because the Ego, true to its inmost nature, takes sides with the outer world it becomes involved in conflict with its own Id.[3]

He stresses that it is not this conflict that brings on illness; illness results from the ego attempting to resolve the conflict by employing an inadequate method: *repression!* He was further of the opinion that *"all decisive repressions occur in early childhood"*.

Despite this grave warning from such an esteemed source, the dominant school of medicine today employs billions of dollars yearly in chemically suppressing the symptoms of neurosis vented by the Id in its attempts to defuse the repressions induced by the world-enslaved ego-self. Repression by suppression is worse confounded.

The Id is not silent. It is the mediator between the Universal Consciousness and the soul, between the collective unconscious and the personal unconscious and between the personal unconscious and the conscious. It flows ever outwards, from the depths to the surface and though unconscious it is imbued with universal consciousness. The power it expresses is lawful, ordered, seemly and beneficent, proffering its primal energy for the arduous ascent of the soul. The Id, 'though it have no tongue will speak with most miraculous organ'.[4]

It alerts the soul to the machinations of the ego-self and does so through dreams, symbols and symptoms. The symbols may appear in the narrative of a dream or may suddenly present through the synchronicity that governs the passage of the soul through life. These are the unbidden promptings that come to protect, direct and guide us; cues that we, unfortunately, so often fail to recognise, dismiss or ignore. The symptoms 'voiced' by the Id are *the characteristic mental and emotional symptoms of the individual*: these are the key to successful therapy.

Like a river seeking the ocean, the Id flows with relentless purpose seeking fulfilment; it is the pure energy creating, vitalising, maintaining, restoring and ultimately dissolving the matter it animates. It is an impersonal, ineluctable force of nature. Striking the flawed prism of the ego/soul complex, it is refracted into morbid patterns, which Freud perceived as a seething chaos of excitement, but passing through the crystal of innocence, it remains unperturbed. In animal life, untouched by human meddling, the Id, in both affect and effect, is always wholesome, appropriate and timely. It is only the free will of the ego-self that can take the immaculate and warp it into warfare and lust.

The Id is in league with the soul. Mythologically, it can be likened to the hero's winged-steed effortlessly bearing the soul through life, serving its needs and firing it with passion and drive for its spiritual quest; a psychic beast in tune with the soul's higher purpose, imparting wisdom from the universal source through dreams, symbols and myth. It is the obdurate opponent of the ego-self: the mountebank, who, in usurping the hero's role, presumptuously mounts the noble animal, and like Freud finds it mettlesome and chaotic, ever threatening to unseat it in the face of life's eventualities. The presence and nature of the imposter is revealed in the symptoms projected outwards in the throes of this struggle.

The pivotal role of suppression of the basic drives of the Id in the production of emotional and physical dysfunction reveals the cardinal importance of two rubrics relating to the central drives of the Id which are associated with aggression and sexuality:

- *Ailments from suppressed anger; ailments from anger with silent grief.*
- *Ailments from suppressed sexual desire.*

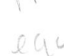 Freud's
ego

The Ego of Freud

Freud conceived the ego (*das Ich*) as having evolved from the Id in response to the modelling influence of the external world. Without the concept of a soul, he ascribed to the ego alone the identity, personality and cognitive attributes of the individual and identified it as the organised and rational, executive manager of the psyche. This equates the ego with the self: a being consciously aware of the encompassing world and possessing both conscious and unconscious functions with which to deal with it. *These functions include judgement, discrimination, organisation of information, reason, analysis, common sense, strategy, control, self-defence and memory.*

The ego's struggle for autonomy is waged on three very demanding fronts, against:

- *The impingements of the external world.*
- *The passions of the Id.*
- *The censure of the superego.*

On this precarious stage, the ego can only achieve a tolerable balance through expedience, compromise and repression. The price is anxiety and tension:

- *Realistic anxiety about life.*
- *Moral anxiety due to the eagle eye of the superego.*
- *Neurotic anxiety over the insistent drives of the Id.*

Coping with these on-going tensions necessitates the development of largely unconscious, *defence mechanisms*: emergency measures that contribute to the dynamic structure of the ego and further distort its perspectives. Common defence mechanisms employed by the ego in the face of anxiety, inferiority, bereavement, guilt, shame and trauma are:

- *Denial.*
- *Dissociation.*
- *Splitting.*
- *Regression.*
- *Suppression.*
- *Control.*
- *Projection.*
- *Compensation.*
- *Rationalisation.*
- *Intellectualisation.*
- *Identification.*

- *Idealism.*
- *Fantasy.*

All of which, in one way or another, are flights from reality and constitute *repression.*

Less commonly, and only in the better adjusted, *sublimation* rather than repression occurs: a beneficial, uplifting response that steadily weakens the ego-structure. When these unconscious survival strategies, identified by Freud and his daughter Anna, are considered in the light of the dynamics of the soul/ego complex, they will be recognised as major hindrances to the progress of the soul.

The common theme of the defensive strategies employed by the ego-self is repression, and *repression is the most potent cause of sickness and disease*: proof, indeed, that the ego-self is the disease from which the soul suffers. Conventional medicine is essentially *ego-medicine*, not *soul-medicine*. When faced by disease, this model acts like the ego-self unable to cope with life; it seeks resolution through suppression. In their knee-jerk response, both the ego-self and medical orthodoxy transgress the dictates of the Id, which demands *expression*! They contravene a law of nature and pit their wits and puny resources against the inexorable might of the Id; such efforts must prove futile, the consequences dire.

In contrast, the principles of homeopathic medicine are perfectly in harmony with the inscrutable workings of the Id (the vital force), which are, without exception, ordered, benign and instinctively intelligent. Homeopathy honours the superior knowledge of the animating force, always selecting remedies, which in their dynamic effect, match the Id's vigour, its direction and the pattern of its externalised phenomena. Even a cursory viewing of the common, protective ploys of the assailed ego-self, reveals the value of certain key remedies in combating their repressive influence: Nat-mur for denial; Lac-can for dissociation; Platina for splitting; Pulsatilla for regression; Thuja for suppression; Ars-alb for control; Anacardium for projection; Lycopodium for compensation; Sulphur for rationalisation, Kali-carb for intellectualisation; Staphysagria for identification, Ignatia for idealisation; China for fantasy; and, overshadowing them all, Carcinosin and Lac lupinum for repression.

In infancy, the Id rules behaviour by asserting the *pleasure principle*: the instinctual seeking of pleasure and avoidance of pain or *un-pleasure* in order to satisfy biological and psychological needs. At this early age, the individual wants all its needs to be gratified immediately and countenances no delay in having its hunger and thirst satisfied. Later in life, this drive for instant gratification becomes focused on sex.

With maturity, the developing ego-self becomes more reasonable, and, while unable to ignore the Id, weighs up gratification in the light of circumstances, social norms and the demands of reality:

> ... it no longer lets itself be governed by the pleasure principle, but obeys the *reality principle*, which also basically seeks pleasure, but pleasure which is assured through taking account of reality, even though it is pleasure postponed and diminished.[3]

The reality principle insists that the ego should consider consequences before deciding to act upon or ignore an impulse. If deemed inappropriate or unwise, the urge will then be repressed or deferred until a more suitable, secure and reasonable time and place is found. This assertion of the reality principle regulates and modifies the pleasure principle of the Id and enables the ego-self to act judiciously with forethought.

All seems well in this scenario, and, would be, if our instinctive impulses were simply biologically driven, monitored by the morality of the soul and untainted by the peculiarities of the ego-self.

The Id is primeval and objective, an instinctively perceiving force which demands harmony, balance and lawfulness. Like the ocean, it is faultless, moving as it must, its tides expressing the homeostatic and creative power of the universe, adamantly voiding unconscious debris onto the shore of the conscious. The Id expresses, the ego-self represses. The repressions of the ego-self, while seeming to repudiate the pleasure principle, invoke the subtler 'pleasures' unconsciously necessitated by the defence mechanisms that the ego-self deploys to counter, or mitigate, its warped perception of life (personal delusion). Life lived through the ego-self is a juggling act, an incessant struggle of appeasement between the instinctive power of the Id, the demands of external reality and the guilt-provoking censure of the bigoted, superego. Anything the ego-self finds threatening to its 'pleasure' – its comfort, security and survival – it represses into the unconscious. The unconscious, represented by the Id, demands that the ego-self shall deal with whatever it has repressed and this causes the unease and tension, which culminates in emotional and physical pathology.

The pleasure and reality principles compete at the divide between the unconscious and the conscious minds, a zone of interminable tension and stress, where the darkness of the intangible and mysterious contends with the light of logic and reason and the insistent Id grapples with the slippery ego-self. This is a region of great therapeutic importance. Certain contrasting rubrics assume great significance, as do the remedies they contain:

- *Darkness aggravates.*
- *Aversion to the dark.*

- *Fear of the dark.*
- *Fear of everything black.*
- *Desire for light.*
- *Fear of night; fear at night.*
- *Shuns the light.*
- *Daylight: aggravation of mental symptoms.*
- *Fear of brilliant objects, the looking glass; shuns brilliant objects.*
- *Fear mirrors in the room* (reflection of light, the ego-self and reality).

To these, must be added, the disturbing influence that some people experience in a world caught between light and dark: the eerie, uncanny, unnerving time of twilight when shadows and imagination loom large and shake the equilibrium of the mind. Such a critical rubric must reveal remedies highly significant to the healing of the ego-disease of the soul. Each remedy will have a special reason for being there. The homeopath has to discern the differences within the similarity that places them in the same rubric.

- *Twilight: aggravation of mental symptoms.*
  Berberis; *Calc-carb*; Causticum; *Phosphorus*; Platina; *Pulsatilla*; Rhus-tox; Valeriana.

Of ominous significance in this small but significant rubric is the presence of Causticum, Phosphorus and Platina. All three appear in the even smaller, unwholesome rubric: *lewdness, obscene: man searching for little girls*: Causticum; Phosphorus; Platina; Verat-alb. Veratrum (white hellebore) is the acute counterpart of Platina. This overlap between the two rubrics indicates the distortion of energy that can be generated at the twilight boundary of Id/ego-self contention. Paedophilia is the most selfish and vile of sexual offences and is rife worldwide.

Not far removed from the twilight remedies are those that *fear both light and dark*. Most important amongst these are the poisonous representatives of the *Solanaceae* family of plants, the nightshades, which for thousands of years have occupied a foremost position in the magic, myth and medicine of various cultures: Belladonna (deadly nightshade) Stramonium (poison apple) and Hyoscyamus (black henbane). All three, in their different, though similar ways, act upon the Id/ego-self boundary and upon the tension between expression and repression. They fear the light and what it reveals, and they fear the dark and what it conceals. In the field of action of the toxic *Solanaceae*, the urges, promptings and repressed emotions of the unconscious well up and enter into conflict with the conscious. The contention is between the two worlds in which we exist: the conscious and the unconscious. The unconscious strives to rise into consciousness to void the warped thinking of generations, the conscious attempts to retreat into the hidden, inner world of the unconscious: to step out of the harsh light of reality. Where the two mental forces interact, strife ensues, and reality and morality may be sacrificed.

In *Solanaceae* illness, the rational mind is overwhelmed by powerful surges emanating from the reptilian brain and the limbic system, those parts of the brain, which together with the right pre-frontal neo-cortex are aligned with the power of the Id. Impulse control is challenged and often sacrificed. The patient is haunted and harrowed by the turbulence of a dark, inner world that warps personality and distorts the vision of life, breaking through into mania, madness and lust. Repression and compensation work hand in hand and are reflected in the action of all three *Solanaceae*, each with its own unique emphasis. The repressed fear of Belladonna converts into fever, anger and rage, the fear of Stramonium into violence and religious fanaticism, and that of Hyoscyamus into jealousy, maliciousness and shamelessness. The complex entanglement of fear, aggression, hatred, religion and lust that beset humanity emerge in the dynamics of these fundamental remedies. Fear repressed becomes anger, anger repressed becomes depression, depression repressed becomes insanity: ever-deepening pathology wrought through repression and compensation moving inexorably inwards according to Hering's law of disease progression.

It must be reiterated that in such emotional seizures, the Id is innocent; it is the ever-flowing river of life flowing towards fulfilment through sublimation. The obstacles to its flow, which produce the turbulence, vortices and cataracts of life, are the intrigues and follies of the ego-self accreted over generations.

The Superego

Simply defined, the superego (*das Über-Ich*) is *the 'conscience' of the ego-self*. It should not be confused with the conscience of the soul. The conscience of the ego-self is acquired by internalising the mores and cultural rules of society, at first, through imprinting derived from the influence, example, beliefs and guidance of the parents – to the degree that the child identifies with the parental agency – and, later, through significant authority figures and idealised role-models experienced by the ego-self as influential and exemplary.

The conscience of the soul, the true-conscience, is the ineluctable voice of the Self, calling to its beloved; it is innate and endowed – the result of many life times of experience. It is testimony to the level of spiritual conscious-ness and the stage of individuation that the soul has achieved and is witnessed in spontaneous empathy, compassion, kindness and generosity and an inborn, unselfish integrity. By contrast, the ethical code imposed by the superego, the false-conscience, is a veneer of correctness modelled on the external world. The ego-self complies with the dictates of the superego to obviate guilt and maintain self-esteem, and, thereby, conforms to consensus propriety and surrenders the soul's sincerity to hypocrisy. Modern-day fealty to *political correctness* has become a ubiquitous example of this sycotic dissimulation.

The superego emerges out of the ego-self as a compensatory structure, just as the ego-self developed as a compensatory structure of the soul. Due to its karmic history, its miasmatic envelope, its descent into a limiting, impinging dimension and the inevitable unreliability of its holding environment during its first years of life, including the prenatal period, the incarnated soul gradually and progressively loses basic trust. This loss of trust extends from the infant's surrounding environment and immediate family to the universe at large and ultimately to the Universal Conscious-ness, regardless of the belief system the child was born into or its conscious perception and evaluation of reality. It loses its connection to a loving, caring, supporting Universe, and, with this, the sense that it is protected, taken care of, understood, loved and valuable. The loss of holding disrupts *the continuity of being*: the unconscious certainty that the soul is an inherent part of the universe and a unique expression of it. Oneness is disrupted, and duality becomes the reality of the soul. It feels separated, not only from everything else in the Creation, but also from its very Origin: it is discon-nected from Being. This is an awful delusion of isolation, abandonment, helplessness and deficiency, which is unbearable. The soul reacts to this seemingly insurmountable difficulty by creating the compensatory struc-ture of the false- or ego-self: a counterfeit-self, founded on a fundamental distrust of reality and a sense of deficiency and inferiority.

The deficiency and inferiority that are implicit to its nature impel the ego-self to invoke a lord and master that will unfailingly impose conven-tional standards of excellence upon it. This overlord, the superego, is largely, but not entirely, unconscious. Freud considered that the emergence of the superego commences at about the age of six, at the start of what he termed the latency period of the ego's development. Most important to this period in both girls and boys is a father figure – not necessarily the biologi-cal parent – who represents for the child: authority, power and strength, and, through performing typical paternal functions, serves as a symbol for identification and attachment. The child ego-self identifies with this idealised, paternal image and internalises it, together with the religious, social and cultural mores it appears to represent. This compound image lays the foundation for the organised, conformist superego that the ego-self needs to give it validity: a harsh and inflexible, inner critic that disciplines it and protects it from the 'unprincipled' and 'socially unacceptable' drives, fantasies, feelings and promptings of the Id. Given this brief, the superego duly sets up the image of an 'ideal-self' by which it measures the ego-self. If the ego-self should fail to live up to this standard through not complying with the superego's moral and ethical rules, it will punish the ego-self with guilt feelings.

Homeopathic philosophy recognises in this convoluted strategy, the anxiety-laden workings of the psoric mind, burdened with pessimism, and the conviction of being incompetent and inferior. The stage is set for disease progression. With maturity, the superego acquires ever-greater authority and forces the ego-self to repress into the unconscious any needs, urges and fantasies that disturb it. The degree to which it succeeds will vary, but when supported by intense ideological persuasion, it can utterly dominate the ego-self.

It would seem that in this scenario the soul is stifled and completely discounted, as it certainly was by Freud, but the emergence of the superego, like the ego-self before it, must be understood as natural and inevitable, and, therefore, essential to the soul's incarnated experience. The superego evolves out of the ego's fear of the Id: a fear that parallels humanity's fear of the forces of nature. Both humanity and the ego attempt to assuage their fears through control and domination. The ego enlists the superego to combat the urges of the Id, the very force of nature that strives for expression and the individuation of the soul. Nevertheless, *the evolution of the superego has purpose.* Although counterfeit and motivated by appearances and propriety, in inducing us to achieve political correctness, fit into society and behave in an appropriate manner, the superego asserts a code of disciplined conduct. Though initially conditional, observed to obviate the pangs of guilt inflicted by the unforgiving superego, *correct social conduct gradually lays the foundation for true morality.*

Shakespeare's acute understanding of human nature enables him to describe the transforming effect of good actions and habits, even when assumed, in incomparably eloquent terms. Hamlet is dissuading his mother, the queen, from returning to the bed of his uncle, the king (the murderer of his father):

> Good night; but go not to mine uncle's bed;
> Assume a virtue if you have it not.
> That monster, custom, who all sense doth eat,

Of habits devil, is angel yet in this,
That to the use of actions fair and good
He likewise gives a frock or livery,
That aptly is put on. Refrain tonight;
And that shall lend a kind of easiness
To the next abstinence: the next more easy;
For use almost can change the stamp of nature,
And exorcise the devil or throw him out
With wondrous potency.[5]

The influence of the superego may be detected in much of our behaviour and particularly in modern, frenetic city-life in the twinges of guilt that afflict us when we are not constantly working and being productive. Often guilt takes a religious slant, the moralistic superego and religion making good bedfellows. The concept of original sin is a typical tool of the superego, burdening even the innocent with guilt and shame, coercing the believer to compulsively seek restitution through observance. The austere, puritanical doctrines of Calvinism, steeped in the dry discipline of piety, industry, sobriety and thrift are characteristic of religious convictions invoked and instilled by the superego.

The superego is ubiquitous; in some, it enforces perfectionism and fastidiousness, or it may fixate on achievement and success; in others, it pricks the conscience to constant acts of charity and self-sacrifice, or it may drive the ego-self to excel in sport, indulge in excesses of physical exercise or strive for some image of physical beauty, which if distorted may even lead to anorexia nervosa. It is a merciless slave driver and since it insists on compliance with an internalised image elaborated from significant people idealised in youth, it adds external layers of borrowed personality that obscure the true-self. Responses to circumstances are ego-based, rigid and programmed, determined by unquestioned assumptions and convictions about reality derived from others. The self-determination and unfolding of the soul are impeded. The relatively fixed and rigid state of the personality and its distorted image of reality, cause the ego-self to attract ever-repeated life-situations. This ego-self stagnation, permitted by the somnolence and inertia of the soul, prevents release and resolution.

Freud's concept of the superego and the Oedipus complex, which we will consider shortly, is criticised as sexist because it exclusively focuses on the role of the father figure in the formation of the ego and superego. He passes over the primary role that bonding with the mother figure plays: a relationship pivotal to the infant's basic trust in the holding environment and to the development of the personality. Nonetheless, as will become clear later, though evidencing patriarchal bias, Freud's thinking is in keeping with colour, chakra and miasmatic theory.

To understand the development of the psychic structures from a perspective devoid of the male prejudices of Freud's early twentieth century background, it is necessary to substitute the term masculine principle for father figure. This principle, like the feminine principle, is not gender related; both are innate to the androgynous nature of all aspects of the creation.

Universally, the maternal principle is always primary. It is symbolised by the colour black – the colour of infinite potential and power. Positive black is enfolding, feminine, intuitive, generative and maternal; and its energy is *yin*. Black is the beginning and the end; out of the darkness all things emerge and into darkness all things return, just as night gives birth to day and day resolves into night. Black is synonymous with the void, the gravid womb of the cosmos from which the material universe arises and to which it will return. At birth, we are born out of the darkness of our mother's womb, and, at the close of life, we slip away into the darkness of mother death. The blackness of the earth and the blackness of storm clouds mutually portray the mothering fecundity of darkness. Mother Ocean, a maternal image more fundamental than Mother Earth, shares the symbolism of black; it is synonymous with the unfathomable depths of the deep unconscious; it is the source of life, the primeval formlessness from which all form arises: limitless, inexhaustible and pregnant with possibility. Black is the undifferentiated force field from which the chakra system takes shape; as its power manifests, black gives birth to red, just as the inky black of coal produces fiery-red embers. This primordial red, black's infant, represents by its long, slow, ponderous frequency, the masculine, *yang*, consciousness and dense, stabilising power of the first, or root chakra: *Muladhara*.

This contemplation of the symbolism of black introduces an intuitive perspective that puts us in touch with the forces that project the material world, and, as in the interpretation of myths and the analysis of dreams, we gain access to mysterious dimensions where Divinity takes on human guise. We retrieve the communion that our remote ancestors enjoyed with nature and the mysterious and sacred aspects of life, and, in a personal way, we become conscious of a science that informs our own: the science of the arcane.

We are conceived and born into the field of black that embodies the loving, maternal power of the Universe. If there were no heritage from spirit, no miasmatic disease, no disruptive impingements from the holding environment and if our parents, siblings and extended family lived in an idyllic, harmonious cocoon of tranquillity, we would luxuriate in the bliss of symbiotic union with our mother, secure in her love, symbolically suckling at the Cosmic breast. But this cannot be, and it is fitting that it cannot be. Even while we float in the warm, enveloping cushion of amniotic fluid within the black haven of our mother's uterus – an organ lying safely in the feminine, *yin*, frequency of the second, or sacral, chakra: *Svadhisthana* – impingements of discord assail us, conveyed to us psychically and nervously through our mother and from our own animal awareness of a wider ambience: flashes of red in the sable of our psyche. During my prenatal life in 1940, Europe was at war, my father was in court, tried as a conscientious objector, his relationship with Arthur Richards had just begun and the Sanctuary in Hunslet was being launched. My mother, still a very young woman, was abruptly thrust from quiet, predictable, Yorkshire-mining-village life into the uncertainty, intensity and spotlight of a joltingly different climate, just as the world was descending into destruction and anarchy. The darkness of my maternal cloister must have pulsed with the ever-flickering glow of red.

Red is *yang*, the colour of warning, of threat and of danger; it arouses the masculine principle, essential to our survival. One with the Id, red animates the foetus and charges it at the quickening. At the onset of labour, the black of the passive womb is suffused with the vigour of red inducing, in concert with its slow, yet, insistent pulse, the contractions of the uterus, impelling the foetus from the sweet, tranquil, dark waters of *Svadhisthana* into the driving red of *Muladhara* and the glaring light of the external world.

Whether boy or girl, this is the path of incarnation: from black to red, from water to earth, from *yin* to *yang* and from the feminine principle to the masculine. First consciousness is seated in the root chakra and that consciousness is the consciousness of the Id; its needs and drives a pressing priority, heedless of the niceties of human society. Like life itself, the Id flows from the dark vastness of the feminine into the sharp actuality of the masculine, which becomes the urgent focus of its consciousness, essential for survival and propagation. The 'woman' in us all, regardless of gender, needs a 'man' and this is the fixation; the 'man' alone possesses the aggression and potency that ensure the material future. 'He' is embodied in the father figure and it is this father figure or male principle, which is instinctively and unconsciously identified as *the* source of safety, security and fertility and is, therefore, idealised and internalised as guide, guardian and 'god': the personifications of the superego! Freud is vindicated!

From the homeopathic perspective, the importance of the male role model in the balanced development of the psyche from birth into adolescence, and the idealisation of the masculine principle and its incorporation into the male or female psyche as the superego archetype, is characteristic of the psoric emotional and constitutional condition. This is easily understood for the development of *Psora* was coincident with human emergence from simple primate life into a nomadic hunter-gatherer culture in the Palaeolithic period. During this prehistoric time, dominant alpha males, like the silverback of a gorilla troop, were the central figures of the small, human bands that grouped together. They were the leaders, responsible for hunting and protecting the members of the group, figures of authority, power and potency, who enjoyed sexual precedence over other males – they were agents of the Id!

References

1 Freud S. *The Wisdom of Sigmund Freud*. New York NY: Citadel Press, 2002. p70.
2 *Ibid.*, pp70–71.
3 *Ibid.*, p90.
4 Shakespeare W. *Hamlet*. London: Oxford University Press. 1968. Act II Scene II. Lines 589–590. p109.
5 *Ibid.*, Scene IV. Lines 160–170.

23

PSYCHOSEXUAL DEVELOPMENT STAGES

Oral and Anal

Having considered Freud's theory of the structure of the psyche, it is timely to contemplate his more controversial theory of the psychosexual development stages that the human psyche passes through during its infancy, youth and adolescence. Whether entirely correct or not, these concepts have become part of the collective myth and have entered into common parlance and idiom. If only by name, the Oedipus complex is familiar to all, and to call a person 'anal', leaves no doubt as to their underlying nature. To every homeopath, the term 'anal' conjures up the image of the Arsenicum archetype (Ars-alb); hence, it is wise for us to know its origin and context. However, on evaluation, Freud's sexually orientated perspective reveals an intriguing world of human thinking, feeling and behaviour that is of immense value in clinical practice and in the study of archetypal behaviour. Nothing happens by chance, and, certainly, neither Jung or Freud happened by chance! Their work is of inestimable value and remarkably, in view of their eventual divergence, they complement one another perfectly.

The beauty of homeopathic philosophy lies in its universal scope and its congruency with all aspects of existence. It provides a trustworthy framework with which to appraise other modes of thought and to know what is of value and what should be discarded. Experience confirms the development of personality profiles corresponding to the five psychosexual stages defined by Freud and these may be recognised in matching homeopathic archetypes.

Because of the fundamental importance, power and potential of the libido aspect of the Id, the unhindered development of the sensual and sexual aspects of the psyche is critical to the health of the personality. In an infant, the Id's aggressive nature is immediately evident in the easily provoked and unrestrained intensity of temper tantrums – *the Chamomilla aspect.* At this age, the sexual element is not as obvious, since, it is concentrated in the sensual delights of mother's skin, her gaze, her scent, her milk and the voluptuous bliss of suckling: the tenderly intimate contact and stimulation of two highly sensitive, erogenous zones: mouth, lips and tongue – breast and nipples – *the Pulsatilla aspect.*

According to Freud's theory every human being passes through a sequence of five stages of sexual development, each linked to a specific erogenous zone. The successful resolution of each stage results in a healthier and more balanced personality, and, equally, failure to do so creates *a dysfunctional personality fixated upon the erogenous zone associated with the unresolved stage.* Later in life, the fixation results in inhibition or overindulgence of activities, sexual or otherwise, related to the particular zone.

The five stages of psychosexual development are:

- The Oral stage.
- The Anal stage.
- The Oedipus/Elektra or Phallic stage.
- The Latency stage.
- The Genital stage.

The Oral stage

This is the breast-feeding stage and extends from *birth to between the age of eighteen months and two years.* During this period, the mouth is the primary erogenous zone. Libido satisfaction is sought through suckling at the mother's breast and by oral exploration of the environment: testing every object by placing it in the mouth. Bottle-feeding, sucking on a pacifier and thumb sucking can provide a substitute means of attaining oral pleasure. Dependency on these substitutes may indicate the development of an oral fixation.

Due to the ego-self not being fully developed, the Id is dominant during this stage and all actions are governed by the pleasure principle, which seeks instant gratification. If the infant perceives the gratification to be either excessive (too much milk, late weaning) or deficient (breast withheld, premature weaning, milk inferior in quantity or quality, milk-intolerance), fixation in the oral stage results and the *'oral' type personality* emerges.

The timing of weaning is critical to this stage. Delay may constitute overindulgence and over-gratification for the infant. Given a singularly, sensitive constitution, a surfeit of nurturing impairs emotional maturation, inducing infantilism, dependency, passivity and self-indulgence. At the other end of the scale, premature withdrawal or failure of the breast thwarts gratification, and, in the sensitive infant, causes feelings of rejection, abandonment and worthlessness.

The oral fixation that results from either extreme impairs normal development and disrupts future behaviour. Since the Id is active from birth, unconscious sexual and aggressive fantasies already exist during the oral stage of development and are capable of powerfully influencing the bias of the oral fixation, which may take on either a sexually-based, overindulged, dependent, *oral-erotic* form or an aggression-based, thwarted, defiant, *oral-sadistic* form. In both, the evolving ego-personality is strongly influenced by the psychological fixation and will focus on activities that involve the mouth. Both types share the fundamental ego-perception of *being forsaken* and alone in a threatening and hostile environment: a delusion that stems from *lack of basic trust*!

In the passive, oral-erotic form, the fixation seeks to recapture the pleasure derived from a surplus of maternal nurturing through comfort and reward eating (sweets, chocolates, salt, starches, puddings, cakes, smoked meats) or through substance abuse (alcohol, tobacco, cannabis, cocaine). Other indications are neurotic loquacity and habitual use of the tongue when displaying emotion.

Those stuck in the oral-erotic phase are immature, passive-dependent, timid, indecisive, naïve and gullible, and, being impressionable, are easily persuaded and influenced by others. They are followers not leaders and avoid responsibility and the limelight. Authority figures, intellectuals and individuals with forceful personalities intimidate them. Due to their low self-confidence and self-esteem, social phobias are common; they prefer the tried and familiar and the company of family or those they know well. They are the centre of their own focus and they know well how to manipulate others into gratifying them. Because of their selfishness, they are possessive, suspicious and jealous of those close to them and also envious of the achievements and possessions of others. Their neediness is expressed in a desire to kiss, cuddle, hug and hold onto the person they are dependent on for love and protection, and, in turn, they need to be kissed, caressed and held.

Tears of self-pity are ever ready to spill over when their desires are not met, whereas, the aggressive oral type is more inclined to throw a tantrum if denied. Although highly emotional and inclined to unashamedly give vent to their feelings through laughter or tears, their emotions though intense are usually shallow and transient. Sympathy and consolation are like chocolates and éclairs to them; they are soon pacified. They lap up fuss, attention and love as if they were suckling at the breast. Being self-absorbed and given to only superficial commitment, they are emotionally and intellectually fickle and cannot be relied upon. They always go where the going is good and easy. The oral-erotic enjoys both giving and receiving oral sex and compulsive masturbation is often symptomatic of their self-love and need for comforting.

In the aggressive, oral-sadistic form, the fixation finds expression in nail biting, biting others and chewing objects (pencil-ends, clothing, etc.) or chewing gum. Like the passive type, they may also smoke and drink and indulge in substance abuse, but their smoking displays macho, masculine affectation and alcohol often triggers their underlying aggressiveness.

The seed of rejection and unworthiness, planted in the mind at this impressionable age due to perceived deprivation, germinates into an unconscious conviction that *they are unlovable and contemptible*. They reject themselves and in turn reject the affection of others and the norms of society. Fuelled by the anger of their grievance, they adopt aggression and defiance as their survival modes. Their neediness is as great as that of the dependent type, but being caught up with underlying resentment and anger, it takes a different path. It is seen in its purest form in the infant or child: a mixture of intense wanting and defiant rejection. The child wants many things; moans piteously or throws tantrums when it cannot have what it wants; but refuses, rejects or throws down the very thing it has clamoured for when it is offered. Likewise, it cannot bear to be touched; it rebuffs any gesture of affection, resents being spoken to or looked at and cannot bear the proximity of others, yet demands to be picked up and carried and screams in rage when put down. In their tantrums they go stiff, struggle, kick, lash out and may bite. Just as they turn away from affection, they are averse to sympathy and consolation. They wish to be seen as strong and self-sufficient.

The sadistic aspect is expressed by way of snappiness, spitefulness and sarcasm; peevish quarrelsomeness and uncivil behaviour; and by emotional and physical cruelty. They have no consideration for the feelings of others and will deliberately enter into a dispute or argument over what they know to be sensitive matters, regardless of the possible outcome. Impatient and intolerant by nature, they are always dissatisfied and complaining, not only with the efforts of others, but also with themselves. Due to their hyper-sensitivity, touch, pain, noise and certain music can irritate them beyond reason, and, similarly, they are incensed by the least interruption and by criticism, contradiction and even trifles. Like their unconscious memory of having been deprived of the breast, any grievance is harboured, and they tend to reflect on past disagreeable occurrences even years later. Their sexuality is both oral and penetrative and they are sexually avid, assertive and selfish. Both orally fixated types desire instant sexual gratification.

As always, when evaluating theories relating to the intangible, mysterious nature of the psyche, it is homeopathy that is able, through the psychical research of its remedy provings, to substantiate or disprove the tenets of such theories. Reciprocally, the theories of Freud and Jung shed light on the dynamics of the homeopathic archetypes. This is true of Freud's psychosexual development stages. The maladaptive signs of fixation at the initial oral stage, point to the fundamental importance of the oral-erotic, passive-dependent Pulsatilla and the oral-sadistic, aggressive, defiant Chamomilla archetypes. They stand at the very base of the archetypal pyramid and in the energy and consciousness sphere of the first or root chakra. Together, they archetypally represent the survival drives of the Id: Pulsatilla personifying the reproductive, libido aspect and Chamomilla the aggressive, survival aspect. Their emotional pictures provide a perfect reflection of the over-gratified, overindulged or thwarted, aggrieved oral personality types. Experience reveals that many oral types swing between the two extremes, at times evincing the passive, weepy, yielding characteristics of Pulsatilla, and, at other times, the active, angry, obdurate disposition of Chamomilla.

In Pulsatilla and Chamomilla, we possess two basic archetypal extremes: the 'wimp' and the 'tyrant'. Both are clearly present within the structure of certain great remedies, e.g. Carcinosin, Lac-humanum, Lac-lupinum, Lac-caninum, Stannum and Anacardium. The union of the two archetypal energies through sublimation (positive expression) can produce the hero (e.g. Aurum – gold); their combination through degradation (repression) can give birth to the villain (e.g. Anacardium – marking nut).

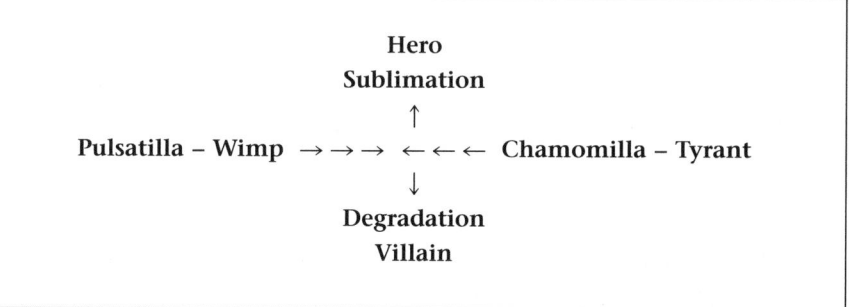

Figure 23.1 *Oral sublimation or degradation*

The Anal Stage

This is the second stage of psychosexual development. It is also referred to as the *potty-training stage, extending from two to four years.* The dominance of the Id is challenged by the emergence of the ego-self. During this period of ego-development, the infant's erogenous zone transfers from the mouth to the lower digestive tract and the anal region. Central to the anal-stage experience is toilet training and this arena presents the first direct contention between the Id and the ego-self. The struggle is between the Id's demand for immediate gratification through the elimination of bowel contents and the ego-self's counter-command to delay or control this gratification until circumstances permit. The potential difficulties involve not only when and where to defecate, but also the nature of the parent's demands and expectations and the issues of neatness and cleanliness. When the parental encouragement is gentle, patient and understanding, the child will generally adjust comfortably to the discipline and learns the value of cleanliness and orderliness, producing a better-adapted adult; but if the demands of the parents regarding toilet training are excessive and too coercive, psychological trauma may ensue causing the development of an obsessive-compulsive personality, too concerned about control, cleanliness and perfection. Erogenous gratification is now fixated on the pleasure derived from controlling and eliminating faeces and by extension on having power and control over parents. The 'pleasure' is now focused on repressing the urges of the Id and on controlling the emotions, the behaviour of others and the order and cleanliness of the environment. The personality that emerges from this dynamic is termed the *anal retentive* and when such values and behaviour are manifest they are described as being '*anal*'. The structures of the ego-self become fixed, rigid and uncompromising and the stage is set for psychopathology. During the anal stage of psychosexual development, the sexual and aggressive fantasies active in the unconscious become more clearly defined.

In those unduly slow to potty train, the Id remains dominant and uncontested by the ego-self. Following the pleasure principle and ignoring the reality principle, the bowels continue to be discharged at will. When parental concern and discipline are neglectful, such spontaneous and uncontrolled yielding to the promptings of the bowel may lead to the development of a self-indulgent personality that fails to develop sensitivity to, and a need for, neatness, cleanliness and order; personal slovenliness and an untidy, insanitary environment result. This type of personality is termed *anal expulsive* and such individuals tend to be highly disorganised, chaotic, undisciplined, unreliable and impulsive, with lack of self-appraisal, inability to take responsibility for their own actions, contempt for order, education and the mores of society and an indifference to the opinion and sensibilities of others.

Homeopathic analysis of the anal archetypes that can emerge during this second stage of psychosexual development reveals two fundamental homeopathic archetypes that perfectly match the anal retentive and anal expulsive personality types: Nux vomica and Sulphur, respectively; and clinically, they are closely related.

Nux vomica

Strychnos nux vomica (poison nut), a medium sized tree of the Loganiaceae family, indigenous to India and Sri Lanka, bears fruit about the size of a large apple with a smooth hard rind or shell, which when ripe is a lovely orange colour, filled with a soft white jelly-like pulp containing five seeds covered with a soft woolly-like substance. These seeds, which are 10 to 30 mm in diameter and 4 to 6 mm thick, have the shape of flattened disks densely covered with satiny hairs, radiating from the centre of the flattened sides and giving to the seeds a characteristic sheen.[1] Internally, they are white and horny. Despite their soft, woolly, innocuous appearance these seeds have an intensely bitter taste and are extremely poisonous due to strychnine, a highly toxic alkaloid that they contain.

The Nux-vom archetype, male or female, is quintessentially *anal-retentive*; a compulsive, ambitious, competitive, achievement driven individual, for whom second best is never good enough. They are perfectionists: A-type personalities, workaholics, who mercilessly drive themselves and others in the pursuit of excellence and success. The goals they set are everything to them; they must be realised whatever the cost, even the sacrifice of morality, the wellbeing of those they command and their own health. Obstacles must be aggressively overcome or swept aside and any hindrance to their forward progress, any thwarting of their ambitions, arouses immense ire, which falls upon their minions, whom they hold responsible and harshly reproach; upon their family, who experience the release of their frustration and irritability; or upon inanimate objects, which they tear, smash or throw. Impatient and hurried, they will not brook the least delay; highly critical and utterly intolerant of inefficiency, incompetence and negligence, they do not suffer fools gladly. Sartorial elegance reflects their fastidiousness and sophistication, which extends to good food, wines, culture and the arts. Their environment is in keeping with their exacting standards: tidy, practical, ordered and aesthetically pleasing. They have the ability to meticulously marshal minutia and also strategize enterprises of vast scope and sway. In their heyday, they have complete confidence in their abilities, they anticipate success and relish being top-dog in whatever sphere they are engaged. This self-assuredness carries over into their inter-action with others, professionally, socially and romantically. They possess poise and presence and are highly articulate, have an excellent command of language and delight in the thrust and riposte of intelligent dialogue and debate.

There is a downside to their superior talents. Their perfectionism and ambitious drive for success are not necessarily attended by moral scruples and empathy for others. They are hard on those who work with them and equally hard on themselves. Extending over years, the zealous and demand-ing intensity they apply to all their endeavours exhausts the nervous system. Often a serious setback, failure or disappointment starts a down-ward slide. They become hypersensitive and over-reactive to all external impressions: noise, music, voices, light, pain and odours. Invariably, the reaction to such unwanted input is intolerance, impatience, irritation and explosive anger. The mind is never at rest, always turbulent and filled with plans, projects and business concerns. Sleep eludes them or is broken and uneasy. They wake typically at 3.00 a.m. and cannot find sleep again. Shortly before it is time to rise, they drift off and sleep their best and then waken feeling drugged, tired and exhausted. Desperate for rest, they may resort to sedatives, creating a vicious cycle of tension and sleeping potions. In order to keep going, many drink copious amounts of coffee and ease their stress with tobacco, wining and dining, sexual encounters and recre-ational substances, especially cocaine.

Major characteristics of the Nux vomica archetype are foreseen in the outstanding features of the plant. Its twisted trunk and its irregular branch-ing pattern present an image of tautness and tension. The strikingly orange fruit speaks with all the eloquence of colour, announcing a dynamic clearly related to the second chakra, Svadhisthana. Orange is feminine red. Whatever red is orange can also be, but usually tempered unless unduly provoked or primed by alcohol. The territorial, tribal aggression and robust, earthy sexuality of red and of the Ferrum archetype have been touched with the feminine and rendered more sophisticated, subtle and refined. Though a warrior at heart and imbued with a love of warfare, Nux is a leader and strategist not a bloodthirsty mercenary or foot soldier. Often the Nux battle-field is the corporate boardroom or the sports-field. Though commonly an opportunistic rake and philanderer, Nux usually has taste and class and though his designs are generally selfish, he is usually an attentive suitor and lover. Orange brings to the passion and ardour of red the eye of the epicure and the connoisseur.

Functionally, the second chakra and the colour orange relate not only to the urogenital sphere but also to the large intestine and especially the sigmoid colon, which stores faecal wastes and gasses until they are ready to be discharged from the body through the rectum and anus. This is the territory of conflict in the anally fixated. Being such a powerful poison, strychnine, the most important active principle of the poison nut tree, imbues the Nux archetype with passion, drive, energy and confidence, but also ensures a tendency to muscular tension, cramps and spasms, not only of the voluntary, skeletal muscles, but also of the involuntary plain muscles of the intestines leading to spastic colon, irritable bowel syndrome and constipation as might be expected in such an anal-retentive archetype.

Number Five archetype

In the soft pulp bed of the mesocarp of the fruit lie not four, not six, but exactly five seeds. Five is the number that designates the human being, often graphically depicted by a man whose head and spread-eagled limbs form a five-pointed star, or, geometrically, a pentagram (pentacle) drawn with lines crossing to the five points. Furthermore, the number stands for the five senses of the animate state and for the five digits of each hand and foot. Hence, five indicates a human being well grounded in the body, hypersensitive to all sensual impressions, possessing an unusual alertness to the environment and those within it, and the mental capacity and dexterity to excel in any intellectual or physical pursuit. Five is also cosmic, denoting the sacred marriage of Heaven, two, and Earth, three; and the five elemental forms of matter: earth, water, fire, air and ether. In step with this universality, the archetype has wide-ranging interests, possesses many talents and has the capacity to master any discipline that draws their attention. This polymath mind is blessed with excellent communication skills, which make them highly accomplished lecturers and teachers. The number is associated with both love and sex, a relationship derived either from five representing the conjunction of masculine three and feminine two or from a more ancient Mesopotamian tradition in which the five-pointed star was an emblem of Ishtar, who, like Aphrodite, was a goddess not only of sexual love, but also of war: a divine dynamic peculiar to the nature of Nux vomica, manifested in the archetype's ambitious, competitive, success-driven nature and highly charged sexuality.

The characteristics of the number five archetype determined by the ancient lore of numerology add further insights to our understanding of the Nux vomica personality. Significantly, orange is recognised as a colour that reflects the normally bright, cheerful, positive nature of a five personality.

The archetype is energetic, highly-strung and volatile and tackles life in a resourceful, enterprising and adventurous way, always welcoming challenge and change. They are daring, unconventional, adaptable, independent and versatile. These positive qualities are enhanced by a sharp intellect, a curious, investigative nature and a rich imagination. Unrestricted freedom to indulge their interests, their passions and their senses, to express their views, fulfil their ambitions, expand their knowledge through new experiences and satisfy their insatiable taste for life, is vital to their wellbeing. To such a free, fast-moving spirit, hindrance is frustrating and intolerable, provoking irritation, anger, resentment and stress, which are released in harsh censure, sarcasm, moodiness or adult temper tantrums. Driving too fast, driving selfishly and abusive road rage are typical of the archetype. They are always buoyant, positive, talkative and vivacious when life is exciting, fulfilling and successful, but setbacks, obstacles, thwarted ambition and betrayal by others reveal a different nature that can be unreasonable, unforgiving, retaliatory, malicious and violent. Despite their wish to play the field, fives harbour an inordinately possessive and jealous streak, which often comes to the fore when they have had too much alcohol. Other weaknesses that may raise problems are having too many irons in the fire; breaking themselves down through the profligate squandering of their vitality; reckless impulsiveness in the heat of the moment; impatience with routine and easy boredom if things are not happening; self-serving fickleness that goes where the going is good; and a flexible morality unashamedly tailored to their needs or objectives.

Weakened Nux-vom archetype

Notwithstanding, the obvious, often abrasive, confrontational maleness of the Nux-vom archetype, its masculine red is absorbed in feminine orange and the hard, horny seeds of the fruit are covered with fine hairs and rest in a soft bed of jelly; both allude to an archetypal softness and vulnerability that is not apparent; it is hidden or repressed. The Nux archetype is at pains to conceal any tenderness that might be construed as weakness. The fundamental, aggressive Chamomilla streak common to humanity is clearly visible; the equally fundamental impressionable, sensitive Pulsatilla picture fails to show until exposed by the erosive action of life. When ambition is thwarted, when freedom of expression is stifled, when their honour is sullied, and their fame and fortune lost, when they have been betrayed by their associates or betrayed in love, when death has taken their dearest from them or when their compulsive and prodigal life has worn them down, their vulnerability emerges. They begin to waver and wilt; their efficiency is impaired, their memory weakened, they make mistakes and are unable to express themselves as they used to; they become indecisive, timid, irresolute, self-doubting, without courage and are beset with worries and fears. Their personal appearance and the order and neatness of their surroundings, which were previously the focus of their fastidious attention and essential to their comfort, fall into neglect. They, who could and would never shed a tear, become weepy and sad. Eventually, their thoughts turn to suicide, possibly by throwing themselves from a window, but they lack the courage ever to do so.

In 1732–33, the English artist, William Hogarth brilliantly captured in a series of eight paintings, entitled *A Rake's Progress*, the decline and fall of Rakewell, a wealthy but spendthrift young man, from a position of affluence and privilege into a state of dissipation, debauchery and debt. He is incarcerated in the notorious, Fleet debtor's prison. Here, his mind gives way and the last canvas depicts him lying almost naked in the celebrated, London mental asylum, Bethlem Hospital (Bedlam), an object of curiosity and entertainment for fashionably-dressed young women. To the last, his neglected and abandoned fiancée, Sarah Young, remains loyal and loving to him, supporting and comforting him in the final, tragic image. While providing a commentary on the dire effects of wasteful, luxurious living, prostitution and gambling, aspects of London society that Hogarth despised, he also displays, in stark contrast, the interplay of the self-absorbed masculine and the selfless feminine archetypes. These paintings could have been created with the Nux vomica archetype in mind.

Sulphur

In contrast, the closely related Sulphur archetype is a classic example of the *anal-expulsive* personality. We shall have reason to discuss this very important archetype in greater detail later. Here, it is sufficient to point out those characteristics that exemplify its anal-expulsive character in childhood and adolescence. The symbol representing the Sulphur archetype is every bit as powerful as strychnine and far more primal: it is the volcano and surely nothing can present a more expulsive or eruptive metaphor. Volcanic activity is characterised by the emission of highly-offensive sulphur-laden fumes through vents in the earth's crust. This activity was at its height during the prebiotic period of planetary evolution when the earth was forming its monumental crust upon a molten ocean of magma. The times were violent, seemingly chaotic and lawless and the terrain that was laid down over those long-past ages was raw and ravaged. Nature wielded her creative hand with extrovert bravura and the results were coarse, harsh and unrefined. The dynamic of Sulphur's remedial action is one with the volcano; it is centrifugal working from the depths onto the surface and from within outwards. It is perfectly coincident with the surge and flow of the Id; both are cathartic!

As much as the Nux archetype is sophisticated, refined and controlled, the Sulphur archetype, in keeping with the volcano and the wild, untamed, volcanic landscape that are its metaphors, is natural, spontaneous, unself-consciously expressive and without pretence. Sulphur subjects often appear feral: unkempt in appearance, coarse, crude and uncouth in speech, un-disciplined in behaviour, slovenly in habit and quite unconcerned about good manners, the opinion of others and the appropriateness of circum-stances. Just as freedom loving as a Nux-vom, the Sulphur archetype flies in the face of rules, regulations and restrictions. They are flagrantly anti-establishment and anti-authority. This lack of respect for those who are in charge and for those who determine what is correct commences in infancy and childhood and may start with resistance to potty training and extend to bathing, brushing teeth, keeping themselves and their rooms clean and tidy and obeying the rules of the house. There is something earthy and primitive about Sulphur; it hearkens back to an earlier period of evolution, before civilisation and all its codes and customs, when humans were in tune with nature, lived in caves and subsisted as hunter-gatherers. An emancipated (anal expulsive), instinctive existence permitting uncon-strained response to spur-of-the-moment impulses.

The Sulphur child is wild and wilful. They are in perpetual motion; mercilessly tease their siblings; are always into everything and at the centre of any mischief; extremely high-spirited; naughty; forever getting into trouble and into fights; disobedient; unheeding and defiant of reprimand. Something must always be happening; they need plenty of action, stimu-lation and excitement. Unfortunately, in this modern consumer age, many are satisfied with experiencing this vicariously, and become addicted to modern technology. Sulphur can be the child who cannot concentrate in school but can play computer games for hours. They have a most remark-able ability to become filthy. No child can become dirtier or more dish-evelled in shorter time than Sulphur or prove so difficult to clean. Their skins appear able to harbour ingrained dirt, which cannot be removed, no matter how they are scrubbed. The volcano is a fire symbol and water is inimical to fire; these fire-children are averse to any serious, sanitary use of water, but delight in using it to make mud, to drench and ruin things. Their hair is in keeping with their volcanic, unruly nature. Unless wet and clinging to the scalp, it is wild, unmanageable and as rebellious as its owner. Its texture is unhealthy, coarse and brittle and it lacks lustre.

To add to their scruffy appearance, their skin is coarse and rough; dry and cracked; red and inflamed-looking; inclined to chap in winter. They often suffer from skin eruptions, styes and dandruff. They bite their nails. They also have unpleasant habits. They are messy eaters. Nasal discharges are conveniently smeared off on the sleeve and whatever they glean from digging around in their noses disappears into the mouth. Sulphurs are great nose-pickers.

Sulphur signifies emergence: the emergence of a habitable planet, the first, sulphur-dependent, biological life form, first man, the ego-self and the intellect, the first tendency to disease, the development of the child and of the adolescent. It is possibly *the outstanding teenager remedy*, for its picture is replete with all the classic characteristics of that time of life: the hang-ups, complexes, prejudices, dissatisfaction, paranoia, selfishness, resentment of authority, rebelliousness, rudeness, arrogance, insolence, sulkiness, laziness, untidiness, lack of hygiene, inability to pick up the feet, bad posture, bad skin, love of the avant-garde, the bohemian and the torn and the ugly, procrastination, lack of manners, lack of discipline, loathing of school, love of play and parties, irresponsibility, love of loud strident music, love of speed, a high sex drive, late retiring and late rising, love of alcohol, tobacco and recreational drugs, especially marijuana. Always looking for the short cut, the quick fix, the Sulphur archetype tries to gate crash heaven by taking mind-altering substances. There are many damaged Sulphur adolescents; often teenagers with attitude and bad habits; rebels without cause, fighting for their independence instead of working for it; non-conformists, who conform to the behaviour and dress of non-conformists. Despite all the above, their parents love them, weep for them and fret and worry over them. While some remain anally-expulsive Sulphurs all their lives, others emerge from this rebellious stage, maturing into more controlled Sulphurs or some related archetype. Homeopathic Sulphur can make the transition from an indolent, easy-come-easy-go shirker to a responsible, productive individual far easier.

While the anally-retentive Nux-vom tends to constipate, often attended by colic and spasms, the anally-expulsive Sulphur is always more inclined towards diarrhoea, a quality it shares with its closely related plant analogue, Aloe socotrina. Sulphur's diarrhoea, like its perspiration is often offensive.

The central position of Nux vomica and Sulphur in the anal stage of sexual development is confirmed by the shift that each can make towards the archetypal picture of the other. The previously immaculate and controlled Nux-vom, when broken down, can deteriorate into a slovenly, dishevelled being, who requires Nux-vom as a remedy, or, possibly, even Sulphur, which follows it well; hence, the unexpected presence of Nux-vom in the rubric, *dirtiness*. The Sulphur archetype can mature out of chaos and disorder into a presentable and ordered person, thus, appearing, seemingly against all odds, in the rubric *fastidiousness*. However, the adult Sulphur taking on the appearance of a bandbox-smart Nux vomica will still invariably betray himself, or herself, in some way: a lack of dress sense or the lack of an eye for matching colours; a frayed cuff, a hole in a sock or underpants, an egg stain; rebellious hair; never standing if they can sit, never sitting if they can recline; inappropriate language and lack of tact; or a proclivity for rationalisation, speculative theorising and fundamentalism. The anal connection of Nux-vom and Sulphur was noted by Margaret Tyler in her essay on Nux-vom in *Homœopathic Drug Pictures*: "One has been told by the old Sisters at the Hospital, that in the older days of Homœopathy, no one dreamed of operating for piles: they used to cure them with *Nux* and *Sulphur* – low – and in alternation."[2]

When the anal-retentive state intensifies, i.e. moves even further to the right, the shift is from Nux vomica towards the pan-perfectionism of Arsenicum album, the most immaculate, fastidious, obsessively-compulsive and 'anal' of all, and towards Arsenicum's chronic counterpart, Thuja, who hides duplicity and degeneracy behind a mask of pristine perfection and correctness. When the anal-expulsive state intensifies, i.e. moves even further to the left, the shift is from Sulphur towards the anarchy and activism of the Ammonium carbonate archetype.

Anal expulsive <– Amm-carb <– Sulphur <–> Nux-vom –>
Ars-alb/Thuja –> **Anal retentive**

The all-encompassing presence of Carcinosin is found in both anally fixated states, as it is in both the oral-erotic and oral-sadistic fixations. It can be either highly-fastidious or very untidy and it can also be a mixture of both, especially when general surroundings and personal appearance are neglected, but the quality of the work that is produced by the archetype is the best possible. Carcinosin is also unable to rest after completing a task until everything is back in its proper place.

Important rubrics in the anal stage of sexual development:

Anal retentive

- *Fastidiousness:*
  *Ars-alb; *Carcinosin; *Pulsatilla; *Thuja.
  Anacardium; Graphites; Kali-carb; Lobelia; Nat-mur; Nux-vomica; Silicea; Sepia; Sulph.
- *Rest: cannot rest when things are not in their proper place:*

Ars-alb; Anacardium; Carcinosin; Lac equinum; Sepia; Sulphur.
- *Conscientious about trifles.*

The black letter and italic remedies, plus those listed under both this rubric and fastidiousness.

*Ars-alb; *Ignatia; *Nat-carb; *Silicea; *Staphysagria; *Thuja.

Baryta-carb; Carcinosin; Digitalis; Graphites; Lachesis, Mag-p-a; Muriatic-ac; Nux-vom; Pulsatilla; Stramonium; Sepia; Sulphur.

- *Always washing hands:*
  Lac caninum; Medorrhinum; Nat-mur; Sulphur.
  Ars-alb; Coca; Curare; Merc-sol; Oscillococcinum; Platina; Psorinum; Sepia; Silicea; Syphilinum; Thuja.
- *Mania for cleanness:*
  Ars-alb; Sepia; Silicea; Sulphur.

Anal expulsive

- *Aversion to washing:*
  Amm-carb; Ant-crud; Lap-mar-c; Physostigma; Psorinum; Sulphur; Tuberculinum.
- *Untidy:*
  Psorinum; Sulphur.
  Adamas; Amm-carb; Androctonus; Arbus-menz; Aurum-ars; Capsicum; Carcinosin; Lac humanus; Silicea.
- *Indifference about personal appearance:*
  *Sulphur; Coca; Kola.
- *Dirtiness:*
  Amm-carb; Capsicum; Graphites; Lac caninum; Platina; Psorinum; Sulphur.

It is a useful exercise to study and compare relevant rubrics in this manner. It is interesting to note that it is not only Nux-vom and Sulphur that cover both forms of anal fixation. Most important in this respect are Lac humanum – the remedy that carries so much of the burden of human emotional trauma due to dysfunctional upbringing and miasmatic inheritance; Lac caninum – man's best friend and the closest remedy to Carcinosin; Graphites – the most fundamental of the carbons and therefore closely related to the formative period; and its carbon ultimate, Adamas (diamond); Silicea – the chronic counterpart to Pulsatilla, a formative remedy as fundamental as Graphites; and Psorinum – the nosode of the primary miasm.

Added to these are the oceanic remedies Nat-mur, Sepia and Phosphorus and the dark remedies Androctonus (Scorpion) and Platina.

A remedy that is missing from the rubric *dirtiness* and must be added, just as Adamas must be added to the rubric *fastidiousness*, is Anacardium, who, pulled and pushed between devil and angel, can be impeccable or unkempt – retentive or expulsive. The number of arsenates (Aurum-ars, Baryta-ars, Kali-ars, Natrum-ars) in the rubric *fastidiousness* indicates the underlying fear and anxiety that drives the compulsion.

References

1 Grieve M. *A Modern Herbal*. London: Jonathan Cape Ltd, 1979. p592.
2 Tyler ML. *Homœopathic Drug Pictures*. Saffron Waldon, Essex: The CW Daniel Company Ltd, 1992. p606.

PSYCHOSEXUAL DEVELOPMENT STAGES

Phallic – Latency – Genital

Phallic Stage

The third stage of psychosexual development is the phallic stage, *spanning the ages of three to six years* during which time the child's genitalia become the primary erogenous zone. This stage is as critical to the development of a balanced, well-adapted and resilient personality as the first two stages, but the dynamics are far more complex.

During this period of development, children become more intimately aware of their bodies and curious about the anatomical differences between boys and girls and between men and women; visual and tactile exploration of their bodies and possibly those of siblings and other children results. The common, instinctive desire to expose the genitalia and participate in 'doctor/patient' games is indicative of this Id induced sexual curiosity and shift in erogenous focus. In addition, the child becomes conscious of gender identity: the different biological and social roles and expectations that are tied to sexual identity.

Boy phallic fixation

Until this time, the mother is invariably the epicentre of the holding environment, the goddess who gratifies every desire; the godlike father is a more remote, peripheral figure, akin to the sky-gods of the ancients. As the all-embracing symbiosis of mother and child wanes and the personal identity takes shape, the physical and emotional separation into a discrete sexual being brings father onto centre-stage alongside mother, and the power of the child's Id becomes focussed upon both parents. This power is fuelled by both aggressive and sexual fantasies that have evolved in the unconscious during the oral and anal stages of development. In the young boy, the libidinal energy of the Id becomes focussed upon the mother (or mother figure) with whom he unconsciously falls in love and about whom he has unconscious sexual fantasies; the aggressive energy of the Id is focussed upon the father (or father figure) whom he unconsciously hates and about whom he entertains aggressive fantasies. The father is now his rival and he is jealous of him because the father psychosexually 'possesses' the mother and sleeps in her bed. The mother is idealised and the father is demonised. In accordance with the pleasure principle, the Id fantasises about killing the father in order to possess the mother, but the pragmatic ego, abiding by the reality principle, represses this desire, not out of innate, moral compunction, but in atavistic submission to the hierarchical precedence and power of the stronger, older, alpha male.

The self-preserving repression of aggression does not resolve the inner conflict, or the hostility; an unconscious fear and wariness of the dominant, male figure in the family remains. Given the nature and behaviour of a specific father, the fear may have a very rational component, but the father's nature, however brutal, is not the primary cause; the fear stems from the built-in beta state of the infantile Id. Freud conceived that once a boy becomes aware of the difference between male and female genitalia, he unconsciously perceives the female to be castrated and his fear of the father becomes an irrational fear of suffering the same fate. However, the Id, unlike Freud and the Lycopodium archetype, does not give such psychological and physical prominence to the male organs, which, even when erect, a very transient phenomenon, are not symbolic of the primitive, hierarchical male power of the Id, which a stag's antlers and a male gorilla's silver-back clearly are. At the heart of the conflict there is certainly fear of loss, but not of the genitals; it is the fear of *loss of power – the power to dominate* (survive, succeed, have) *and the power of identity* (value, significance, respect), attributes essential to self-esteem and self-confidence. Repress or remove these, and one is, indeed, castrated: a state of mental and emotional disempowerment! Because dominance in primate and early-human bands granted the alpha male sexual precedence, the contention has sexual and jealous overtones, which in the presence of miasmatic distortion can turn to abiding hatred and the unconscious desire to kill.

In the light of these atavistic dynamics inherent to the phallic stage of psychosexual development, certain repertory rubrics are significant and particular archetypes that nurse the unconscious feelings identified above need consideration: *desire to kill*; *jealousy*; *jealousy with sexual excitement*; *hatred*; *hatred and revenge*.

Girl phallic fixation

A young girl between the age of three and six has the same potential for sexual and aggressive fantasies derived from the Id as a young boy, but the attraction that triggers the Id response in a girl is directed towards her father, whom she unconsciously falls in love with and wants to sexually possess. The mother becomes her rival. The father is idealised and the mother is demonised. The same issues of hierarchical, dominance exist for the girl as they do for a boy, but the power struggle is between herself and her mother for the favours of her father. The girl's infantile Id is in beta mode, she therefore fears and is wary of the dominant, alpha female in the home and submissively acknowledges her right to possess the father psychosexually and sleep in his bed. The price is jealousy, hate and aggression, unconsciously felt towards the mother (consider Lac humanum, Thuja).

Emotional castration

When power is wrested from a child of either sex during the phallic period of development, either through authoritarian domination by the same-sex parent, whom the child hates, or through rejection by the contrasexual parent, whom the child adores, emotional 'castration' occurs. This constitutes the disempowerment of the masculine principle within the psyche: an energy that is essential for self-esteem, the assertion of will and self-protection. Fixation is ensured and the scene is set for future psychosexual and relationship problems. All phallic stage fixations involve imbalance between the masculine and feminine aspects of the ego-self. 'Castration' implies weakness of the masculine, which in male or female produces a non-assertive, diffident, submissive archetype.

Resolution

In general, as the child matures through the phallic stage it comes to realise unconsciously that it is wiser and safer to identify with either the father, in the case of a boy, or with the mother, in the case of a girl, in order that he may survive to one day marry a woman like his mother or she a man like her father. This shift removes the tension of competitive rivalry, defuses the jealousy and aggression felt towards the same-sex parent and moderates the possessive desire felt for the opposite-sex (contrasexual) parent; processes that must reach full resolution in the later stages of sexual development for psychic homeostasis to be achieved. Full resolution implies the capacity for authentic relationship with others of either sex without the prejudice of idealised or demonised, parental archetypal images imprinted in the unconscious. This natural unfolding is a process of sublimation; the power of the Id is released to freely expand, create and achieve.

Ongoing fixation

The emotions, ideas and fantasies revolving around a child's desire to usurp the position of the same-sex parent or to sexually possess the contrasexual parent are held in the unconscious by dynamic repression. If they remain unresolved, continued repression distorts reality, adding to the complexity and dysfunction of the emerging psyche. The filters imposed by the perspectives of the ego fixated in the phallic stage prevent the soul from forming relationships uncontaminated by gender programming installed during this highly impressionable, immature period of life. Since, complete resolution is the exception rather than the rule, varying degrees of resolution and fixation are to be expected, determined by endowed and inherited characteristics innate to the individual; not least of all miasmatic influences.

Idealisation

Major fixation in the phallic stage of development is apparent when during the teenage, genital stage and the years of high libido that follow (a critical time when sexual relationships assume great importance and often play a major role in the way life unfolds) the desire to sexually possess the contrasexual parent has persisted and is still inextricably linked to the idealised image of the parent formed during the immature phallic stage. This image persists in the unconscious in a form unmodified by mature evaluation, discernment or judgement as a hero or heroine archetype; a glorified, magnetic, mythical being that can exert irresistible attraction when its living counterpart seems to appear in the individual's life. As we shall consider in detail later, the idealised image is incorporated in the anima (the eternal, universal archetype of the feminine) of the young man's unconscious as an exquisite goddess or in the animus (the eternal, universal archetype of the masculine) of the young woman's unconscious as a radiant god, and is projected upon the person of the 'beloved' rendering them irresistible; a fatal attraction born of infatuation, romanticism and wishful thinking and not based on knowledge of or concern about who the 'beloved' truly is. This is often a recipe for disappointment, disillusionment and disaster.

The temperament and character of the parent from whom the idealised image is formed will always possess weaknesses: human frailties unfit for modelling. Sometimes, the majority of idealised characteristics prove wholesome enough and despite the attraction being based on fixation in the phallic stage, the possibility of a mutually beneficial relationship may still exist. Unfortunately, it is most often the discordant traits of character, those which stand out most starkly and impinge most intensely and often traumatically on the consciousness of the young child, which tend to be mirrored. Who would imagine that the selfish, cruel, foul-mouthed alcoholic or misogynist father, who abuses the mother and beats the child; the waster and the dropout; the murderous activist for whom life is cheap: or the histrionic, self-absorbed, socialite mother; the cold, aloof martinet; the immature hysteric; or the sensual libertine, whose infidelities mortify her children, could possibly provide a model for idealisation? Yet, given innate potential in the young psyche (karmic and miasmatic) and phallic fixation, it is even so! The aberrant archetype becomes a template for recognition of the 'ideal' male or the 'ideal' female; its flawed nature mythologised in the unconscious and imprinted in the amygdala: the primitive mammalian memory-brain.

Here, sensitivity to the presence of the mythical archetype is harboured: an innate alertness and keened perceptiveness, likened to animal, olfactory, memory intelligence, which instinctively recognises friend, foe and potential mate and will then activate appropriate, behaviour responses. The energy pattern of the idealised archetype is also installed in the consciousness of the lower chakras. These energy centres both transmit and attract frequencies with which they resonate; activities that contribute to the unfolding reality of the individual. Given time, that reality gains force and form, inexorably and fatefully drawing the idealised archetype within the ambit of the fixated, vulnerable psyche, which has unconsciously been broadcasting its longing. Through resonance, the archetype, thus summoned, is charged with irresistible potency.

Recognition is instinctive and immediate, even when the negative traits of the parental template upon which the archetype is modelled are as yet only latent. A bond is established, which is cemented, especially in the instance of a girl or young woman, or a young man with a strong, romantic, feminine aspect, by sexual intimacy. Sooner or later, the young girl or woman realises that she has, indeed, 'married her father', warts and all! Too late, she discovers that the courteous, caring and considered behaviour of her lover, partner or husband hides attributes with which she is all too ominously familiar. Against all the promptings of common sense, prior-experience and her instinct for self-preservation, and, in some cases, even disregarding the safety of herself and her children, the spell holds! She stays in the relationship, rationalising that "she will change him", or out of desperation, or from wishful thinking, believing his protestations of remorse and promises that "it will never happen again". She can even become habituated to her victim state, helplessly caught in a spider web of her own weaving.

Characteristic of such phallic-stage fixation, even in the very early stages of romance or relationship is the deafness to advice, especially parental, and blindness to warning signals: incompatibility, selfishness, arrogance, possessiveness, jealousy, immaturity, chauvinism, misogyny, laziness, lack of ambition, womanising, infidelity, excess alcohol and the use of recreational substances. The stronger the aversion parents have towards the subject of her fascination, the stronger the attraction becomes and the more stubbornly it is adhered to. Parental disapproval and opposition is often the spur that ensures disaster.

Fixation in the phallic stage is the evil spell of the wicked fairy – the spindle that induces inertia – the narcotising prick of the needle that spirals the victim into a state of psychic slumber, at the total mercy of circumstances and another being. Even when, for some reason, the relationship is sundered, the spell still binds her; her internalised image of the 'knight in shining armour' remains paradoxically intact to haunt and possess her. She has escaped the clutches of 'Tom' only to find herself in the grip of 'Dick', and, if nothing changes, 'Harry' is waiting around the corner. The dynamics of her life seem bound to repeated cycles of inescapable attraction to toxic men who contaminate her life. The kiss of the prince is needed to awaken her, release her and spirit her to safety. 'He' may be in the form of her own masculine principle that empowers her to break free; a critical saturation point of grief and pain; a real-life prince who gives her the kiss of true love; an esteemed guide or mentor; the well-selected homeopathic remedy.

Idealised mother figure

Needless to say, in the above scenario, the genders may be reversed, with the male being irresistibly attracted to women, whom he unconsciously and instinctively identifies as possessing the characteristics of his idealised, mother figure. For a man who still needs a mother rather than a partner, a relationship based upon this affinity may seem satisfactory. Nevertheless, the attraction is based on ego-self fixation in the phallic stage and not on soul consonance. Self-determination and mature, unprejudiced judgement are impaired. The mother-fixation seldom provides a sound foundation for a mutually satisfactory and creative adult relationship. In effect, the man fails to leave the nest and fully grow up. He too has pricked his finger and falling under the spell of the spindle, succumbs to psychic slumber. Like his female counterpart, he may constantly end up being attracted to domineering, self-centred partners, who wear the trousers and keep him under their thumb: 'hen-pecked' and submissive. If the woman he chooses to replace his mother is not of a forceful, assertive nature and does not take control of his life, his first loyalty may always remain with his often manipulative, possessive, selfish mother. Neither of these scenarios proves a recipe for marital success.

Demonised 'good' father

There is invariably an underlying humour in life, which expresses itself through paradox and can be either light or dark. The fixation on the parental figure can be inverted. Taking the daughter-father fixation as an example, the inversion is most common when a kindly, upright, disciplined, educated and successful father is experienced as critical, disapproving and rejecting and the fixated child is defiant and rebellious. The qualities of the conservative and correct father, upon whom the daughter is fixated, and by whom she feels rejected, are demonised, and she is irresistibly drawn to men who display archetypal traits that are the antithesis of those of her father. One such young lady informed me that if nine young men were paraded before her, all exemplary by conservative standards and social pedigree, and a tenth was of dubious background, dishevelled, unshaven, tousle-haired and tattooed, impolitely lounging against a door frame with cigarette hanging from his mouth, thumbs in belt and a sardonic smile on his face, a modern-day James Dean, it would be he who attracted her attention: different and dangerous, not boring and predictable like her monotonously 'grey,' disapproving father. While acknowledging that behind a conservative and outwardly correct veneer, a villain or pervert may lurk, and that the shabby and feral may mask a rough diamond, or even a saint, nevertheless, this inverted fixation more often than not leads down a tortuous and uncertain path that too often brings heartache to daughter and parents alike. Sometimes, through hardship and grief, the inversion is reversed but without fixation, for life has brought about healing and the ego-self has lost much of its power to subvert; the daughter gains insight into her own rebellious and defiant nature and perceives the virtues in her critical father and his concern for her.

Fixation victims

For both genders, the majority of bad relationships due to phallic-stage fixation result in the abuse of the feminine principle by the masculine and this dynamic tends to be self-contaminating, leading to a repetitive cycle of victimisation from which the sleeping soul fails to escape. This holds equally true for homosexual relationships founded on such fixation. Even after a break-up and a taste of freedom, against all common sense and previous emotional pain, the enslaved ego-self is characteristically drawn back into the same sick relationship or will find someone else to abuse it.

Phallic-fixation archetypes

The correct homeopathic remedy can prove a revelation, releasing the bonds of fixation and victim consciousness that trap the ego/soul complex in damaging relationships. The nosodes, Psorinum and Carcinosin, must always be considered in such situations, either as *the* constitutional remedy or as an adjunct to assist others; both suit the captive victim-state. Medorrhinum is often effective when the dynamic is homosexual. The C-type Carcinosin is ill-equipped to deal with the stresses, demands and decisions of everyday life and in the face of challenge or trauma freezes and dissociates from feeling and even identity. This state of emotional apathy or inertia is characteristic of the stunned, numbed, defenceless state of the fixated ego-self and is manifested through denial, self-sacrifice, compromise, expediency, procrastination and rationalisation. All of which keep them shackled in their misery. The definite therapeutic relationship that exists between the cancer nosode and the victimised feminine principle, long established by clinical experience, sharply highlights the role that such subtle or blatant abuse plays in the development of malignancy, especially when the abuse extends over years and is aggravated by infidelity. The rigid, controlled, repressed nature of the afflicted C-type ego-self ensures that the impingement implodes, inducing cellular anarchy beneath a veneer of stoic fortitude.

The *Ranunculaceae* plant family provides us with three remarkable remedies for the narcotised state of phallic stage fixation. These are Pulsatilla (meadow anemone), Staphysagria (stavesacre) and Cimicifuga (black cohosh). Each covers its own unique picture of fixation. As indicated by their alternative common names, Staphysagria (louse-wort) and Cimicifuga (bugbane) are insect repellents. Analogy indicates that these two botanical cousins must prove excellent remedies for those who are particularly open to victimisation or parasitisation. This correspondence guides the wise shaman, who prescribes them for those who are burdened by a victim consciousness that draws them into abusive relationships from which they lack the strength to escape. Other well-known insect repellents that may be called for in the treatment of victims of physical, emotional or sexual abuse are: Agaricus (fly agaric), Anatherum (vetiver), Camphor, Cocculus (Indian cockle), Ledum (wild rosemary) and Thuja (cedar).

Since ancient times, the plant juices of either Staphysagria or Cocculus have been employed to stupefy and catch fish by adding them to pond water. The stupefied state of the fish simulates the protracted soul-slumber of phallic fixation, but more alarmingly also the helpless condition of a victim of date-rape, when the abuse has been facilitated by alcohol or the surreptitious administration of an incapacitating drug such as Rohypnol. The after-effects may require treatment with one of these two remedies or possibly the psychotropic remedy, Stramonium, which when used clandestinely removes memory of both the violation and the perpetrator.

The human breast is the very symbol of the female principle; hence, it is not surprising that Carcinosin, the nosode prepared from carcinoma of the breast, stands at the pinnacle of remedies called for in the treatment of the abused feminine principle, often a victim situation brought about by fixation in the phallic stage of psychosexual development. This pathogenetic affinity naturally extends to the Lac (milk) remedies since they are prepared from the distilled maternal virtue of the breast. This is especially true of Lac-can (bitch's milk), the remedy closest to Carcinosin. Although all Lac remedies must be considered in this light, some deserve special mention: Lac humanum, because it corresponds to so much human suffering, Lac defloratum (skimmed cow's milk) and Lac ovis (sheep's milk) because they suit fixated beings who either submit to their plight with docile, bovine acquiescence or possess an easily manipulated, follow-my-leader, sheep-like nature.

Two remedies stand out above all others for the treatment of severe bruising of the breasts, an injury which must be considered analogous to deep trauma of the feminine principle: Bellis perennis, the common or English daisy, a manifestly feminine symbol, and Conium maculatum (poison hemlock), the poison that was administered to Socrates after he was condemned to death by the patriarchal bureaucracy of Athens, for being a 'gadfly' to the conscience of the State. Deep contusion of breast tissue can provoke the development of breast cancer in a constitutionally vulnerable subject; this is a field covered by these two remarkable remedies, linking them strongly to Carcinosin. Their cancer preventing power extends beyond physical trauma as the initiating cause; it protects against the psychic blows to the inner feminine that most often lie at the root of cancerous change. Both Bellis and Conium are important remedies for young girls and women caught in phallic stage fixation. They will be discussed in detail in *Healing the Soul* volume 3 under *Carcinosis*, the cancer miasm.

A constellation of remedies for the fixated and bruised psyche orbit around Carcinosin. The most important were recognised by Donald Foubister, who was responsible for the pioneer work that defined the initial picture of this great nosode. These were: Bellis perennis, Sepia (cuttlefish), Lac caninum and Folliculinum (ovarian follicle). To these leading remedies, we may add Ignatia, Nat-mur, Aurum-mur-nat, Berberis, Staphysagria, Causticum, Lycopodium, Thuja and Conium and also two acute remedies for intense trauma: Aconitum and Stramonium. Beyond these central remedies lie others.

Relevant rubrics in this regard are:

- *Ailments from: abuse.*
  - *Sexual abuse.*
- *A history of long domination by others.*

Oedipus myth

Freud wisely turned to Greek mythology for a well-known tale to illustrate his hypothesis of the unconscious, incestuous love of a son for a mother and the desire to overthrow, supplant or kill the father, for myths are ever the purveyors of intuitive and received wisdom and often do so in an impelling and unforgettable way. He found what he required in the famous story of Oedipus (*Oidipous* in Greek). The myth has many versions, but the one best known is that related by Sophocles in his play *Oedipus the King* (*Oedipus Rex*).

When Labdakos, the King of Thebes died, his son, Laios, was still an infant. For a number of years, his great-great uncle Lykos ruled as regent in his stead; but subverted by the corrupting comforts and authority of regal power, he usurped his nephew's position and declared himself king. Once achieved, he lost no time in fulfilling a vow of family vengeance made to his dying, elder brother Nykteus against his daughter Antiope, who, with her husband Epopeus, the King of Sicyon, had defied Nikteus and earned his hatred. Intent on honouring this fraternal vow, Lykos marshalled his Theban forces and marched upon Sicyon where he defeated and slew Epopeus. He brought his captive niece Antiope back to Thebes and kept her imprisoned in his palace.

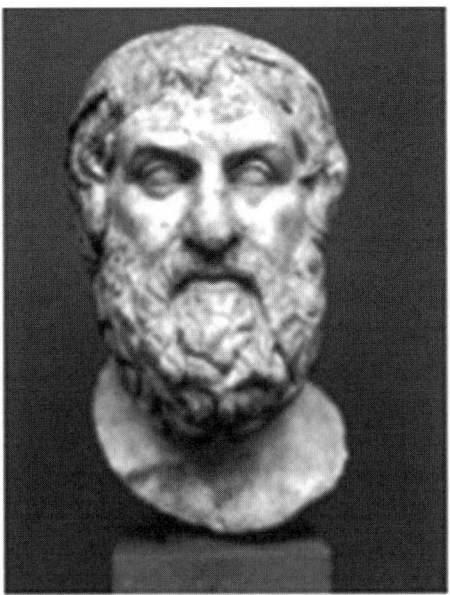

Figure 24.1 Bust of the playwright Sophocles. A Roman copy of an earlier Greek original. c270 B.C.E

After many years, Antiope contrived her escape from her uncle's clutches. Once reunited with her twin sons by Zeus, Amphion and Zethos, now, no longer children but grown men, she successfully conspired with them to bring about the downfall and death of the tyrant, Lykos. Amphion and Zethos then claimed the throne of Thebes for themselves, and, to secure their position, banished Laios, the rightful heir, into exile.

Pelops, the king of Pisa kindly offered the disinherited prince a safe haven in Elis, in the north-western Peloponnese. Whilst a guest at the court of Pelops, Laios taught the king's young, illegitimate son, Chrysippos, the art of charioteering. The tender youth, dearly loved by his father and cherished even above his legitimate siblings, was exquisitely handsome in form and feature. Laios conceived an irresistible passion for him. Foolishly, in transgression of his protector's hospitality, a tie held sacred in the ancient world, Laios abducted Chrysippos with the intention of either seducing or ravishing him. The young man did not share his tutor's passion and adamantly refused to yield to his advances. Consumed with longing, Laios would not be deterred and tried to take by force what he had failed to achieve by tenderness. To escape violation, Chrysippos killed himself with his sword. By the time his father, Pelops, heard of this tragedy, Laios had departed for Thebes to reclaim his throne, which had been left vacant at the death of the usurpers, Amphion and Zethos.

With Laios beyond his might, the anger of the distraught father reached out to him and all his progeny from afar in the form of a most terrible curse, which would be held responsible for all the disasters and tragedies that subsequently descended upon the royal house of Thebes.

In time, Laios married Iokaste, a distant-cousin of peerless beauty, who was scarcely nubile. When months had passed without sign of pregnancy, Laios decided to secretly consult the Delphic Oracle for guidance and to hear whether his child-bride would ever conceive. Apollo, the God of Prophecy, who presided over this most sacred shrine, gave him answer through the priestess of the oracle, the Pythia, or pythoness. Gifted with psychic powers, the priestess was able to commune with the god, usually giving supplicants advise in cryptic or ambiguous terms, just as the collective unconscious informs the psyche through the medium of dreams. The god's answer to the Theban king, however, was direct and coldly unequivocal; he presaged only tragedy and disaster. In his introduction to *Oedipus the King*, Sophocles provides us with the dread words uttered by Apollo:

> I will give you a son, but you are destined to die at his hands. This is the decision of Zeus, in answer to the bitter curses of Pelops, whose son you abducted; all this did Pelops call down upon you.[1]

The dire warning chilled Laios's passion for Iokaste. Without a word of explanation, he withdrew from her and ceased all intimacy. Distressed and fearing that he no longer desired her, one night, she plied him with drink, and, when he could no longer resist her charms, enticed him into her arms and seduced him. Apollo kept his word: she fell pregnant and duly produced a son.

Laios was aghast. Could he thwart the god's prediction? Would any mortal dare such presumption? Laios had no doubt or scruple, he seized the infant from its mother's breast and delivered it to a trusted shepherd in his service, with the instruction to abandon it upon Mt Cithaerona, tethered by an iron pin driven through its feet: a cruel act born of superstition and fear that the baby might be spirited away and spared. The shepherd did as he was bidden, but, as he was about to leave the baby to perish, the power of Apollo and human compassion overcame him; he retrieved the child, bore it home and tended its wounds. Fearing the wrath of his king should he discover the child still lived, he begged a fellow shepherd from Corinth to take the child beyond the borders of Thebes and raise it as his own. As it happened, the Corinthian was a servant of Polybos, the King of Corinth. Hoping to find a home more suited to the station of the infant, the shepherd presented the baby to his master and mistress. The royal couple, still childless after many years of marriage, recognising the baby's noble birth by its rich, swaddling clothes, gladly received it as a gift from the gods and adopted it as their own. Due to the wounds to its feet, the royal couple named the infant Oedipus (*swell foot*).

Oedipus grew to manhood as the much-honoured Prince of Corinth, the beloved son and heir of King Polybos and his queen, Merope. The loving and protective foster-parents never told him that he was adopted. It seemed that fate smiled upon the young prince and that his future would be blessed with every advantage, but the dark curse of Pelops hung over him and turned the wheels of destiny with remorseless intent. It waited only for him to come of age.

The unexpected appearance of a baby in the lives of the long-barren, royal couple caused rumours to circulate that the child could not possibly be their own. With the passing of years, these whisperings died away and no word ever came to the ears of the young prince; but there were those who remembered and secretly sneered at him. One fateful evening, at a banquet, a drunken guest, with whom he had an altercation, taunted Oedipus with not being the true son of Polybos. Shocked at his accuser's temerity and shamed by the presence of others, who had heard his words, Oedipus appealed to his parents for the truth. They hastened to reassure him, but a seed of doubt had been planted. For the first time, he earnestly scrutinised his features, hoping to find a family likeness. He sought in vain. Although confident of his parent's love for him, Oedipus was alarmed. He feared they were concealing a terrible truth. Without a word to anyone, he set out for Delphi to consult the oracle.

The urgent question of his parentage drew no response from the priestess. She remained silent, as if scrutinising not only his future but also his very soul. When she addressed him, her words were heavy with portent. They shook Oedipus to the core. She prophesied that he was destined to kill his father and marry his mother with whom he would father children. Oedipus was horrified, for, to the ancients, incest was the gravest of sins. Assuming, because of the god's silence on the matter, that Polybos and Merope were the father and mother the oracle spoke of, Oedipus vowed never to return to Corinth while ever they lived. He would foil the terrible prediction! 'Again, as his parents had done, he sought to give the lie to the oracle'.[2] On leaving Delphi, he turned his back on his birthright and dressed as an unarmed peasant set off on foot on the road to Thebes. It was a fateful decision. Through the words of Oedipus to his mother and wife Iokaste, many years later, Sophocles relates what happened in a narrow defile on that ill-fated journey between Delphi and Daulis:

> When I came to the place where three roads join, I met a herald followed by a horse drawn chariot, and a man seated therein . . . the leader roughly ordered me out of the way; and his venerable master joined in with a surly command. It was the driver that thrust me aside and him I struck for I was angry; the old man saw it, leaning from the chariot waited until I passed, then, seizing for weapon the driver's two-pronged goad, struck me on the head. He paid with interest for his temerity; quick as lightening, the staff in this right hand did its work; he tumbled headlong out of the chariot, and every man of them I killed.[3]

Apparently, little has changed during the 2500 years since this was written. Road rage seems to be a basic masculine (not necessarily male) weakness. In those distant times, however, violent consequences were more common. In this famous instance, the curse of Pelops exacted vengeance. The old man Oedipus slew was Laios, his father.

Oedipus continued on his way to Thebes. Since his destination was still uncertain, the terrain difficult and he had only his feet to carry him, the journey took considerable time. He arrived to find the city in confusion and in the grip of fear. The Theban king had been killed by brigands on the road to Delphi. This was the tale fabricated by the only surviving bodyguard of the five that had accompanied Laios. Seeing the ease with which Oedipus dispatched his comrades, he had slipped away unseen and on returning to the city concealed his cowardice by relating how they had been set upon by a band of well-armed assailants rather than a lone wayfarer bearing only a staff.

Upon the death of the king, Kreon, the brother of Iokaste, had taken on the role of regent. He was at once faced by a terrible threat to his people. Hera, the Goddess of Marriage, had sent a savage monster, a she-devil, called the Sphinx (the throttler) out of the wilds of Ethiopia to terrorise the city in punishment for Laios's abduction of Chrysippos.

In its Greek form, the Sphinx was one of its kind; a unique, merciless demon of destruction that ravened for human flesh; it had the head of a ferocious woman, the fangs and eyes of a cat, the claws and body of a lioness, the wings of an eagle and a constricting, serpent-headed tail. It lay in wait at the entrance to the city; only permitting travellers passage if they could answer a riddle. Those, unable to answer, she immediately strangled and devoured. Many died in this manner, including Iokaste's nephew, Kreon's son Haemon (*Haimon*), whose very name foreboded a 'bloody' end. After the prince's death, the evil escalated; the Sphinx began to prey on the city at large, like a serial killer, taking one victim after another at random. Thebes became a city of terror and despair. In desperation, Kreon offered both the throne and his widowed sister, Iokaste, to anyone who could free the city of the monstrous predator. Iokaste was in her early thirties and exquisitely beautiful. Many were the heroes and suitors who staked their lives on the chance of possessing such a fine city and such a beautiful woman. All came to a miserable end, their bones bleaching white before the gates of the city. This was the situation that awaited the young traveller as he approached the walls of Thebes.

Oedipus came upon the voracious beast as it was tearing apart and devouring its last victim. Unsated, ever-greedy, it rose up before him, wings spread wide, and *'o'ersized with coagulate gore'*, glowered at him with baleful, slavering malevolence. The young prince gripped the staff that had recently served him so well at the crossroads and intrepidly demanded passage. With a ghastly grimace the Sphinx menacingly fixed its glaring yellow-green eyes upon him, and, in a high-pitched scream that rent the air, shredding his every nerve, posed the riddle that heralded death.

"What being with but one voice, of all things treading the earth, has sometimes four-feet, sometimes two – yet sometimes three – and is weakest and slowest when it has the most?"

Oedipus did not hesitate. "Man," he answered. "Because, as an infant, he crawls on all fours, stands and walks freely on two feet as an adult, and leans upon a staff in old age."

Mortified by the disclosure of her precious conundrum, the Sphinx flew to the top of Mount Phicium and flung herself onto the rocks below. Thebes was released from the scourge and Oedipus was received within the walls with all the triumph and tribute given a conquering hero. Kreon was as good as his word. He stepped down from the throne in favour of Oedipus and gave him his sister Iokaste as bride. Thus, the word of Apollo was fulfilled and the curse of Pelops enmeshed mother and son in incestuous union.

The tragedy of Oedipus played out in various ways, but the most familiar account, established by Sophocles, was that he and Iokaste had many prosperous years of devoted marriage together as the honoured and respected King and Queen of Thebes, during which Iokaste gave birth first to two daughters, Antigone and Ismene, and, then, two, irreconcilably feuding sons, Polyneikes and Eteokles. However, despite their love and contentment, the demon of destiny, the insatiable curse of Pelops, still brooded over the couple, ever poised to destroy their happiness and inflict bitter reparation. Inevitably, the truth about the birth of Oedipus, the death of Laios and the marriage of mother to son came to light; confirmed, with no malicious intent, by the very shepherd, who, so many years before, had taken pity on the rejected and condemned infant. Iokaste, was the first to hear the appalling truth. Distraught with guilt and grief, she fled to her chamber and there, in utter despair, hanged herself. She was already dead when Oedipus, in turn, faced the irrefutable proof. Sophocles captures the moment in stark, powerful verse:

> Alas! Alas! All is out! All is known, no more concealment!
> O Light! May I never look on you again.
> Revealed as I am, sinful in my begetting,
> Sinful in marriage, sinful in shedding blood.[4]

Oedipus hastens to Iokaste's rooms and finds the doors bolted. When no answer greets his cries for entry, dreading the worst, he hurls himself with superhuman strength against the barrier, and, bursting the bolts from their sockets, stumbles into the apartment beyond. The Chorus, who are cast as observers and commentators, describe the terrible scene and the horror that follows:

> We saw a knotted pendulum, a noose,
> A strangled woman swinging before our eyes.
> The King saw too, and with heart-rending groans
> Untied the rope and laid her on the ground.
> But worse was yet to see. Her dress was pinned
> With golden broaches, which the King snatched out
> And thrust, from full arm's length, into his eyes –
> Eyes that should see no longer his shame, his guilt,
> No longer see those they should never have seen,
> Not see, unseeing, those he had longed to see,
> Henceforth seeing nothing but night . . . To this wild tune
> He pierced his eyeballs time and time again,
> Till bloody tears ran down his beard – not drops
> But in full spate a whole cascade descending
> In drenching cataracts of scarlet rain.[5]

The imagery of the poet is vivid and distressing, sparing the audience nothing of the grim drama, the anguish and the self-loathing: a detestation of self that sought, not the escape of suicidal oblivion, but cruel retribution through the agony of punctured eyes and a life of darkness.

Revelation from the past brought not only personal tragedy and blindness to Oedipus; it caused his political downfall. He was banished from Thebes in accordance with a decree he himself had passed against the unknown slayer of Laios and in obedience to a directive given by the Delphic Oracle. As the sons of Oedipus and Iokaste were still minors, their uncle, Kreon, once again ruled as regent.

Analysis

I have retold this famous myth in some detail not only because it is a tale worth telling, but more importantly because it permits us to enter into the realm of mythical thinking, which is also the metaphorical world of our dreams and the obscure regions of our unconscious minds. Another persuasive reason is the facile ease with which many invoke the psychopathology of the "Oedipus complex" without fully understanding its origin and why Sigmund Freud originally coined the term.

The tale is replete with archetypal imagery. The curse of Pelops passing through the generations of the royal house of Labdakos of Thebes – exacted as the price for decadence, corruption and internecine strife and redolent with cruelty, greed, envy, jealousy and vengeful hatred – mirrors the heritage of miasmatic disease coursing through all human constitutions. A morbid legacy that has even contaminated innocent animal life.

Sent by Hera, the Goddess of Marriage (and relationships), the Sphinx in all her horror, personifies the hateful anger, indignation and resentment nursed within the abused feminine against male domination, persecution and exploitation. Though female, as with militant feminists, the Sphinx, paradoxically, expresses the deleterious force of the masculine principle within women. She embodies an amalgam of archetypes central to such energy, the cat (Lac felinum), the lioness (Lac leoninum), the eagle (Aquila chrysaetos), the snake (Lachesis) and woman herself (Lac humanum). The correct answer to her riddle – "Man!" – is the answer the fixated, feminine does not wish to hear or accept: that the object of her addictive fixation and unconsciously held rage and hatred; the cause of her suffering, from childhood to old age; is the masculine principle, typified in her own father. Rather than bear the truth, she casts herself onto the rocks of self-sacrifice.

Oedipus is the sensitive male whose feminine energy knows the truth and answers well. But, as Hahnemann was first to realise, even in the most honourable, the pervasive taint of miasmatic legacy persists until it is made good. Working always with the forces of destiny, the 'curse' inexorably fixates Oedipus' libido energy on the imprinted image of his mother and 'draws him into 'madness'. The mesmerising image must be erased, must be lost to the vision of the fixated ego-self. The soul, facilitated by the indicated homeopathic remedy, blinds the ego-self to that 'which should never have been seen' – and – that 'which it still longs to see' so that 'henceforth it sees nothing but the night' – the inner, authentic vision of the Self.

The paradox of the relative plane foretells that that which causes will cure: disease itself works inexorably towards the fulfilment of this law. It is the destructive energy of syphilis, which particularly attacks the vision of the inflated, self-absorbed ego-self: ocular syphilis can involve all structures of the eye from conjunctivitis to uveitis, retinitis, optic neuritis and atrophy.

Homeopathy penetrates the veil of symbolism, taps into the wisdom of the collective unconscious and through the power of the potency raises from the depths the archetypal images fitted to the myth. Oedipus, in the intense grip of his emotions, seeing the pins securing Iokaste's broaches and acting on the impulse, snatches them up and with syphilitic zeal plunges them repeatedly into his eyeballs from which gouts of blood spurt.

At the word pin, or needle, the homeopath's ears should prick; certain archetypes arise before the mind's eye. The rubric *fear of pins – of sharp, pointed things* contains remedies related to the Oedipus saga and phallic stage fixation: Alumina, *Apis*, Ars-alb, Bovista, Lac felinum, Mercurius. Nat-mur, Platina, *Silicea*, *Spigelia*. A small, but highly significant rubric related to a pivotal myth, pointing to the importance of the remedies it contains and suggesting relationships between them. The fear may encapsulate a fear of hypodermic syringes and operations, especially to the eyes, face and head, but there are deeper psychosomatic reasons for this peculiar fear relating to early life psychosexual fixation pinned to the memory-board of life. This was born out in the most singular life of the mother-fixated Isaac Newton, whose constitutional archetype was Silicea!

Confirming the universal nature of the wisdom intrinsic to myth, two remedies within the rubric immediately demand attention: Mercurius and Arsenicum album (Ars-alb), mercury and white arsenic, the two elements employed extensively and often heroically by the dominant school of medicine in the treatment of syphilis before the advent of penicillin. Two remedy archetypes of remarkable compass, being equally suited to most serious pathology and to many acute conditions met in everyday practice.

Psychosexual fixation, the theme of the rubric, is a condition in which circumstances and constitution conspire to blight the personality with traits detrimental to psychic homeostasis. The distortion is imprinted on the structure of the ego-self like the effect of a pervasive and persistent poison. Significantly, no elements, other than phosphorus and lead, have been as responsible for chronically contaminating humanity than mercury and arsenic; their toxic effects linger for a lifetime. Of ominous significance, is the knowledge that these two archetypes, that announce their psycho-sexual fixation via fear of pins and sharp-pointed objects, are two of the most malicious and murderous archetypes in the materia medica.

While only Mercurius and Silicea are noted for dreaming of pins, two other archetypes must be remembered when considering psychosexual fixation: Lac lupinum (Wolf) and Androctonus (Scorpion) and this is born out in very significant dreams experienced by these archetypes; dreams that are graphically reminiscent of Oedipus' self-mutilation.

Wolf: *Intruders got daughter. Black magic, voodoo needles in eyes, calling 911, my children are being hurt.*

Scorpion: *murdered grandfather by poking a knitting needle through one of his eyes.*

Clearly, Lac-lupinum should be thought of in instances when a person believes that they are being subjected to psychic abuse, 'voodoo', black magic or evil spells. The possibility of a dark occult connotation must be remembered in all archetypes fixated on or fearful of pins and needles. The practice of sticking pins in a voodoo doll representing a hated individual, with the vengeful desire of doing them harm, has become idiomatic, and, therefore, must be within the metaphoric range of the pin and the needle. Isaac Newton's vindictive anger was relentless, the passing of a lifetime left it unadulterated: an example of the pin's relationship, not only to Oedipus fixation, but also hatred and revenge. Those born under the sun sign of Scorpio are known for their suspicion, jealousy and desire to get even with those who hurt or offend them. The dream of the archetype is explicit in this regard and the archetype's vindictive nature is further symbolised by the animal's 'sting in its tail'.

* * * * *

While Mercurius deserves more attention concerning the dire effects of psychosexual fixation, the Hermes/Mercurius archetype has been given much consideration in *The Wolf* and I am, therefore, reserving further elaboration of this most important 'dark' archetype for a later date and a different book. In the instance of Arsenicum, however, the recent case of Dr Harold Shipman, the mother-fixated medical serial-poisoner is sufficiently alive in our memories to justify a consideration of the homicidal role of the Arsenic archetype – the arch-poisoner!

Arsenicum album – white arsenic

Arsenic – the very word on the tongue conveys a sense of lethal potency and in the mind conjures the image of a stealthy, cowardly poisoner and a victim's sudden or lingering death. Though employed as a poison in antiquity, arsenic's notoriety stems from the French and Italian Renaissance when it was the preferred poison used for political assassination and domestic murder. Before the Middle Ages, poisoning was by means of arsenic's vividly coloured sulphides, yellow orpiment and red realgar, which were much in demand as colouring agents and for use in cosmetics. Their bright colours and strong taste required great cunning on the part of the poisoner; but help was on hand. Working in his laboratory, the eighth century Arabic alchemist Jabir ibn Hayyan, discovered the colourless, odourless crystalline arsenical compound, arsenic trioxide, which became popularly known as "white arsenic".[6] It was a boon to the poisoner; it was potent and discreet. In small or large doses, it produced symptoms that mimicked various naturally occurring sicknesses prevalent at the time, particularly gastro-enteritis, dysentery, typhoid, and cholera. Slow-poisoning could resemble heart or kidney disease or malignancy.

The ruling classes welcomed it with gratitude and were soon using arsenic to murder those who opposed them. In the fifteenth century, the Italian de' Medici family that ruled Florence, became proficient in its use: a craft that Catherine de' Medici (1519–1589), took with her to France when she married Henry of Valois, who was to become Henry II. It was to prove of value to her, when, after the death of her husband, she became queen-regent and later when she was the power behind the throne of each of her three weak and ineffectual sons (Francis II, Charles IX and Henry III). It was an age of constant civil and religious strife and Catherine's shrewd ruthlessness was critical to the survival of the Valois dynasty. However, the most infamous of all were the Borgias, Pope Alexander VI (Rodrigo Borgia) (1431–1503), his son Cesare (1475/6–1507) and his daughter Lucrezia (1480–1519). Although the family name has become synonymous with political murder and arsenic poisoning, much of their notoriety probably stemmed from the allegations of rivals and the exaggeration of popular rumour. Of Cesare, however, there can be no question, he was always ready to eliminate anyone who stood in his way, but the case against the Pope, though suggestive, is less certain and despite a common myth that she possessed a hollow ring with which she readily poisoned drinks, there is no historic basis for the accusations levelled at Lucrezia.

However, there can be no doubt about the culpability of many who followed in the Borgias' footsteps in the following centuries. Though large doses of arsenic would kill within a few hours or days, often the preferred means of poisoning was by small, repeated doses, permitting the poison to work slowly and insidiously without rousing suspicion: evidence of pitiless premeditation, hatred and revenge, since the victim suffered a wretched and protracted death. Records reveal that it was particularly women trapped in unhappy or abusive marriages that resorted to the poison – proof of the insidious masculinisation of the abused feminine principle, witnessed in less lethal form in Ignatia, Nat-mur, Sepia, Staphysagria, Causticum, Lac-lupinum and Carcinosin and fully realised in Arsenic.

Aqua Tofana

In the late 1600s, a beautiful, enterprising young Sicilian woman Giulia Tofana, an apothecary's assistant in Palermo, saw the opportunity of helping hapless women get rid of their husbands by putting to profitably use what she had learned about mixing potions. She was a radical feminist and resented the inferior standing of women and the general prevalence of misogyny. She set about concocting a colourless, tasteless, odourless arsenic-based solution, which could easily be added to water, wine or cosmetic creams. This became her much-famed *"Aqua Tofana"*. She soon prospered, receiving many referrals from satisfied customers. Such was the demand for her services that she moved her business first to Naples and finally to Rome. For over fifty years she practiced as a professional poisoner; the awe and regard in which she was held always keeping her one-step ahead of the law. During her tenure, it was not only husbands that were at risk; the powerful and wealthy among the nobility had reason to be circumspect about accepting invitations to dine-out.

Finally, a would-be client turned informant and revealed her whereabouts to the Papal authorities. When the police came looking for her, she was alerted by the locals and under their protection made her escape to a nearby church where she was granted asylum. A rumour was quickly stirred-up by those wanting to lay hands on her that she had poisoned the waters of Rome. Using this as justification, the police violated the sanctuary of the church and seized her. Under torture, never a guarantee of truth, she confessed to being implicated in the deaths of some 600 men during her time in Rome. Tofana, her daughter and three assistants were duly executed by hanging; then, in a gesture of male bravado and defiance, her body was contemptuously thrown over the wall of the church that had given her safe haven. She was seventy-years-old when she died.

The dark masculine

Considering the archetypal patterning of this piece of Arsenic history, it is apparent that the substance has extremely dark connotations. It is essentially a masculine archetype embodying the energy, drive and focus of the masculine principle in either man or woman. Tofana was primarily a purveyor of arsenic to jealous, neglected and abused women. However, murderous intent in a woman stems not from her abused feminine aspect, but from the indignation, rage and hatred harboured in her frustrated, trapped masculine aspect. Lacking the physical strength and social standing to redress her grievances or escape her misery, she resorts to poison: her masculine fist, club, knife or gun. In Rome, both the murderer and the murdered exemplified the aggressive and destructive nature of the un-adulterated masculine principle.

In this arsenic vignette, Giulia Tofana, herself an archetypal Arsenic feminist with a pitiless hatred of males was in effect prescribing crude arsenic for an Arsenic state of mind existing in both client and victim: the jealous or trapped woman, driven to murderous intent through abuse, and the arrogant, selfish, unfaithful misogynist responsible for her rage. The same archetype was persuasive in the elite who killed for political gain, a title or a fortune. The archetypal nature of a substance may be deduced from its properties, uses and history in human affairs and defined from its homeopathic provings and clinical evidence of its efficacy.

The Arsenic homeopathic potency used in proving trials and in therapy is a unique energy frequency derived from the archetype and carrying its physical and esoteric nature. In the trialist or patient constitutionally tuned to the archetypal image, the high potency touches and activates both the personal and collective unconscious. It elicits a concordant response, expressing the reality behind the form and evoking a healing event capable of addressing the soul-ego conflict. In the trialist, the archetype is revealed; in the patient, the archetype is sublimated; both constitute healing. Emotional and physical symptoms revealed or erased in either process are indicative of the archetype. In the story of Tofana, the arsenic archetype is revealed in all the role players, including the poisoner herself.

Rubrics for marital murder

The murderer:

- *Desire to kill:*
  - **Sudden impulse to kill.*
  - **Impulse to poison.*
  - *Loved ones (and by extension: members of the family: husbands, wives, rich or titled relatives etc.).*
- *Morbid impulses.*
- *Jealousy (and envy): between men and women; between women; between men, between children.*
- *Love of power.*
- *Ambition for fame*
- *Desire for money.*
- ***Avarice.***
- *Kleptomania.*

- *Embittered.*
- *Ailments from:*
  - *Anger with grief; anger with indignation.*
  - *Betrayal – disappointment, deception – infidelity.*
  - *Humiliation.*
  - *Family discord.*
- *Estranged from family: she from her husband – he from his wife.*
- **Forsaken feeling – of not being loved by parents, husband, wife, family, friends.*
- *Sensitive to reprimands, reproaches and criticism.*
- **Escape: attempts to escape.*
- **Fear of killing (fear of the impulse).*
- **Rage leading to deeds of violence.*

An important rubric that must be added to this list is: *hatred and revenge*, an awful alliance that festers in the heart of the dark Arsenic.

The murderer and the murdered:

- *Cruelty, brutality, inhumanity* – and **cruelty to animals* (here, include 'cruelty' to *husbands* or *wives*).

The murdered:

- *Boaster, braggart.*
- *Selfishness, egoism.*
- *Haughty.*
- **Censorious, critical.*
- **Dictatorial, domineering, dogmatic, despotic.*
- *Abusive, insulting – husband insults wife in front of children, or vice versa.*
- *Fear of being murdered.*
- *Delusion: others are conspiring to murder him.*
- *Delusion: he will be murdered.*

The poisoner's rubrics:
Considering Tofana herself: within the rubrics we find a step-by-step chronicle of her life:

- *Desire to kill: impulse to poison.*
- *Want of moral feeling; disposition to become a criminal without remorse.*
- *No sense of honour.*
- *Desire for money.*

– and most revealing:

- Delusions (imaginings or fancies):
  - *Contaminates everything she touches.*
  - *There are conspiracies against her.*
  - *She is a criminal.*
  - *She has committed a crime.*
  - *Unpardonable, she has sinned away her day of grace.*
  - **She is being watched.*
  - *Pursued by the police.*
  - *Policemen coming into the house.*
  - *About to be arrested.*
  - *Doomed.*
  - *About to die.*
  - *Sees persons hanging – beckoning to be cut loose.*
- *Fear of suffocation.*
- *Dreams of death.*

Add: *Fear of men and hatred of men*: core symptoms of the abused Arsenicum archetype.

These rubrics, gleaned from provings of white arsenic, bear startling resemblance to real life situations and to human behaviour: proof of the archetypal patterning which choreographs our lives. The archetype can overshadow a country, city, the times, events and people: the drama of their lives, their eccentricities, their thoughts, impulses, desires, fears, imaginings and dreams. We exist within the narrative of a myth; whether our role be heroic or humble, it will be crucial to the outcome.

A pennyworth of poison

The nefarious intrigues of the Medici and the Borgias and the sinister skills and witch-like reputation of Tofana surrounded arsenic with a mystique that fascinated, intrigued and repelled the public. Imaginative tales regarding its mysterious, magical qualities abounded, often magnified to supernatural proportions. This mythology persisted into Victorian times when arsenic's lethal effects enjoyed a revival in popularity. Inexpensive and easily available, it was now no longer the preserve of the aristocracy, but well within the reach of the lower classes. Most general stores held supplies of white arsenic and sold it indiscriminately over the counter as a rat poison to anyone who placed it on their shopping list. This casual indifference, apart from inviting murder, created a public hazard because the crystalline oxide of arsenic was a colourless, odourless, innocent-looking white powder, which could easily be mistaken for sugar or flour. This led to a number of deaths due to it being mistakenly used in the preparation of food.

As in earlier times, embittered women found that the white powder provided a perfect solution to marital misery. It was also of value to those impatient to benefit from an inheritance or a relative's insurance policy. But more shocking by far was the use of arsenic by the poor to poison mouths they could no longer feed. At a time when mortality amongst infants and children was high, often due to gastro-intestinal infections, arsenic's ability to simulate such illnesses could be put to murderous use with little fear of detection. Further temptation sprang from the many burial policies that were available to ensure against the ignominy of a pauper's grave. By enrolling a child in several of these so-called 'burial clubs', the profit derived from their death could be handsomely multiplied.

Mary Ann Cotton – "Mother Death"

The most infamous of all infanticides bent on financial gain was Mary Ann Cotton (Robson) (1832–1873) a very attractive woman born into crushing poverty. Until the advent of Harold Shipman more than a century later (see

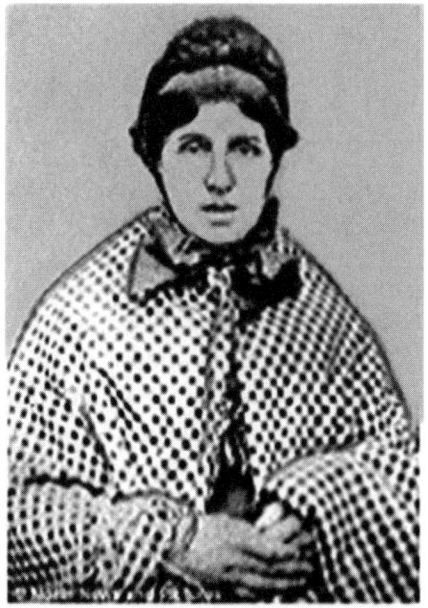

Figure 24.2 *Mary Ann Cotton (1832–1873) Britain's first serial killer*

below), she was the most prolific serial killer in British history, notching up 21 victims, most, if not all, by arsenic poisoning. Numbered among these was her mother, three of her four husbands, a lodger (shortly after he revised his will in her favour), most of her stepchildren, and eleven of her own thirteen children. Each murder, apart from that of her fiancé, resulted in Mary Ann collecting insurance pay-outs. Although the sums she accrued were relatively meagre, they were substantial for a woman from a poor mining community in County Durham. The only husband to escape her ministrations was James Robinson, her third husband, who refused to insure his life in her favour and eventually threw her out when she accumulated debts and stole money from him. Unfortunately, this was only after she had managed to poison two of his children and her own daughter from her first marriage; all within the month of April, 1867 – a particularly bad year in which six of Mary Ann's children fell ill and died. Her last husband, a Northumberland collier, Frederick Cotton, and his children all died, like the rest of her victims, from an intestinal disorder, loosely diagnosed as 'gastric fever'.

How Mary Ann Cotton's activities remained unsuspected by her family, those who knew her and the insurance companies, remains a mystery. Her uncanny fortune held out until the death of Charles, the last of the Cotton children, aroused suspicion; this lead to an inquest, a trial, her conviction and the death penalty in 1873. Although she was spared public execution (the law had been changed in 1868) she was unfortunate to have her execution conducted by William Calcraft, the most celebrated and controversial hangman of the time. Originally employed to administer floggings to juvenile offenders held in London's Newgate Prison, when appointed hangman, Calcraft brought his malicious sadism to bear on his new craft. Rather than the traditional method of having the criminal's neck broken instantly by the weight of the body falling through the gallows trapdoor, Calcraft favoured a short-drop method of no more than 3 feet by which the condemned literally 'hung by the neck until they died': a process of slow strangulation, awful to witness and lasting minutes. This was Mary Ann Cotton's fate and her archetypal destiny. The innocuous white powder that gave her control over life and death insidiously poisoned her spiritually, robbing her of her maternal nature and feminine morality, leaving a monstrous, greedy ego-self, devoid of humanity and love; her soul strangled to silence by the coils of the ego's constricting masculinity.

Hidden within this sordid image of human decadence lies *a mute death wish*, the last remaining impulse of the soul to escape a ruined life and sabotage the uncontrolled ego-self. Chatting to a local grocer Tomas Riley, who also happened to be an assistant coroner, Mary Ann asked him if she could put her stepson Charles into a workhouse. When Riley said no, she coolly replied "Perhaps it won't matter, as I won't be troubled long. He'll go like all the rest of the Cotton family."[7] Five days later, Charles Cotton was dead. Remembering her words, Thomas Riley went to the police and insisted on an investigation before the issue of a death certificate. At the inquest, Mary Ann defended herself by saying that Riley's accusations were due to her having repulsed his sexual advances. Although the jury returned a verdict of natural causes, journalists following up on the story discovered the trail of death that marked her past. Suspicions were once again aroused and forensic tests performed on Charles Cotton's exhumed body revealed that he had died of arsenic poisoning.

Yet again, the rubrics of Arsenicum album accurately reflect an archetypal template. The histories of Tofana and Mary Ann illustrate the link between the Arsenic archetype, money, murder and hanging (death by strangulation). Though neither poisoner consciously sought such a death, it was the inevitable consequence of their unconsciously programmed, voluntary actions; it stemmed from an underlying *desire to be killed*. The specific rubric *suicidal disposition* in the Ars-alb remedy picture highlights a marked dichotomy within the emotion; a contradiction that typifies the conflict between the ego-self (fear of dying) and the soul (suicidal disposition); a conflict which Mary Ann Cotton's soul finally won by betraying her own murderous ego-self:

Suicidal disposition:

- *By hanging* (*Ars-alb; Aurum; *Belladonna*; Carbo-veg, [add Carcinosin], Helleborus; Nat-sulph; Terebinth).
- *With fear of dying.*

Both rubrics are in the highest type, indeed, Ars-alb is the only black letter remedy in the rubric *suicide by hanging*.

Other means of destroying themselves are:

- *To set oneself on fire.*
- By gas.
- *With a knife.*
- By poison.
- Throwing oneself from a height – *from a window.*

In the light of Mary Ann Cotton's terrible history, the rubric *desire to be killed*, in which Ars-alb appears, acquires meaning and can be better understood. Only a handful of remedies are listed in this strange rubric: *Ars-alb*; *Aurum; Belladonna; Carcinosin; Coffea tosta; *Phytolacca*; Stramonium.

Harold Shipman – 'Dr Death'

On 13th January 2004, Harold Frederick Shipman, the British serial killer and medical doctor responsible for killing at least 215 of his patients, committed suicide by hanging himself with bed sheets from the window bars of his Wakefield Prison cell. The following day he would have been 58 years-of-age. Sentenced to life imprisonment in 2000, he had been in custody for just over four years. Death of a poisoner by strangulation, whether by execution or suicide, is archetypal and is suggestive of the Arsenic archetype. Shipman did not use arsenic to commit his murders; he injected patients with lethal doses of diamorphine, but his profile conforms to a distinct form of the Arsenic archetype standing close to Sulphur. Fixation is pivotal to the psychopathology of both Mercurius and Arsenic. Shipman followed this pattern; he had an intense mother fixation, which, together with the syphilitic miasm that gave it birth, led him to murder for self-gratification.

Harold Shipman was born in Nottingham, England, in 1946, second of the four children of Harold Shipman, a lorry driver, and his wife Vera, who were both devout Methodists. Fred, as his parents knew him, was the favourite child of his domineering mother, Vera, who instilled in him a sense of superiority, which would estrange him from his contemporaries at school, at university and later from his medical colleagues. Although he was an accomplished athlete, performing well on the football field and in track events, he remained strangely aloof, a loner, his sense of superiority keeping him at a distance, preventing him from socialising and bonding with others. His early promise as a pupil was not sustained at high school

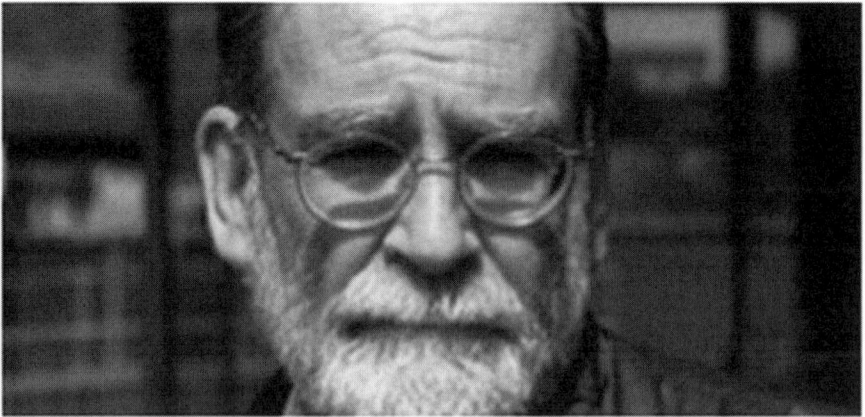

Figure 24.3 *Harold Frederick Shipman (1946–2004)*

where he achieved average grades by dint of determination and hard work rather than intellectual flare. This contrasted sharply with his intellectual evaluation of himself.

Harold senior did not provide a strong father figure with whom he could identify. In consequence, Shipman failed to differentiate his own personality from that of his authoritarian mother, whom he adored. This Oedipal fixation and his failure to integrate into society compromised the dynamics of the psyche, resulting in a poorly developed superego and a weak, impressionable, narcissistic ego-self, inflated with arrogant conceit imparted by a doting mother. Sexual and aggressive fantasies from the psychosexual development stages were neither repressed, resolved, or sublimated and could be lived out without the constraints of conscience. The Arsenic foundation was laid and needed only an appropriate trigger for the archetypal patterning to play out. This came at 17 when Shipman's mother, the source of his identity and object of his adoration, was diagnosed with terminal lung cancer. He suffered vicariously with her as she steadily wasted and declined and experienced and welcomed in his own being the relief morphine afforded her during the final stages of her disease. This would become his craving need and modus operandi when he commenced murdering his patients.

He resolved to study medicine. After failing his first attempt, he gained entrance to Leeds University Medical School, progressed well with his studies and qualified in 1970. It is of interest that both at school and university, he remained a grey, inconspicuous figure, barely remembered by fellow students and teachers, other than for his pretentious, condescending arrogance. In 1974, he joined a medical practice in Todmorden, West Yorkshire, and seemed to emerge from his shell. He was more outgoing and his enthusiasm and commitment to his work made him respected by colleagues and patients. But, warning signs of his innate narcissism were apparent: his derogatory remarks, rudeness, sarcasm and confrontational manner that brooked no contradiction or criticism and demanded things be done his way even when faced by senior colleagues. *He always needed to be in control!*

In 1975, he was caught forging prescriptions for Pethidine, a synthetic opium-like analgesic, for his own use. In the light of his mother fixation and his indelibly imprinted image of her release from suffering through the action of morphine, this was an ominous sign of a need to quell his own inner turmoil in a similar way. This would transform into an insistent craving for the vicarious satisfaction he had experienced during his mother's dying; driving him to selfishly re-enact the event through his elderly, female patients; robbing them of life, but temporarily relieving his insatiable fantasy.

When his colleagues challenged him, his mask slipped, revealing an underlying aggression they had never suspected. He first pleaded for a second chance, but when this was refused, he became enraged, violently threw a medical bag to the ground and unrepentantly stormed out of the room. He refused to resign and had to be forced out of the practice.

After a brief period of rehabilitation, which saved him from being struck off the medical register, he moved to Hyde in Cheshire where he joined a general practice. His new colleagues found him competent and hardworking, but with a tendency to be arrogant and patronising towards patients. In 1993, Shipman broke away to start his own one-man practice, freeing himself from accountability to his colleagues. Outwardly, he was a respected member of the community: a caring, competent family doctor, especially valued for his willingness to make house calls. Nothing seemed amiss until in March 1998 a funeral parlour expressed concerns to a Hyde doctor about the high death rate among Shipman's patients, the large number of cremation forms he needed countersigning and the fact that his patients, almost all female, were invariably found fully clothed and either sitting up in an easy chair or lying on a settee, whereas, elderly, sick patients who died were usually found in night attire and in bed. A covert police investigation was initiated, which proved superficial and desultory, revealing nothing untoward. Unaware that for a short time he been the object of police scrutiny, Shipman continued to kill, poisoning three more victims before he was eventually arrested in September of the same year.

As with Mary Ann Cotton, the hidden conflict between the soul and the compulsive, out-of-control ego-self achieved resolution through a 'stupid act' of self-betrayal: the childlike forgery of a high-profile patient's will. *At soul level, Shipman wanted to be caught!* Acting against the self-preserving instincts of the ego-self, from deep within the maimed psyche, the soul achieved its goal! *Desire to be killed* (Cotton) can be extended to *desire to be apprehended* (Shipman) in the Arsenicum picture.

His final victim was Kathleen Grundy, a wealthy, vigorous 81-year-old, a prominent member of Hyde society and ex-mayor, who was found dead at her home on June 24, 1998. Shipman, the last person to see her alive, recorded her death as being due to 'old age' and on his old typewriter forged a will in her name, excluding her family and bequeathing £386,000 to himself. With unconscious determination, spurred on by his narcissistic sense of impunity and his greed, he had engineered and ensured his own downfall.

Kathleen Grundy's daughter, Angela Woodruff, a lawyer, convinced that the will was a forgery and that her mother had been murdered by Shipman, alerted the police. Mrs Grundy's body was exhumed and a post-mortem proved that she had died from a diamorphine overdose. A raid on Shipman's home brought to light altered medical records, the incriminating typewriter and a small hoard of jewellery. Shipman's years of murder had come to an end; he was arrested, tried and convicted to life imprisonment!

Detective Chief Inspector Mike Williams said:

> He was an arrogant type of individual to deal with. And I don't say that lightly. I've listened to the interviews, and he certainly wanted to control and dominate the interview and the officers, at times belittling them. He was treating this as some sort of game, a competition, pitting what he considered his superior intellect against those of the officers who were interviewing him.

The South Manchester coroner, John Pollard, who knew and worked with Shipman, had his own theory about the doctor's motives:

> The only valid possible explanation for it is that he simply enjoyed viewing the process of dying and enjoyed the feeling of control over life and death.[8]

This was certainly true, but the nature of the 'enjoyment' and the reason behind it were far from simple. It was complex, distorted and miasmatically sick, displaying the darkest face of the Arsenicum archetype, utterly selfish, controlling and devoid of conscience; a serious deviation in an archetype usually dominated by an imposing superego.

The motive of male serial killers is invariably sexual and aggression is implicit in the act of killing. The positive aggression and libido aspects of the Id are perverted by miasmatic disease and warping of the psyche into a craving for sadistic, sexual pleasure. Although not overtly sexual, Shipman's serial killing had to possess the same components. The libido aspect linked and timed the murders: a build-up of tension fuelled by fantasy of the orgasm-like dissipation of anxiety, stress, pain and suffering vicariously experienced by a sexually fixated 17-year-old, reaching irresistible proportions and demanding release in a fixated, stereotyped way. The gratification intensified by a narcissistic temperament and the sense of power an Arsenic archetype derives from being in control and calling the shots – even over life and death. As after a sexual killing, the release was followed by a refractory period: an interval in which fantasies begin once more to mount until they demand another death. Through habituation, the intervals grow shorter and the tension builds more rapidly, relief is shorter lasting; caution may be cast to the winds. The recessive, therefore, veiled, sexual component lay in the fact that all his victims were elderly women, counterparts for his dying mother upon whom his Oedipal sexual longings were fixated.

His prison diaries contain some insights into his thinking while in captivity. They reveal a state of deep despair and concern for his wife and her finances and the effect of his incarceration upon his family. He repeatedly alludes to the possibility of suicide:

> 13 April 2001: If I was dead they'd stop being in limbo and get on with their lives. I'll think a bit more about it. I'm desperate, no one to talk to about it who I can trust. Everyone will talk to the PO's (police officers) then I will be watched 24 hrs a day and I don't want that.

> 26 June 2001: . . . As near suicide as can be, know how and when, just not yet.[9]

Relevant rubrics are:

- **Anxiety:** *about his family.*
- **Fear of poverty.**
- **Despair:** *of life.*
- **Weary of life – loathing of life.**
- Delusion, imaginings: *his time has come to die.*
- **Thoughts of death.**
- Delusion, imaginings: *wants to hang himself.*
- Delusion, imaginings: **that he is being watched**.

Shipman was anally retentive and highly secretive. He confided in no one, not even his wife Primrose. Under police questioning, when not providing some implausible explanation for his actions, he remained supercilious, obstructive, taciturn and monosyllabic. He was devious and made up his transparent lies extemporaneously. In the face of incontrovertible evidence, he continued to profess his innocence, even after conviction and when in prison. He remained an enigma; psychologists and criminologists could only speculate on why he killed repeatedly without obvious motive. Kathleen Grundy seemed to be an exception, but knowing the killer, the forged will that was to spare more lives was undoubtedly an opportunistic add-on, just as was the stolen jewellery; irresistible pickings for a magpie Arsenic.

The anally fixated Arsenicum is invariably immaculate, impeccable, fastidious and perfectionistic, but when police searched the Shipman house, to their surprise, this doctor's dwelling place was a mess, dirty and untended, strewn with dirty clothing and old newspapers; much like the lair of an anally-expulsive Sulphur. Shipman's be-whiskered face, unruly hair and general appearance were certainly Sulphur-like. As in the relationship between Sulphur and Nux-vom, this paradox evidences how deterioration of the psyche can produce a shift of archetypal expression, not indiscriminately, but to a closely related and in this case more primitive archetype: Ars-alb to Sulphur, while retaining the outstanding character traits of Arsenicum: his overweening arrogance, selfishness and cruelty.

The repertory accurately reflects his tell-tale idiosyncrasies

- *Aversion to persons around him.*
- *Contemptuous.*
- *Haughty.*
- *Love of power.*
- *Insolence, impertinence.*
- **Dictatorial, domineering.*
- *Intolerance.*
- *Impatience.*
- **Disposition to contradict.*
- *Anger from contradiction – intolerant of contradiction.*
- *Answers curtly.*
- *Indisposed to talk, desire to be silent, taciturn.*
- **Avarice.*
- *Cruelty.*
- *Unfeeling, hard-hearted.*
- *Unsympathetic, unscrupulous.*
- *Abusive, insulting.*
- **Malicious, spiteful, vindictive.*
- *Mocking – sarcasm.*
- *Desire to kill; impulse to poison.*
- *Deceitful, sly.*
- *Foolish behaviour.*

* * * * *

Continuing our consideration of psychosexual phallic-stage fixation, it is necessary to consider Freud's prejudiced attitude towards homosexuality, his understanding of phallic fixation in girls and Jung's modification to this understanding through his concept of the *Elektra complex*.

Homosexual fixation

Homosexuality is not caused by phallic fixation as Freud and others theorised, but homosexuality and bisexuality may certainly expose the ego-self to the dangers of phallic-stage fixation. Freud's conclusions were made at a time when homosexuality was regarded religiously, secularly and clinically as an aberration and a perversion of normal sexuality. Consistent with this prejudice, psychopathological reasons were sought to explain its basis. As the gentle, loving bonobo have shown us, homosexuality is as natural and normal as heterosexuality and utterly consonant with the androgynous nature of the Universe. As with heterosexuality, its emergence in an individual can be facilitated and modified or distorted by conditioning and by constitutional and miasmatic influences, but the sexual orientation itself is inherent, not aberrant. The homosexual has most commonly a syco-tubercular miasmatic constitution and is particularly liable to fixation in the phallic-stage of psychosexual development. In both heterosexual and homosexual subjects, it is this fixation combined with conditioned imprinting and miasmatic influence that may lead to sexual peculiarities and perversions e.g. sado-masochism, fetishism, paraphilia, bestiality and paedophilia.

Freud's sexual fixation

Initially, Freud used 'Oedipus complex' solely to denote a young boy's unconscious attraction and desire for his mother and his consequent unconscious aggression towards his father. Later, he affirmed that girls like boys also initially experience sexual desire for mother and aggression towards father and termed this unconscious dynamic the 'feminine Oedipus attitude or the 'negative Oedipus complex'.

In counterbalance to a young boy's presumed 'castration fear', Freud, by a process of convoluted thinking, giving the male genitals prime importance for both sexes in the phallic stage, proposed 'penis envy' in young girls: anxiety experienced (approximately between the ages of 3 and 6) when a young girl's unconscious sexual impulse focuses on her mother and she realises that lacking a penis she cannot heterosexually express this. The only solution seems to lie in the acquisition of her father's penis: a focus that develops into an unconscious sexual desire for her father. She imagines that it must have been her mother who castrated her as punishment for the attraction she now feels for her father. This conclusion turns her sexual focus even more towards her father and matures into a desire to replace her mother in the affections of her father. De-fusion of these tensions is achieved first through identification with mother in order to better replace her and finally through displacement of her sexual focus from father to men in general. This final shift, if free from fixation, brings resolution.

I think it is true to say that most minds first contemplating Freud's theories of 'castration fear' and 'penis envy' that place the male genitalia centre stage, find them odd and uncomfortable. They possibly reflect a phallic fixation in Freud himself. If, however, the male genitalia are understood to metaphorically represent the masculine power of the Id, present in both sexes, Freud's theories reveal a dynamic that is in keeping with the natural hierarchical and ritualistic tensions existing between dominant (alpha) and submissive (beta) individuals found in primates and animals that live in packs e.g. wolves. It is distortion of this dynamic that leads to psychopathological fixation in miasmatically fraught *Homo sapiens*.

Elektra

Carl Gustav Jung disagreed with Freud in his assertion that the libido of a young girl is first focused upon mother and only subsequently on father. Jung believed that the initial libido prompting in both sexes was directed towards the contrasexual parent and that in consequence young girls harbour unconscious sexual desire for their father rather than their mother, coupled to aggression towards their mother rather than their father (Lac humanum). Since this dynamic was inconsistent with the narrative of the Oedipus myth, he introduced the term, 'Electra complex', to define the daughter-mother rivalry for psychosexual possession of the father – a change in terminology that annoyed his senior colleague.

In doing so, Jung's reference was the 5th-century Greek myth of Elektra, who, with her brother Orestes, plotted matricidal revenge against their mother, Klytaimnestra, for the murder of Agamemnon, their father. The story, which is the final chapter in the lamentable saga of the ill-fated house of Atreus, was made famous by all three great tragedians of the time, Aeschylus, Sophocles and Euripides, each giving to the common theme his own poetic interpretation.

Agamemnon, the son of Atreus and King of Mycenae, was overlord of the Achaean army during the Trojan war: a ten-year conflict waged on behalf of his brother Menelaos, King of Sparta, whose wife Helen, the most beautiful woman on earth, had been abducted by Paris, the son of Priam, King of Troy. During the long absence of her husband, Klytaimnestra took Aigisthos, her husband's cousin, as lover and fellow-regent.

In Aeschylus's great work, *Agamemnon*,[10] Klytaimnestra hates her husband intensely and with good reason. Before the war, Agamemnon ordered the sacrifice of their daughter Iphigineia to appease the goddess Artemis (Roman: Diana), who had becalmed the Achaean fleet in the port of Aulis; preventing it from sailing for Troy. The anger of the goddess had been aroused by Agamemnon's blatant impiety: while hunting in the area, he had thoughtlessly shot a stag sacred to the goddess and then arrogantly boasted that he was a finer hunter than Artemis herself. Tradition had two versions regarding the fate of Iphigineia: Aeschylus is straightforward and has her sacrificed on the altar; Euripides, in his *Iphigineia in Tauris*,[11] has the virgin princess spirited away by Artemis, at the very moment of sacrifice, to become her mortal priestess in the land of the Taurians. In either case, Artemis relented, the Achaeans secured fair winds for their voyage and Klytaimnestra lost her daughter.

With the fall of Troy, the conquering forces set sail for home. Warned of Agamemnon's imminent return, Klytaimnestra, motivated by deep hatred and a lust for revenge, plots his murder. On his arrival, she receives him with feigned joy, inveigles him into a soothing bath to ease the fatigue of his travels, incapacitates him with garments she casts about him in the water, and, as he struggles in alarm to gain his feet and escape their hindrance, stabs him to death with three savage blows of a knife. She is exultant in her triumph and in a further catharsis of vengeance murders Kassandra, the Trojan princess that Agamemnon has brought with him from Troy as a prize of war. The bloody deeds done, Aigisthos emerges from his hiding place rejoicing at the destruction of the house of Atreus. He and Klytaimnestra marry and continue to rule Mycenae. Elektra, knowing the craven, vicious nature of Aigisthos and fearing for her much younger brother's life, has Orestes sent away to the safety of the court of their maternal uncle, Strophius, the King of Krisa.

In the *Odyssey*, Homer tells us that eight years elapse before Orestes returns to Mycenae to avenge his father. The detail of events in the build-up to the fulfilment of this act differs in the various tragedies, but the theme is consistent. Orestes gains entrance to the palace, makes himself known to Elektra and with her help first kills Aigisthos and then Klytaimnestra. Elektra's involvement in the murders ranges from acting as an accomplice, luring the unsuspecting victims to their fate (Sophocles), to eager and aggressive participation (Euripides), goading her hesitant and less resolved brother to plunge his sword into their mother's heart: exemplifying the masculine in woman – oft-times more fearsome than in man – just as he reveals the feminine in man – an oft-times repressed energy.

This well-known story from classical times, particularly as pictured by Euripides, held the emotional ingredients that Jung required. Love of the father – no matter his nature and deeds – and – hatred of the mother – no matter how justified her emotions and behaviour – and fixation in this state: a portent of emotional dysfunction and future problems, if not disaster!

Freud's concept of the phallic stage of psychosexual development and the associated Oedipus complex aroused much controversy and criticism among fellow psychoanalysts with varying degrees of acceptance and rejection, producing debate that persists to this day. However, Jung's substitution of the Elektra complex for the phenomenon in girls was not a repudiation of Freud's basic phallic theory; it was a modification that in effect bestowed Jung's seal of approval. When the masculine principle and its assertive and aggressive drive are perceived as central to Freud's theory and the male genitalia as simply symbolic, the true value of his thinking becomes clear and proves of inestimable value in clinical practice.

Latency Stage

After the highly charged phallic stage of psychosexual development, so fraught with fantasy and conflict between erotic attraction, resentment, hatred, rivalry, jealousy and fear, at *5 to 6 years-of-age* the psyche enters what Freud called the latency stage that lasts until puberty. Although the sexual aspects of the psyche's development appear to be dormant, the dynamics are still present, but now hidden due to sexual thoughts and unconscious fantasies receding or being repressed. Character traits developed during the first three stages, including any fixations that remain unresolved, are carried forward and consolidated or modified by conditioning, circumstances, constitution, miasmatic influences and the level of balance established between the inveterate rivals: the soul and the ego-self. Ever-present is the outward flow of the irresistible Id. The drive of the repressed sexual aspect of the libido being ungratified is channelled or sublimated into external activities such as schooling, acquiring new knowledge, friendships, play, communication skills, sport and hobbies. These activities are largely shared with children of the same gender. By socialising successfully, the child, or pre-pubescent, develops vital qualities for a healthy, adult emotional life, namely, reciprocity, sharing, empathy, moral and ethical values and the development of an internal conscience or super-ego.

This stage is as vulnerable to impingement and fixation as are the earlier stages. While many factors may disrupt the balanced development of the psyche during this impressionable period, certain elements are particularly damaging. Of critical importance are failure to adequately resolve the conflicts and fixation of the Oedipus/Elektra stage of development; failure to comfortably manage the socialisation process; and the absence of a positive father figure with whom to identify and from whom a strong ego-self and a principled super-ego can be modelled. A strong (not inflated) ego-self is a psychic structure capable of incrementally incorporating soul qualities, a process of sublimation that ultimately leads to the subsuming of the ego-self by the soul and the attainment of individuation or Spirit.

Failure to bond with the mother or the primary caregiver in the earlier stages of psychosexual development is a critical factor in psychic dysfunction later in life and in either gender will compound the effect of any developmental failure in the latency stage. This cannot be sufficiently emphasised and points to the prime importance of the Lac (milk) remedies, Carcinosin and those remedies particularly connected to the breast and its functions.

In a young boy, failure to differentiate his own personality from his mother's; failure to socialise successfully; lack of a positive father figure; and a poorly developed super-ego (little or no conscience) are ingredients for trouble, as evidenced by the Mercurius and Arsenicum archetypes (see Shipman above). A young man blighted by such a deficient latency period is emotionally handicapped. The ego-self is weak and fearful; it has a poor self-image, fears society and grasps for external supports rather than soul qualities to sustain it. To survive emotionally, the inadequate ego-self employs defence mechanisms that are psychologically damaging, robbing them of happiness and hurting those who care for them. The primitive sexual and aggressive fantasies and instincts are not controlled or repressed. When coupled to an absence of conscience, this psychic configuration holds the potential for antisocial behaviour, cruelty and physical, sexual and emotional abuse.

A girl is similarly affected when she identifies with a weak, mother figure and has no positive father figure with whom she can identify and from whom she can model a balanced, moral super-ego. A weak, vulnerable, self-serving ego-self develops, motivated to survive whatever the cost to themselves and others.

Genital stage

The final period of psychosexual development is the genital stage, which extends from *puberty through adolescence into adult life*. Although this stage, by definition, encompasses most of the person's life, it is the adolescent period that is particularly crucial to the type of individual that will advance into mature, adult life. The chance exists to resolve childhood conflicts and issues resulting from fixations during the previous stages. During the teenage years, as in the phallic stage, sexual orientation returns and is centred upon the genitalia. However, it is now no longer infantile and solitary; it seeks gratification through sexual relationships, which are adult and consensual. The personality is more evolved and the primary, instinctive drive for sexual gratification, which promotes adolescent sexual experimentation, is generally tempered by secondary needs that seek satisfaction, not only sexually, but also emotionally, intellectually and symbolically (e.g. marriage). These secondary considerations should assume increasing importance with maturity and bring about successful resolution of the genital stage through a settled, mutually fulfilling relationship. They embrace friendship, companionship, shared interests and responsibilities and eventually the joy of a family. Integral to this stage should be the development of psychological independence from parents. When a well-adjusted and balanced personality emerges from this final stage, the aggressive and libido aspects of the Id can be directed intellectually and creatively towards achieving fulfilment through love, work, art and play, while benefiting society and life.

Reflecting the patriarchal perspective and prejudice of his time, Freud considered heterosexuality to be the proper outlet for the adult sexual instinct. Putting this aside, together with his misconception that homosexuality is a sexual perversion, fixation and its associated conflicts can certainly lead to deviant sexuality. Less serious, but clinically important: fixation in the early stages of psychosexual development may leave a woman in the clitoral phase of sexuality rather than the mature vaginal phase that should be reached during the genital stage. This results in sexual orgasm only being achieved through clitoral stimulation and the absence of vaginal orgasm. Less serious fixation may be indicated when a woman experiences occasional vaginal responsiveness leading to orgasm.

Differentiating the orgasmic potential in a woman is of value in ascertaining the presence or absence of a psychosexual fixation and when present, its degree of severity. This is of help in determining treatment and monitoring response. In a mature woman, the emergence of vaginal orgasmic potential, even if at first only occasional, is an indication of movement away from fixation and of improvement in the overall health of the constitution.

References

1 Morford MPO, Lenardon RJ. *Classical Mythology*. Oxford: Oxford University Press, 2007. p406.

2 Sophocles. *The Theban Plays*. London: Penguin Books, 1974. p24.

3 *Ibid.*, p48.

4 *Ibid.*, p58.

5 *Ibid.*, pp60–61.

6 Whorton JC. *The Arsenic Century*. New York NY. Oxford University Press Inc. 2010. p18.

7 Mary Ann Cotton. *Wikipedia*. Available online at: en.wikipedia.org. (Retrieved 27.03.2018.)

8   BBC News website: *Harold Shipman: The killer doctor.* Last updated: Tuesday, 13 January, 2004. http://news.bbc.co.uk/1/hi/uk/3391897.stm (Retrieved 27.03.2018.)

9   BBC News website: *Shipman's despair revealed in jail diary.* Last updated: Friday, 26 August 2005. http?//news.bbc.co.uk/1/hi/uk/4187198.stm (Retrieved 27.03.2018.)

10 Pearson AC (ed), Headlam W (trans). *The Agamemnon of Aeschylus.* Cambridge: Cambridge University Press, 2010.

11 Theodoridis G (trans). *Eupides' Iphigeneia In Tauris.* Available online at https://www.poetryintranslation.com/PITBR/Greek/IphigeneiaTauris.php (Retrieved 09.03.2018.)

25

SYMBOLISM OF THE PIN

Study of the symbolism of the pin and the needle takes us beyond psycho-sexual fixation and the Oedipus myth and beyond what we have already deduced about the pin's connection with inveterate emotions and vindic-tiveness.

In pursuing this metaphor, we need to explain why Silicea: a highly refined, sensitive and spiritual archetype, and Mercurius: a cold, heartless, morally depraved archetype – both *dream of pins and fear pins* but differ in that Silicea obsessively *searches for pins* and Mercurius, quite unlike Silicea, *dreams of swallowing pins*.

Why the difference? What does it mean? How may we interpret such an odd preoccupation and such a peculiar dream? The fear of what is sharp and hurts, cannot account for either. Does the difference in some way reflect their morality?

The answer lies in the interpretive approach used in dream analysis. Knowing from homeopathic experience, the close, yet antipathetic, relationship existing between the Silicea and Mercury archetypes, we can presume that the *symbolism of the pin* in the rubrics *searching for pins* and *dreams of swallowing pins* has a similar theme, but a diametrically opposed purpose.

In mystical thinking, the pin or needle directs us to the point or dot at the centre of a circle. The circle, like the *ouroboros*, is the symbol of totality, unity and eternity – an image permanent, but dynamic. The central pin, marker or dot, denotes the source and origin of all manifestation: a symbol of primordial, creative power, infinitely compressed and concentrated at an infinitely circumscribed point – so dense, yet, so un-manifest, that it can only be conceived of in an immaterial way – as a hole or void: the utterly, formless principle from which everything animate and inanimate origi-nates. This pinhole void is the sacred symbol of the Cosmos in potential form prior to manifestation: a poised state of absolute equilibrium and harmony. Indeed, in Chinese thought, the needle presents an image of the functional balance and synergy between *yin* and *yang*, between the feminine and masculine principles; the eye of the needle symbolising the feminine and the shaft of the pin the masculine.

In astrophysics, this immensely dense, infinitely small point of absolute power is termed a *singularity*. At the moment of the "big bang", its vast potential is released to create the expanding universe. At the end of a cosmic cycle, the contracting universe resolves back into the void of infinite potentiality. In the image of the pin and its hole, ancient philosophy, meta-physics and the discoveries of atomic physics find correlation.

Expanding the esoteric perspective, the central point of the symbolic circle is the source of emanation or departure from Oneness; it is also the point of termination on the return to Oneness; a unity brought about by spiritual integration through the resolution of opposites: the very goal of individuation and the destination of the Hero's path.

In Sanskrit, *bindu* is the word for a point or dot. Used in its feminine form, *bindi*, it refers to the small ornamental, devotional or mystical dot applied to the forehead of Hindu women. In the same spiritual tradition, *yantra* means a mystic diagram, which, like the mandala, can be used to balance the mind or focus it on spiritual concepts. The hexagram, the six-pointed geometric star comprised of two equilateral triangles, as in Judaism's Star of David, is such a diagram. In this *yantra*, which in Hinduism depicts the union of the god Shiva (masculine principle) and the goddess Shakti (feminine principle) in the root chakra of the energy system of the body, the *bindu* is the most sacred point at the centre of the star. *Here, the dot represents the undifferentiated godhead, Brahman,* in whom the feminine and masculine principles are entwined in perfect equilibrium. This symbolism accords with the pin (point, dot or hole), being the metaphor for Divinity as both source and objective. The dot is, furthermore, the sign of the sacred monosyllable, Om, which in Hinduism represents both the un-manifest (Brahman) and manifest (Ishwara) aspects of the Absolute or Supreme Consciousness. Finally, the dot is the central starting point for the development and elaboration of any mandala: a *yantra* or diagram representing the Cosmos. Here, it is the 'seed', 'sperm' or 'drop' from which all else emerges; imagery which is consonant with the pinpoint being the 'source'. The central point of the mandala surrounded by a circle indicates the Universal Divinity. When the mandala is visualised as the psyche, the innermost circle represents the indwelling Divinity: the Spirit-self – the Atman!

In the light of this excursion into metaphysics, the *searching for pins*, uniquely witnessed in Silicea, no longer merely points to eccentricity, meticulous perfectionism, futile endeavour (looking for a pin in a haystack), relentless resentment or pricks of conscience – all of which are facets of the crystal archetype – but can be interpreted as an innate drive towards spiritual unfoldment and sublimation. In searching for pins, Silicea is yearning and striving for the centre of the *yantra*, the *bindu(i)* that marks the bulls-eye of spiritual endeavour. The very structure of the quartz crystal, made up of ever-repeated tetrahedrons, which always culminate in a crowning pyramid, the ultimate symbol of spiritual ascent and final transcendence, signifies the noble aspiration of the Silicea archetype.

Mercurius does not search for pins – far from it – it *dreams of swallowing them*! Clinically, this strange dream confirms the link between Mercurius and the remedies Hepar-sulph and Silicea, both of which may be indicated for inflammation of the throat, characterised by a sharp pain on swallowing, as if a splinter (pin) or fishbone were caught in the throat (a symptom also true of Alumina and Nat-mur, both in the *fear of pins* group). Esoterically, dreaming of swallowing pins has great metaphorical significance. A pin is a singularly sharp object, capable of inflicting painful injury. Swallowing pins in a dream, reveals an unnatural response to life, fraught with painful and damaging consequences. It depicts an act contrary to the highest meaning of the pin, which ultimately stands for the Supreme Consciousness and the Spirit, or Self.

The great usurper and miscreant, the false- or ego-self, epitomised at its worst in the dark aspect of the syphilitic archetype Mercurius, in asserting its dominance within the psyche, 'swallows' the true- or soul-self, stilling its voice and rendering it impotent to employ its higher perspective and realise its sacred goal. In the process, 'God', the pin's highest metaphor, is 'swallowed' or eclipsed and the ego-self makes materialism its shrine. The goal of individuation, for which the pin is a metaphor, is subsumed (swallowed) by the ego-self. In 'swallowing' God and Spirit, Mercury blinds the soul to its purpose and destiny. Like Oedipus, the soul is blind and banished – estranged from humanity and love!

Aptly, the cover of my copy of Oedipus the King by Sophocles[1] is illustrated by a detail from *Oedipus and Antigone or The Plague of Thebes*, by Charles Francois Jalabeat, which depicts the blind Oedipus being led away from the chaos of Thebes on the arm of his daughter Antigone; metaphorically depicting the need of the soul, blinded by the materialism of the ego-self, for guidance from the feminine principle – the only force that can restore its vision and place it once again upon the Hero's path.

Whereas, the Silicea crystal is the very image of shape, structure and order and is often worn as a protective talisman, Mercury, the only liquid metal, is not what it seems, silvery-pure, clean and innocent; it exudes corruption and death and from its shiny, convex surface reflects a distorted reality, warning of an archetypal potential – selfish, heartless, cruel, perverse and clandestine. In contrast to the stable, solid and refined Silicea, Mercury epitomises formlessness and instability; it is a shape-shifter, elusive, nimble and agitated; touch it and it quivers, drop it and it scatters into a myriad of droplets each as slippery, tricky and evasive as the others, adhering to the noble metals – 'going where the going is good' – but cohering only to other droplets – 'birds of a feather flock together' – a symbol of deviousness, opportunism and treachery – the archetype of the tyrant, the mobster and the murderer.

Small wonder that Mercurius and Silicea are incompatible clinically and cannot be given together or in sequence; the action of either has to be followed by Hepar-sulph before the other can be freely utilised. Devil and angel cannot consort!

On the most superficial level, the fear of pins in Silicea is also clearly related to it remarkable ability to expel foreign bodies such as splinters of wood, iron filings, tiny shards of glass or thorn points, all of which feel as if a pin were embedded in the flesh.

* * * * *

Pins and needles archetypes

Fear of pins and needles.
Alumina; *Apis*; Ars-alb; Bovista; Lac felinum; Mercurius; Nat-mur; Platina; *Silicea*; *Spigelia*.

Dreams of pins or needles.
Androctonus, Lac lupinum, Mercurius, Silicea.

In conjunction with the *pins and needles* rubrics, *pain as from a splinter (fishbone) in the throat* should also be considered in the light of phallic-stage fixation.

Throat: pain as from a splinter.
Alumina, Apis, *Arg-nit, Berberis, Calc-carb, Causticum, *Chelidonium*, *Dolichos, *Hepar-sulph, Ignatia, *Kali-carb, Lac-can, *Lachesis*, Mag-carb, Mercurius, *Nat-mur*, *Nit-ac, Physostigma, *Silicea*, Solanum-nig.

A degree of overlap is evident, and a number of other major archetypes are drawn into the phallic-stage fixation fold. Two lesser archetypes in the throat rubric are of interest: Physostigma (calabar bean) which has a specific affinity for the eyes, especially the vision, inducing night-blindness – an action apposite to the Oedipus theme; and Dolichos (cowhage) a right-sided remedy with pronounced liver and skin symptoms: its splinter in the throat sensation on swallowing is below the right angle of the jaw. The right side is the masculine, ego-self side and the skin, which is the external target of Dolichos action, in psychological terms, represents the persona, the mask that the ego-self wears to further its ends. This picture of negative masculine energy and an ego-distorted façade (skin manifestations) in an archetype that has a splinter in its throat, ties in with the slang word prick (pin), which used in its vulgar sense means penis (phallus) and in its pejorative sense denotes an obnoxious or despicable man – a misogynistic abuser.

Note that Hepar-sulph, the archetype that can mediate between the devil Mercurius and the angel Silicea, has the thorn or fishbone in the throat symptom a sign confirming the relationship between the three archetypes.

The esoteric imagery of the pin and its symbolic connection with phallic-stage psychosexual fixation gives the pins and needles rubrics the stature they deserve and as with Silicea and Mercurius, the means to better evaluate associated archetypes.

Even when fear of pins seems to relate to fear of the pain they can cause, e.g. fear of the doctor's hypodermic, there may well be deeper psychological reasons for the fear, often more related to the symbolism of the pin than it simply being a sharp object. It may signify a fear of penetration and this can be expanded to a fear of sexual, *phallic* penetration – *fear of sex and fear of rape* (a common fear noted in singularly few remedies).

The fear of pins, can equate with fear of *"the slings and arrows of outrageous fortune"*: fear of the seemingly arbitrary, random and unpredictable life events that can puncture peace and complacency. The phobia may also allude to the pangs of guilt and conscience that can afflict even the hardest heart:

> . . . leave her to heaven and to those thorns which in her bosom lodge to prick and sting her.[2]

There is no time to consider and compare all the archetypes in the three rubrics, but it is worth giving a brief look at the remaining archetypes in the *fear of pins* rubric.

Arsenicum

The pin has a special relationship to Arsenicum for common usage makes the pin a symbol of cleanness and neatness: *as clean as a new pin; as shiny and bright as a new pin; as neat as a pin*: all indicative of Arsenicum, the pan-perfectionist; possibly the most anally-fixated archetype of all, but often the victim of phallic-stage fixation, e.g. Harold Shipman.

Arsenic and mercury are, apart from phosphorus and lead, the most potent bio-accumulative, environmental toxins posing a danger to planetary life. Psychosexual fixation of these two malevolent archetypes in the phallic-stage poses a similar danger to society, where the two are capable of the worst sexually orientated crimes. This will be a future topic for consideration.

Apis

The rubric, *fear of pins*, also contains Apis mellifica, the honey bee, and Bovista (*Calvatia gigantea*) the giant puffball, two closely related remedies. Apis is highly complementary to Mercurius and its salts; it shares their characteristic burning, stinging pains and similarly singles out the kidneys for attack, producing, and, therefore, curing, acute glomerulonephritis, especially when due to ß haemolytic streptococcal infection.

Common idiom that attaches bee characteristics to human behaviour reveals intuitive recognition of the existence of a bee archetype e.g. *as busy as a bee; to make a beeline; a bee in the bonnet; the bee's knees*. Study of the mythology and natural history of this remarkable insect, so critical to the homeostasis of the planet, provides us with insights into the psyche of the Apis-type individual; a picture which is fleshed-out by homeopathic provings of the insect and its venom. It takes little imagination to visualise the mature, strong Apis female as a powerful, matriarchal figure, a queen

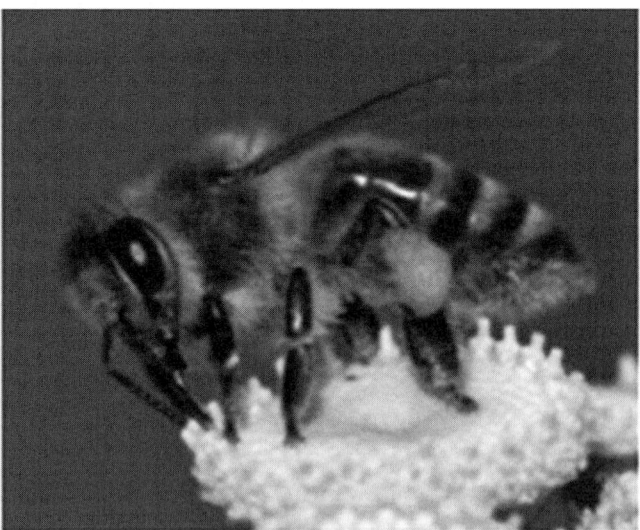

Figure 25.1 The Western honey bee (Apis mellifica)
(Wikipedia)

bee, whose controlling assertiveness and regal dominance assure the homage of husband and of sons and daughters and their partners. She is pivotal to the dynamics of her family, holding court and meddling in everyone's affairs. In nature, the efficiency and integrity of the beehive depends on the submission of the female workers and the male drones to the controlling authority of the queen exercised through the influence of her pheromones. The archetype is set-up for mother-fixation and this tendency is reproduced in the human Apis archetype – but extends to either parent. The fear of pins and sharp, pointed objects is to be expected in an insect whose survival centres round a sting. As important as the sting is to the worker and the safety of the hive, it is of even greater importance to the queen. No sooner has a young princess emerged from her special birth cell than she will fight to the death with any other of her royal sisters that has hatched at the same time. She has a smooth, un-barbed, curved sting that she uses to kill her siblings – indicative of an archetypal penchant for extreme, even vicious, sibling rivalry and jealousy. Unlike the workers, the young queen-to-be does not lose her sting after use and can fight again and again.

Androctonus – fattail scorpion

When pins and needles feature symptomatically, Androctonus (fattail scorpion) must be considered, for although it is not yet listed in the rubric

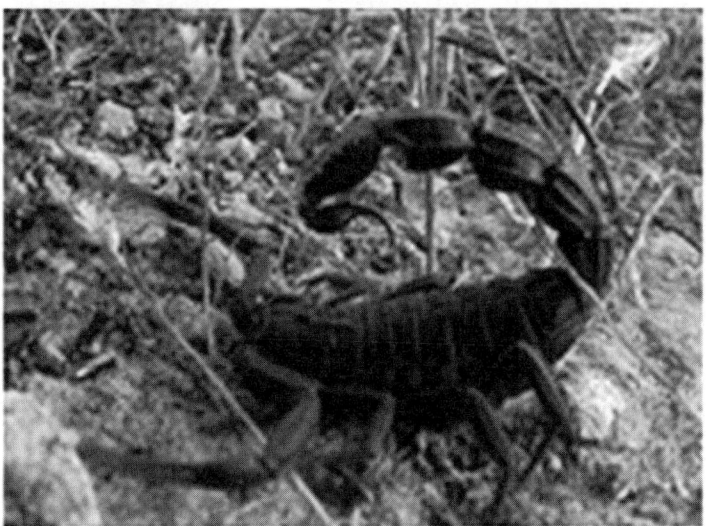

Figure 25.2 *The fattail scorpion (Androctonus crassicauda)*
(*Wikipedia*)

fear of pins, it has the very relevant and ghastly dream previously noted: *murdered grandfather by poking a needle through one of his eyes.*

Bovista

The giant puffball, Calvatia gigantea, known to homeopathy as Bovista,[i] is a very impressive mushroom, whose fruiting body can reach relatively immense proportions, up to 150 centimetres in diameter and 20 kg in weight. The mature puffball contains trillions of tiny, dry spores, which are forcefully ejected as a black powder when the fruiting body ruptures. When this powder is burned, it produces a smoke, which is intolerable to bees and drives them away from their hives.

This traditional use of the powder provides a clue, which homeopathic use confirms: Bovista is closely related to Apis and should be remembered whenever Apis symptoms come to the fore. Apart from the *fear of pins and sharp pointed things*, the two remedies share other symptoms and signs: *awkward; everything falls from the hands, especially pre-menstrually*; pitting oedema and urticaria; ovarian cysts; aggravation of symptoms from hot weather and getting warm. Bovista is a feminine remedy and its suitability

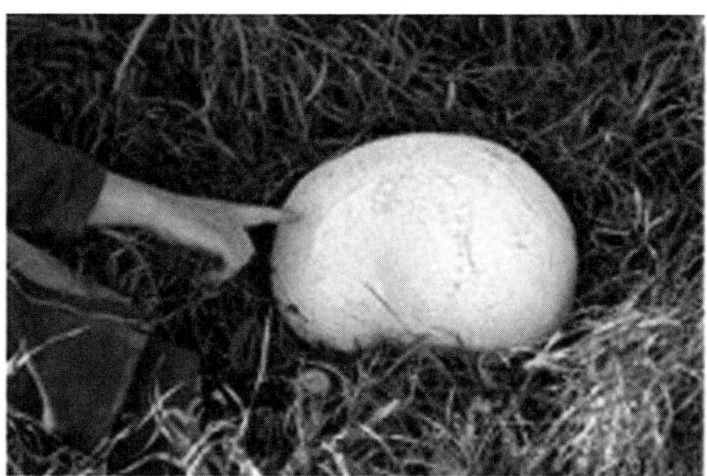

Figure 25.3 *The giant puffball (Calvatia gigantea)*

(Wikipedia)

---

[i] Bovista is a genus of fungi commonly known as the true puffballs. Reference to the genus has appeared in several 19th-century textbooks on homeopathy (Wikepedia). However, the fungus used in homeopathy, though referred to as Bovista, is actually the giant puffball (*Calvatia gigantean*). See Vermeulen F. *Prisma Reference: Ultimate Prisma Collection*. Volume 4. Glasgow: Saltire Books, 2017. p306.

for abuse is revealed in: *dreams*: *anxious dreams about animals biting them*; *of being bitten by snakes*; *of vermin*; *of worms creeping*.

The temperament may be inflated like the puffball itself: extrovert, loud, indiscrete, voluble, vivacious, hurried, irritable and quarrelsome; a big puffed-up ego, full of opinion and attitude, ever looking for a fight, whose pride is easily slighted and who takes everything amiss: *a flimsy egotism, puffed with conceit, punctured by the least jibe*. The contrary is true, matching the flabby, deflated puffball after its spores have been ejected: a timid, intro-verted, secretive being, lively in company, but sad, depressed and not interested in anything when alone (Sepia; Conium); stolid, apathetic indifference; so absent in mind that, even with great exertion, is unable to pay attention to what is being said or done; stares vacantly into space (navel-gazing – the empty, vacuous contemplation of nothing); irresistible drowsiness as if intoxicated or drugged; inefficiency – loses way in familiar streets, makes mistakes in speech and writing; indolence worse after eating. Whereas Apis is worse for suppression of sexual desire, Bovista is deflated after sex: staggering, confusion and numbness in the head.

Bovista's connection to the Oedipus myth extends beyond the pins/needles symbol to the blood that the poet vividly etches into our memory. Bovista is a remedy for bleeding wounds and a haemorrhagic diathesis (a constitution that tends to bleed easily). In folk medicine, Bovista powder is still used as a styptic to staunch bleeding. Other arche-types dream of snakes, but characteristic of Bovista's dream is the extreme aggression of the snake that pursues them; it sinks its fangs most frequently into their ankle or calf and leaves an open, bleeding wound. This bleeding reveals that Bovista's syphilitic miasmatic energy has evolved into the tubercular miasm (pulmonary tuberculosis is characterised by the coughing up of blood and an unusual tendency to bleed is indicative of a dominant tubercular miasmatic state).

The phallic-phase fixation of the Bovista archetype is exemplified by the structure of the giant puffball, which is attached to the soil by means of a fungal root that resembles an umbilical cord. The archetype, in like manner, is tenaciously attached to the subject of its fixation, like a baby to its mother; it resists the severing of its emotional, umbilical lifeline. The typical Bovista relationship is tempestuous and despite its dependent quality, fraught with disruptions – quarrelling and fighting. Communi-cation is reduced to heated disputes and disagreements in which flashes of emotion are richly embroidered with profanity. Such outbursts may be followed by sulky moroseness and taciturnity, quite at odds with the usually vivacious personality, never at a loss for words and opinion.

Alumina (aluminium oxide)

The spores of Bovista are intensely dry and like the spores of Lycopodium (club moss) may be used as a dusting powder. The ash of the puffball is extremely rich in Aluminium; a fact that links the two as remedies. They share a remarkable spread of symptoms and both are excellent for dry, intolerably itchy eczema. However, it is the symptom *fear of pins* that confirms the singular energy running through all the remedies in the rubric. In Alumina, the symptom achieves a heightened form: *suicidal tendency* or *violent homicidal impulses when seeing a knife, a sharp object or blood.* The study of the Alumina archetype and its aetiology highlights many of the causative factors contributing to phallic fixation and its consequences. The archetype lacks defined boundaries, lacks a sense of identity and personal worth and needs to identify with others to achieve some sense of being. Often, history reveals that there was no strong authority figure or role model to give substance to the ego-self, or the child's self-esteem was broken down by parental scorn, criticism and domination; or their self-determination was lost through religious or political indoctrination. They have been 'castrated' and in the knife (pin, needle), the lost phallus, their masculinity, is symbolically resurrected, to be clasped and wielded destructively with all the force and intent of the repressed rage, humiliation and hate pent up within them. It becomes a penis substitute to thrust repeatedly into the object on which they wreak their wrath. The same copulative action is seen in the ghastly self-mutilation of Oedipus. With similar symbolism behind it, the colour red representing the aggressive, *yang*, power of the Id, concentrated in the first chakra, acts like the sight of a knife to the disempowered Aluminium archetype and prompts violent impulses which can spill over into acts of violence, based on weakness of the ego-self, not strength.

Natrum muriaticum

Nat-mur (common salt) is so close to Apis it is referred to as its chronic. This refers to the fact that when Apis has proved successful in the treatment of an acute manifestation of disease, Nat-mur will frequently prove to be the long-term archetypal remedy for that patient. They are both well suited to the atopic state (allergy), both are indicated for water retention and conditions characterised by oedema, both display curious awkwardness or clumsiness and tend to drop things; Nat-mur is also inclined to inadvertency, knocking things over and tripping over things. Together with the *fear of pins* common to each, these unusual characteristics also draw Bovista into the close Apis/Nat-mur relationship – a fact that can be of great help clinically. The very nature of Nat-mur is fixated – fixated in emotions and often in co-dependent relationships. The archetype is closed-off, private and insular; over-conscious of correct, proper behaviour; their grief and guilt crystalize instead of reaching resolution. The final act of Sophocles' play depicts Oedipus (even his name indicative of oedema) in an extreme Nat-mur emotional seizure, consumed with shame, grief, guilt, self-reproach, wounded honour, humiliation and shock. The vision of Nat-mur is thrust inwards and blinding itself to any excuse or mitigation, the arche-type continuously plunges culpability into its conscience.

Spigelia

Spigelia anthelmia (pinkroot or wormbush) is a small herbaceous annual of the *Loganiaceae* family of plants. As its species name, *anthelmia*, and its common name, *wormbush*, imply, it is a remedy for worm infestations, a property which indicates archetypally that it is a remedy for victimisation and abuse

It is a plant that markedly affects the nerves, causing sharp stabbing pains and pains that are violent and burn like hot needles or wires; primarily in the region of the head, eyes, face, teeth and heart. Spigelia has a

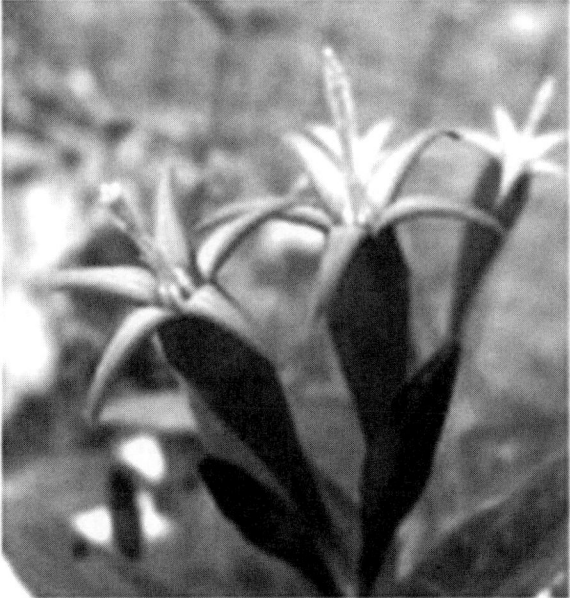

Figure 25.4 *Pinkroot or wormbush (Spigelia anthelmia)*
(Wikipedia)

particular affinity for the heart causing violent palpitations and violent sticking or compressive pains in the heart, which may radiate up into the neck and throat and extend into one or both arms. Cardiac symptoms are very much worse for the least movement or bending double and are better for drinking warm water, which they crave. Symptoms, especially the neuralgias, are more left-sided. The eyes are particularly targeted with severe pain in and about the eyes, such as Oedipus must have felt as he plunged the needle repeatedly into his eyes.

- *Ciliary neuralgia; supra orbital neuralgia.*
- *Severe pain, in and around the eyes, extending deep into the socket, worse thinking of them.*
- *As if needles were thrust in the eyes.*

Spigelia is more a woman's remedy; a gender relationship inferred by its alternative common name *pinkroot*, and its more left-sided symptomatology. The Elektra phallic-stage fixation may lead a Spigelia girl down a rocky road, fatally attracted to men like her father, often despite his serious drawbacks. The archetype shares with Silicea the highest degree of sensitivity to *steel points being directed towards her* (4), especially towards her eyes (Lac felinum) and *fear of pins and pointed sharp things* (4); so much so, that she even imagines seeing them when they are not there: *delusion of pins.*

Although unwise in love, Spigelia is a highly intelligent young lady, with plenty of drive and ambition, committed to making her way in the world; and, in keeping with her affinity for pins, bringing to her aspiration, a sharp enquiring mind that can focus one-pointedly on a chosen goal. Like an archer with her bow, the mind of Spigelia is always looking to the future and aiming at nothing less than the bullseye. Once decided on a course of action, particularly in the choice of a career, she is determined and will not be deterred from achieving her objective. This may point her towards a profession or towards the performing arts. In either, she sets her mark high; she wants to shine, like a 'new pin', and be noted as outstanding and exceptional.

- *Ambition – much ambition.*
- *Craves attention, wants to be seen, and become an actress.*
- *Desire for challenge in becoming an actress.*
- *Insists on carrying out her plans.*
- *Absorbed, buried in thought about the future* (unique).
- *Thoughts, profound, about her future.*
- *Anxiety about the future.*
- *Industrious, mania for work* (2).

- *Conscientious about trifles.*
- *Ideas abundant, clearness of the mind.*
- *Seriousness.*

A defining quality of the Spigelia archetype is the striking disparity between her intellectual and emotional intelligence.

Like Nux-vom and Ignatia, Spigelia belongs to the *Loganiaceae* family of plants, and psychologically she portrays a mixture of the traits of both. Intellectually, she resembles Nux vomica: the outstanding example of the A-type personality, driven to succeed; but, emotionally, she is like Ignatia: the temperamental easily-infatuated romantic-idealist. In Spigelia, marriage of the two, creates a high-flying, executive-level young woman, noted for her astute far-sightedness, initiative and enterprise, or an accomplished and very cerebral actress, who diligently researches every role she plays – but the private lives of both are a disaster, due to their lamentable lack of caution and judgement when choosing the men they invite into their lives (*heedless, careless*). Spigelia is the princess, who has pricked her finger on the evil witch's spindle of psychosexual fixation (*fear of evil*): her intellect and common sense fall asleep and she welcomes her 'ill-gifted father' into her bed!

Unlike Nux vomica and Ignatia, Spigelia contains no strychnine; its active constituents are cardio-active alkaloids (ryanoids). Nonetheless, the *Loganiaceae* family tendency for passion and intensity is still present in the Spigelia personality. They bring this to bear in all they do. They are charged with energy: *high-spirited, cheerful, excitable, exhilarated, hyperactive, restless, vivacious* and never feel better than when they are intensely occupied; bringing all their resources together in a single-minded effort to achieve their chosen objective: 'seal the deal' or 'play the role'. An arrow, stiletto, bodkin, needle or pin are ideal metaphors for their unswerving trajectory.

The aggressive fire of the Id can be discerned in the vigour and urgency of their commitment. Small wonder they *dream of fire* and have illusions of fire. Their riveted focus will often elicit inspiration: likened by the poets to a bolt of lightning illuminating the mind (*dreams of lightning; of being struck by lightning*). There is no room for flippancy, joviality or trivialisation regarding their commitment (*averse to jesting; cannot take a joke; indignation; easily offended* [2]); they cannot even break off to enjoy themselves with others without feeling they are shirking their duty (*unable to enjoy herself with others, without feeling sad*). Like Nux vomica, they are aggressively competitive, like Ignatia, they are over-emotional. The combination has consequences. As much as they are elated and cheerful when progress is smooth and successful, they become angry, irritable, ill-disposed, quarrelsome and verbally abusive when someone or something gets in the way, or their efforts fail. Then, some of their worst traits come to the fore, directed against those they feel have hindered or thwarted them, or those who have succeeded where they have failed. In their envy, anger and indignation, they stoop to denigrating and 'foul-mouthing' them.

- *Indignation with slandering.*
- *Ill-disposed: envious contemptuous, impatient, insulting, slandering.*
- *Cursing and swearing.*
- *Anger (2); face suffused and red.*
- *Being beside oneself (2).*
- *Easily offended (2).*
- *Violence, vehemence.*

However, her true danger lies in the other limb of the Id: the libido aspect, which has intensity and passion equal to the survival aspect. This, married to her phallic-stage Elektra fixation, spells even more trouble, for Spigelia can be as sensual and sexual as Platina. Indeed, where many a Platina 'promises much, but delivers little', being more sensual, provocative and seductive than sexual, Spigelia has a naturally high sex drive. When the young Spigelia girl is irresistibly attracted, by her psychosexual fixation and her animus projection, to a man whom she unconsciously and instinctively identifies as possessing the characteristics of her idealised, father figure, and the relationship is consummated by sexual intimacy, she finds herself caught inextricably in a web of fixation-desire and sexual lust. The obsession becomes morbid!

Despite her sharp, penetrating mind, Spigelia can be willingly led by her chosen male along a precarious and decadent path of distraction and debauchery: the libido energy, that makes her such a gifted and creative being, deviated towards sexual excesses and substance abuse. Aiding this downward path are her innate sexuality and the transient emotional and physical relief that diversion and escapism afford her. This is a sad and familiar picture in the corporate and entertainment worlds where predatory 'wolves' abound.

- *Ailments from debauchery.*
- *Ailments from sexual excesses.*
- *Lasciviousness, lustfulness.*
- *Dreams lewd, lascivious, lustful.*
- *Dreams amorous with orgasm.*
- *Alcoholism (2)*, always a very real danger for Spigelia, even to *delirium tremens.*

- *Occupation or diversion relieves.*
- *Thinking – complaints worse thinking of them.*

Faced by such a case and all the abuse and emotional suffering that can result from a relationship based on ego-self fixation and bonding to a selfish, dictatorial or misogynistic man, the homeopath may be prompted to prescribe one of the *Ranunculaceae*: Pulsatilla, Staphysagria or Cimicifuga, but fortunately, so often in these Spigelia cases, a simple physical symptom and not a 'mental' saves the day. The physician is gifted a telling Spigelia 'physical' that gives it preference over other 'victim' cases. The characteristic pains often supply the clue, but associated eye complaints and the tendency for emotions to cause strong palpitations and flushing of the face are indicative. Further clues may be a great fear of the 'medical needle', the hypodermic syringe: *fear of injections* and the inability to look at open scissors, knives, blood or an open wound. The fear of injections is a symptom shared with Silicea, which is Spigelia's chronic counterpart, just as it is of the three *Ranunculaceae* ladies. Another indication of the Spigelia/Silicea relationship is evidenced in a characteristic headache shared by both: *pain extending from the left occiput to above the left eye.* When Spigelia has done its work, the remedy that is most often needed to address the deeper aspects of the case is Silicea.

Lac felinum

Phallic-stage fixation, due to unresolved psychosexual competition for the opposite-sex parent, can induce a girl to develop into a woman, who is instinctively driven to dominate men (see 'penis envy' below) either as an unusually seductive woman, who is vain and conceited and has a sense of superiority and entitlement, or, paradoxically, as an unusually submissive woman, who is insecure, feels inferior, lacks self-esteem and is self-effacing (boys will show this same polarity, being either aggressive, vain and over-ambitious: father-fixated; or passive, submissive and excessively diffident: mother-fixated). These contrasting states are both mirrored in the archetypal pictures of two closely related remedies Lac felinum (the domestic cat) and Platina (platinum): both of which appear in the rubric *fear of pins, etc.*

Lac felinum (milk of the cat), like all the Lacs, provides a remedy suited to each stage of psychosexual fixation. It is multi-miasmatic, but particularly suited to the tubercular and cancer miasms, sharing many symptoms with the miasmatic nosodes, Tuberculinum and Carcinosin. The fear of sharp, pointed objects (needles, knives, scissors) is understandable in a creature that utilises sharp canines and vicious, needle pointed claws to assert or resist dominance. Reminiscent of the horror of the Oedipus imagery, the archetype cannot tolerate anything sharp-pointed anywhere near the eyes, which, in catfights, are highly vulnerable to injury (cat's eyebrow whiskers give early eye-closing warning when touched). Lac felinum people instinctively pull back when a finger or some sharp object is pointed at them or when a hand or object comes close to their face, out of fear that their eyes might get hurt. They also, like Silicea and Spigelia, cringe at the thought of a hypodermic needle being thrust through their skin into their flesh; a thought which is far more disturbing than any fear of the pain it might cause.

Lac felinum can be a mysterious and seductive woman who uses her potent charms to ensnare her lovers in bonds of infatuation and irresistible desire; her combination of sultry sensuality and disdainful aloofness driving men (or women) to distraction and obsession. She is a *femme fatale* – a deadly woman – who exercises a hypnotic power over her victim and is sadistically cruel in toying with an admirer's emotions, taking pleasure and pride in the anguish of unrequited longing and love she can arouse; a delight she cruelly prolongs, playing hot then cold, flirtatious and fickle, like a cat with a mouse. Behind the beauty, charm and magnetic allure lurks a phallic fixation that desires to control, dominate and manipulate men. The Lac felinum man may have an underdeveloped masculine aspect and in consequence be caught up in a tenacious Oedipal 'incestuous' bond with mother or some other mother figure. An above average number of Lac felinum males are either homosexual or have a strongly developed feminine aspect; they are romantic, idealistic, artistic and creative and often excel in the arts, design, literature, music, drama and dance. This is to be expected for the cat is nocturnal and lunar, archetypal attributes that are essentially feminine. The dog by contrast is diurnal and primarily solar, though it also has important lunar aspects.

Lac felinum must be added to what we may term homosexual rubrics: *Love-sick with someone of the same sex* and more specifically:

Love sick with her own sex: Calc-carb; Calc-phos; *Lachesis*; *Lac felinum*; Medorrhinum; Nat-mur; Phosphorus; *Platina; Pulsatilla; *Sulphur*; *Thuja.

Love sick with his own sex: *Lac felinum*; Medorrhinum; Nat-mur; Origanum; Phosphorus; Platina; Pulsatilla; Sepia; Staphysagria; *Thuja*.

These rubrics feature a number of the central remedies of the materia medica, but like many key rubrics must be regarded as incomplete. The absence of Lac felinum is only one example. Silicea, which is the chronic counterpart of Pulsatilla should be in both rubrics, as should Staphysagria, Calc-phos and Calc-carb. Of interest to our theme is the presence of Platina, especially highlighted in the female rubric.

Platina

Platina, must always be considered in tandem with Lac felinum; it too is lunar and therefore feminine in its expression, hence, pre-eminently, but not exclusively a woman's remedy. It is a lustrous, grey-white metal possessing a wonderful, cool, bold, elegance and sleekness that often serves better than gold to complement the glittering fire of diamonds. Wondrously rare, far more expensive than gold, it adorns the throats, wrists, ears and fingers of the wealthy, famous and fashionable. It is associated with glamour, refinement and ostentation. Greta Garbo, the Swedish film actress and icon of Hollywood's silent and classical periods, holding a platinum cigarette holder with sophisticated affectation, provided an image of languid elegance and refined, feminine sensuality that personifies the archetype. Howard Hughes intuitively picked up on this energy when he recognised the star potential of Jean Harlow, who eclipsed other stars of her era to become the platinum blonde sex symbol of the 1930s. Platinum, like Lac-felinum, can be a *femme fatale*, an archetype frequently depicted by these two film stars. As noted, these remedies appear in the small rubric *fear of pins*, as do Apis and Mercurius, both outstanding remedies for acute glomerulonephritis and chronic nephritis. Both Harlow and Garbo died of kidney disease: Harlow, in 1936, while shooting *Saratoga* with Clark Gable, from nephritis probably consequent to scarlet fever she had contracted earlier in her life, she was only 26 years of age; Garbo died from kidney failure after a supportive period of dialysis treatment in 1990, at the age of 84.

These links and relationships are not arbitrary or coincidental; they are proof of the universal archetypal patterns held in the collective unconscious. When we contemplate certain key rubrics, we are looking at the blueprint of life. When we incorporate classical mythology in our understanding of archetypes and the universal patterns written into life events and add to this the special mythology of homeopathic provings, we enter a magic world of correspondences and connections, which offer irrefutable evidence of an unwavering order and unity underlying apparent chaos and diversity. Therefore, looking at the path we have just walked – phallic-stage psychosexual fixation, the cancer miasm and related remedies, the myth of Oedipus, the significance of the sphinx, the appalling self-mutilation with a broach-pin, the rubric *fear of pins* that includes Lac-caninum and Platina, both *femme fatale* archetypes, and, from that connection, the charismatic film stars Greta Garbo and Jean Harlow, who both portrayed irresistible 'deadly women' and died of nephritis – we should not be surprised, when studying the life of Garbo, that although so unique and special, she, nonetheless, fitted an archetypal mould, fashioned miasmatically and by phallic-stage fixation, which determined her eccentric nature, her exquisite features, her remarkable career, her rare genius and the dread diseases that finally afflicted her.

* * * * *

Greta Garbo (1905–1990)

Greta Garbo was born Greta Lovisa Gustaffson and her childhood in Stockholm, Sweden, was spent in harsh, psoric circumstances surrounded by poverty and the drab, grey ugliness of a city slum. Yet, this deprived and humble setting did not hold the inner vision of this sensitive, imaginative young girl captive.

From an early age, she dreamed of one day becoming an actress and whilst still at school directed her friends in make-believe performances. At 13, due to the necessity of contributing to the meagre family income, she left school to seek work. Many years later, she confessed to having an inferiority complex because of her lack of high school education. In 1919, the deadly influenza epidemic that had swept through Europe in the wake

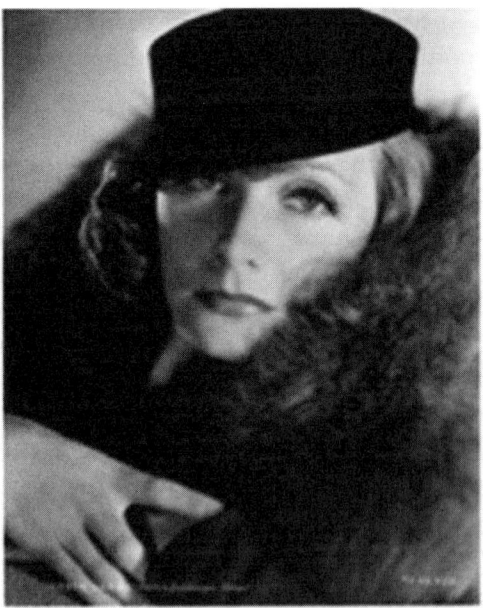

Figure 26.5 *Greta Garbo (1905–1990)*
(MGM)

of the Great War reached Stockholm and her father, with whom she was very close, fell critically ill. During his protracted illness, which led to his death in 1920, it was his 14-year-old daughter, Greta, who stayed at home, tended him and accompanied him to hospital for treatment.

In this small cameo lifted from a person's life, an archetypal picture emerges, which though steeped in *Psora* – poverty, disadvantaged circumstances, lack of education, inferiority complex – reveals a rich, venturesome fantasy life, aspiration, focus, leadership qualities, stage ambition, strong paternal bonding, compassion, early responsibility and an urge to nurse others: ingredients that must lift that person out of straightened, limited circumstances and transport them into a better and more creative life. So, it was with Garbo! Analysing these historic details archetypally, miasmatically and homeopathically, it is apparent that other miasmatic forces overlaid the psoric foundation. The rich imagination, sensitivity and desire for expression through acting point to the presence of the Tubercular miasm, but when the sense of inferiority at not being fully educated, the compassion, the assumption of responsibility at an early age, the commitment to nursing a loved one and the enduring grief of a daughter for a father lost are added, a mixed miasmatic state emerges indicating *Carcinosis*, the cancer miasm and more specifically the C-type, psora-dominant Carcinosin archetype (see *Healing the Soul* Volume 3); an archetype which despite great ability often suffers from an inferiority complex, especially concerning their intellect and their education. The following rubrics show how clearly Carcinosin matches the life situations depicted.

- *Fantasies, imaginations*: *exaltation of*: Belladonna; Cannabis indicus; Carcinosin; China; Hyoscyamus; Lachesis; Opium; Stramonium and Sulphur all in highest grade.
- *Responsibility*: burdened with at too young an age: Calc-carb and *Carcinosin in italics*; Lycopodium in lowest grade
- *Over responsible*: Aurum; *Calc-carb; *Carcinosin*; Ignatia; Kali-carb; Nat-mur; Nat-sulph.
- *Compassionate*: *Phosphorus and Calc-phos; *Carcinosin*; Causticum; Dulcamara; Ignatia; Nat-carb; Nat-mur; Nit-ac; Nux-vom *all in italics*
- *Anxiety about family*: Acetic-ac; Ars-alb; *Calc-carb*; Calc-silicata; *Carcinosin*; Hepar-sulph; Petroleum; Phosphorus; Pulsatilla.
- *Night-watching* (the bedside vigil): *Carcinosin; Causticum; *Cocculus; Cuprum; *Nit-ac*; Selenium; Zincum.
- *Nursing of others*: Bryonia; Calc-carb; Carcinosin; Cocculus; Phos-ac; Phytolacca; Pulsatilla; Sepia; Silicea all in highest grade.

- *Grief at the death of a loved one*: Calc-carb; *Carcinosin; *Causticum; Gelsemium; *Ignatia; *Kali-brom*; Lachesis; *Nat-mur; Nux-vom; Phos-ac; Platina; Staphysagria; Sulphur.

Such a study is always of value to the analyst because not only does it confirm the intuitive gut-feelings about a case, it also brings into focus related remedies that may be required.

Despite her celebrity, Garbo was a very private person, who never married or had children, largely lived alone, enjoying only the company of close friends and acquaintances, had a fear of strangers, mistrusted the media, suffered lifelong melancholia, and maintained her 'elusive mystique' to the very end. These reclusive, introspective traits coupled to her mesmerising beauty and her incredibly eloquent eyes and expressive features, which could subtly portray the innermost feelings of a character by the slightest of movements, fitted her ideally for the silent screen. It was in this genre that she established herself as one of the greatest actresses Hollywood had ever produced.

Her eccentricities soon became evident. During a shoot, she would forbid all visitors on set and insisted on having surrounding screens to prevent extras and technicians from watching her whilst acting. When taxed about the necessity for these, she replied: 'If I am by myself, my face will do things I cannot do with it otherwise.[3]

She slipped with ease into the era of sound and some of her most famous roles followed. She became an icon, a cult figure, and 'Gabomania' became a worldwide phenomenon. Significantly, in the light of her private life and her archetypal nature, she became associated with a famous line from her film *Grand Hotel*: "I want to be alone; I just want to be alone". Commenting later on whether these words also reflected her inner feeling, she remarked: "I never said, 'I want to be alone'; I only said, 'I want to be let alone.' There is a world of difference."[4] This reflects an important ambivalence, evident in the actress and in the archetype, a desire for privacy and solitude, aversion to the intrusion of strangers and the general public, yet a need for the company of someone well known or someone close (this particular ambivalence is suggestive of Conium, a major remedy of the cancer miasm)

Her career came to an unexpected and unheralded end in 1941, when she was only 36 years-of-age. Although preceded by indecision and uncertainty, her eventual withdrawal from the limelight was out of choice, not necessity. Although she was subsequently offered many roles, she never completed another film. She had grown tired of Hollywood life, which had never suited her; her desire to act was played-out; and she longed for a life away from the public eye. Although reclusive by nature, she never became a total hermit. She always enjoyed walking, either alone or with a companion, and on the streets of New York, she became a familiar, casually dressed figure wearing conspicuously large sunglasses. In her final years, she became increasingly withdrawn and in 1984, six years before her death from pneumonia and renal failure, she received treatment for breast cancer.

She became a legend, a charismatic being, exalted and idolised by her public, whom she was at pains to exclude from her life. It was said of her that she did not act; she lived her roles. She accessed the emotions of the character she was portraying within her own being and gave them expression, most importantly through the wondrous eloquence of her magnificent eyes: the windows of her soul. One with the collective unconscious, this remarkable actress was able to intuitively and instinctively touch the frequency of the fictional archetype and authentically bring it to life. This was so intense and meaningful that the stature of her performances consistently overcame the inadequacies of plot and dialogue that plagued most of the mediocre productions she starred in. Her acting was psychic mediumship, a communion with a deeper dimension of experience, which gave entrée to the full spectrum of human emotion; a gift imparted by the multi-facetted cancer miasm that was dominant within her and consonant with her own inner being. Its artistic vent closed, and its energy pooled within the narrow confines of a controlled, insular, depressed psyche, the miasmatic pattern finally achieved physical expression in malignancy of a breast that had never suckled or found maternal expression.

The connections between Garbo and the Oedipus/Elektra complex are remarkable. In the study of *mystic homeopathy*, no matter which way one turns magical associations rise up before the enquiring mind. A thread, like that of Ariadne, presents and by following it we move from difference into unity. The clue in this instance was the act of self-mutilation perpetrated by Oedipus: it fixed the attention on eyes and on needles, indicated miasmatic and remedy connections and led to Garbo. Her life reveals the playing-out of archetypal patterns in heroic proportions. The eyes are pivotal to the myth of Oedipus and to the myth of Garbo; her eyes were the focus of her genius and her magnetic power, and she occluded them, denied them artistic expression and later veiled them behind the protective shield of sunglasses. Her life after retirement, by comparison with what she had attained, was desultory and aimless; she herself often described it as "drifting." She had put out her eyes!

Characteristic of her underlying miasm, her artistic flare sought vicarious satisfaction in acquiring works of art and she expended repressed creative energy in the joy of walking (Carcinosin loves to dance). But age cannot contend with the inexorable advance of miasmatic disease, particularly when urged forward by the unresolved grief of a daughter for her father and a nature subject to depression. The theme of the Oedipus/Elektra complex that threaded her life is revealed in the cancer of the breast that developed and also in evidence unearthed by biographic researchers that she was bisexual and had intimate relationships with male and female lovers. A final touch to her portrait is the name given to this inscrutable, reclusive woman of mystery by the press: *the Swedish Sphinx*!

References

1 Sophocles. *Oxford World Classics; Oedipus the King.* Oxford: Oxford University Press, 1998.
2 Shakespeare W. *Hamlet.* Oxford: Oxford University Press, 1968. Act I Scene V. Lines 86–88. p79.
3 Paris B. *Garbo.* New York NY: Alfred A Knopf, 1994. p320.
4 Shapiro FR. *The Yale Book of Quotations.* New Haven CT: Yale University Press, 2006. p299.

26

FEMININE AND MASCULINE PRINCIPLES

The Spiral: The Sacred Archetypal Form

The fundamental symbol of the wholeness of the creation is the spiral, which since ancient times, in all cultures, has been perceived as a positive, dynamic representation of the universal, life-force flowing through all aspects of existence, cosmic and microcosmic. It is seen in the far-flung spiral arms of a star-laden galaxy, the elliptical orbits of heavenly bodies, the force of a cyclone, the vortex of a whirlpool, the whorls of a nautilus shell, the spiral arrangement of petals in a blossom and leaves on a stem, the furling of a fern frond, the coils of a snake, the print of a finger, the double helix of DNA and the path of electrons spinning about the nucleus of every atom. The vortex forces of wind, water and fire manifest the swirling energy that drives the cosmos.

The spiral symbolises the evolution of the universe, the expanding motion of cosmic energy rotating outwards from a fixed point of origin, continuously extending, reaching out to infinity. It equally symbolises the involution of the same energy returning to its origin, and the vast pulse that cues cosmic expansion and contraction. It depicts the unbroken unity of all forms, the sequential flow of cause and effect, the co-existence of past, present and future and the majestic celestial cycles of generation, preservation, destruction and regeneration. The wheeling momentum of the spiralling circle witnesses the punctuation of time and the cyclic rhythms of the cosmos – galactic, stellar, solar, lunar, planetary, seasonal, tidal and physiological: the cardiac, respiratory, menstrual and waking-sleeping-dreaming rhythms.

The clockwise uncoiling-spiral is overt and denotes expansion, centrifugal manifesting-power, ascent and masculine energy; the counter-clockwise coiling-spiral is covert and denotes involution, centripetal potentiating-power, descent and feminine energy. Hence, the double spiral, which represents these extremes, is not only a universal image, but also a

caduceus as symbol of health

potent fertility symbol. As exemplified in the twin wreathing of serpents around the rod of the caduceus, the staff of Hermes (Mercury), adopted as the symbol of medicine, it captures the polarity and balance of opposing principles or contrasting cosmic currents; it expresses the paradoxical nature of existence, and, simultaneously, the cohesion and compatibility underlying opposition. This profound enigma is demonstrated in the healing power of illness, the initiatory role of suffering and birth through death.

Yin-Yang symbolism

The intertwining and communication between opposites, the synergy of attraction and repulsion and the conjugation of male and female energies, embodied in the double helix, are also clearly depicted and wonderfully expressed in the differentiated, yet embracing, black and white configuration of the Chinese *Yin-Yang* symbol. This well-known, *universal image of balanced dynamism* depicts how contrary principles and forces are interconnected, interdependent and complementary in the relative world. It illustrates the presiding Oneness that underlies and supports the illusion of duality; Heaven and Earth are fused in mutual embrace. *Yin* is dark and *Yang* is light, yet each contains the essence or seed of the other. Every mode must contain the germ of its antithesis. In the darkness of material ignorance glows the light of Divinity; in the light of Universality broods the darkness of individuality. Like the double spiral, the *Yin-Yang* symbol denotes the creative tension, alternation or fusion, between the inseparable opposites, *Yin* and *Yang*, which generates change and motion, expansion and contraction, evolution and involution.

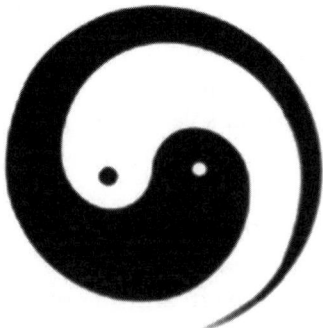

Figure 26.1 Yin-yang symbol

Yin is primary; out of the darkness all things emerge; it is feminine and lunar, associated with the moon, the earth, water, the sea, the night and the unconscious; it is characterised as slow, soft, yielding, enfolding, cold, moist, diffuse, passive, receptive and nurturing; it is enigmatic, imaginative, inspirational and intuitive.

Yang is secondary: consciousness emerging from the ocean of the unconscious; the light of the intellect emerging from the shadows of instinctive life; it is masculine and solar, associated with the sun, the sky, fire, the mountains, the day and consciousness; it is characterised as fast, hard, inflexible, resistant, hot, dry, focused, active, creative and aggressive; it is unambiguous, rational, logical and empirical.

Within a simple, yet dynamic, androgynous symbol, the Chinese have encompassed and concentrated the deepest philosophy, which expresses the arcane structure of the universe and the spirit domain; it brings opposites together and engenders perpetual motion, transformation and continuity amidst apparent inertia, contradiction and separateness. In its central state of poised equilibrium, in which all contrasts are counterbalanced, the symbol represents that state of inner stability and serenity in which all motion ceases, calm prevails, and the soul transcends suffering. It denotes the centre of life's labyrinth, the focal point of individuation. Like the caduceus it is, therefore, also a symbol of spiritual, emotional and physical health based upon balance, harmony and the unification of opposites.

It is significant that the primal symbol of the unity of diversity and the inseparability of the male and female principles – the double spiral, implicit in the *Yin-Yang* motif, is manifested in the basic unit of life: the cell. The double-stranded molecules of DNA (deoxyribonucleic acid) that hold the genetic information that programmes function, determines gender and passes hereditary characteristics or genetic traits to offspring is a spiral polymer of nucleic acids held together by base pairs of nucleotides, twisted to form an extended double helix. Its coded convolutions, comprising the genome of species, archive the continuity and oneness of all life and display this unity through the ultimate symbol of the cosmos: the double spiral.

Kundalini

The fundamental importance of the double spiral as the ubiquitous image of the twin forces of the universe was recognised by the Rishis, the seers of ancient India, more than three thousand years ago, and documented and defined in the oldest Sanskrit texts of Hinduism: the Vedas. Through our Divine Essence, Being, or true nature, we are in constant, unbroken union with our infinite Source, one another and the entire Cosmos. This means that each one of us possesses the unbounded power of the Creation in potential form: it is our spiritual birthright. This limitless, latent energy coiled within the energy counterpart of the physical body, known in esoteric teachings as the 'subtle body', is concentrated in the region of the sacrum and coccyx and was visualised by the ancient seers either as a goddess or as a sleeping she-serpent (the unrealised female creative energy) wrapped three and a half times around a smoky-grey lingam (the unrealised male creative energy), together representing the totality of Creation in a state of dormancy. In this context, the serpent and the lingam are synonymous with the Chinese *Yin* and *Yang* respectively, and the female principle is again recognised as primary. Each coil is said to symbolise one of the three *gunas*, or *'operating principles'* of the manifest universe; at the base, *tamas*, or *'inertia'*; in the middle *rajas*, or *'activity'*; and lastly, *sattva*, or *'balance.* The final half-coil at the apex of this triangular region of immeasurable energy, signifies the soul's transcendence and release from these principles.

The primordial, cosmic energy visualised in this way was called *Kundalini* by the Rishis, which in Sanskrit denotes, *'coiled.'* It is seated within the first *chakra*, which is called *Muladhara*: the *'root'* chakra, anterior to the sacral, or sacred, bone. The triangle of Kundalini, pointing upwards, superimposed upon the inverted triangle of the sacrum, forms a hexagon, or six-pointed star, a powerful and ancient mandala signifying the congruous union of the macrocosm (the Universe) and the microcosm (the Self). This union is conjured in the Hermetic phrase: *'as above, so below'*, and further portrayed in the Hermetic symbol, the *caduceus*, the winged staff with two snakes spiralled about it in opposite directions. In keeping with the *Yin-Yang* symbol, in the hexagon, the macrocosm and the microcosm are portrayed as one; each contains the other. Implicit in the symbol is the knowledge that through understanding the Self comes understanding of the All. To the Rishis, the downward triangle symbolised the goddess *Shakti*, the sacred embodiment of femininity, and the upward triangle symbolised *Shiva*, the sacred embodiment of masculinity and consciousness free from the bonds of mortal desires; yet again pointing to the inextricable unity of the universal feminine and masculine principles. In more modern times (the 17th Century), the six-pointed star, created by the combination of two equilateral triangles, has become the sacred symbol of Jewish identity and of Judaism. In this context, it is the symbol of Basic Trust – trust undeterred by the severest trials – trust in God!

The Chakras

The *chakras* (also referred to as lotuses) are the multiple, animating energy centres spread throughout the body, which are confluent with the force fields of the Creation: the power of the universe flows through us. The Sanskrit word *chakra* means a *'wheel'* or *'disk'*; accurate metaphors for the spiralling vortices of energy that constitute these concentrated centres of vital force. There are seven major or core chakras in the subtle body arranged at intervals along the length of the spinal cord and the central nervous system starting at the coccyx and ending at the vertex or crown. The lower five are intimately related to the important nerve plexuses of the body, the upper two to the central nervous system and the cerebral cortex. In the first chakra, the energy is most dense and of lowest frequency, in keeping with the most physical level of the organism and the grosser or lower organs (the skin and its appendages, large intestines, the muscles and bones, etc.) with which it is associated. Within each successive chakra, the ascending energy is ever finer and of higher frequency, until at the seventh or crown chakra (*Sahasrara*) it is as ethereal as pure consciousness. Together, the chakras form an energy pyramid or spiral with the first chakra forming the base and the seventh chakra the pinnacle.

The vital force of the universe, which permeates all aspects of the creation, expresses its various qualities through colour. The colours of the spectrum equate with the ascending loops of the sacred spiral that symbolises the spiritual journey of the soul towards Self-realisation or individuation; metaphorically, a rainbow that ends in a pot of gold. Each of the seven colours, ranging from primordial black, within which all colours are potential, to transcendent white into which all colours merge, embodies the light and dark attributes of the level of soul consciousness to which it is related. These spectral colours are universal, eternal and archetypal and coincide with the energy levels of the seven major chakras.

The first chakra, which is located at the base of the spinal column, in the region of the coccygeal plexus of nerves and the *cauda equina* (the nerve roots and rootlets attached to the end of the spinal cord) and has its peripheral point of activation in the perineum, is associated with red, the colour of the visible spectrum that has the longest wavelength, the lowest frequency and the slowest vibration. The highest chakra at the crown corresponds with the colour violet, which has the shortest wavelength, the highest frequency and the most rapid vibration. Between these poles, the other primary colours of the spectrum are found, each associated with a specific chakra, according to vibratory frequency. Each chakra influences the function of specific body regions, systems and organs and the entire system forms a keyboard for the thoughts, feelings and emotions of the psyche. Thus, chakras, colours, organs, functions, thoughts, emotions and soul evolution are interrelated, and the importance that Dr Letari and my father gave to colour therapy can be better understood. Indeed, knowledge of these relationships is invaluable to any physician who seeks to heal.[1]

As we shall consider later, energy is subject to mind, hence, emotions can impact on energy and influence the function of the chakras. For optimal function, the energy pattern of a chakra should be in perfect equilibrium. Human nature and life's circumstances do not permit this; there is always some degree of aberration. The deviation is usually chronic, associated with long-continued, persistent, habitual thoughts, emotions and tendencies or the insidious effects of miasmatic and chronic disease, but the impact of sudden, severe, and intense emotional upsets, such as shock, fright or bereavement and acute illness can also disturb normal chakra function. In response, a chakra may become excited and overactive or inhibited causing sluggishness or inertia. The former may be termed a too open or vulnerable state of the chakra and the latter a too closed or blocked state. The material body, being subject to these changes in the energy patterns of the chakras, responds accordingly, its functions erring either towards excess or deficiency; if persistent, such disturbed function will lead to physical pathology. The colour remedy corresponding to the specific chakra imbalance given in appropriate potency (high for over-activity and low for under-activity) can prove of great value in modifying chakra imbalance and facilitating the action of the indicated homeopathic remedy.

The Aura

While the physical body is enclosed and limited by its external envelope, the subtle or energy body is not; it radiates beyond the confines of the physical vehicle. This radiance can be seen by psychic mediums gifted with clairvoyance and is known as the psychic aura. The seven colours of the primary chakras are visible in the aura: red, orange and yellow, corresponding to the first three chakras, are visible in the lower half of the aura; green, corresponding to the fourth chakra, in the centre of the aura, radiating from the level of the heart; and blue, indigo and violet, representing chakras five, six and seven, in the upper half of the aura. According to the physical and emotional health of the individual, the auric spectrum will manifest specific changes in shade, intensity and purity, enabling the trained psychic to diagnose both physical and emotional problems. Current emotions evoke corresponding colour changes in the aura. Intense, hateful anger may be seen as crimson-red spikes of intense energy amidst broiling clouds of black. Residual and habitual emotions, until transcended, become permanent features of the auric colour display, each according to the nature of the emotion.

Spirituality and purity of soul brings a brilliant radiance, which like the halo of the saints depicted in religious works of art extends beyond the aura as magnificent rays of gold and white. When called for, my father was able to read the aura of patients who consulted him. This psychic vision was a great aid to diagnosis and the assessment of progress. Sometimes, however, he would become aware of striking features in the aura of complete strangers. On a number of occasions, he drew my attention to someone passing by and commented on their health or psychological state from what he perceived in their aura. While detecting auras is evidence of psychic awareness, it proves of little value if the psychic is unable to read this map of the soul. Without such insight, the psychic is like a person in the street confronted by an MRI scan: unable to interpret what they see. For reasons such as this, Dr Letari and my father stressed the pressing need for psychics to be trained in the science of their art.[2]

Energy channels – the Nadis

From the first chakra, Muladhara, a network of energy channels extends through all parts of the subtle body linking all the primary and secondary points of concentrated energy, which constitute the chakra system. These subtle channels, are called the *nadis* (single: *nadi*: Sanskrit for *'channel'*, *'stream'* or *'flow'*). Their all-encompassing reach can be likened to the circulatory and lymphatic systems of the body. Through these invisible conduits, the universal creative energy, known as *prana* (*'vital force'*) courses and flows, vitalising and sustaining the subtle body, which in turn animates and maintains its physical counterpart in harmonious equilibrium. This life-sustaining energy, comparable to the Chinese concept of *qi*, or *chi*, permeates and links us to one another and to the Cosmos. It is within us and about us; a cohesive and functioning force imbued with Cosmic Intelligence and intent. It achieves its greatest and most complex expression in 'living' forms. The nadi network spreads through the body along specific immaterial channels or meridians, which bear the organ related points used in the practice of acupuncture. In the iris of the eyes, palms of the hands, soles of the feet and the convolutions of the ears, the energy meridians terminate in clearly defined zones or reflex areas, which, when both sides are combined, represent a complete image of the body. The zones correspond to all the systems and organs and can be precisely charted. This permits the iridologist to evaluate the health of a patient through studying the changes in the colour and fibre pattern of the iris caused by ill-health, much as the psychic can analyse the aura; and enables the reflexologist to balance organ function through pressure therapy administered to the appropriate areas of the soles or palms.

From the immense, latent energy of the coiled Kundalini arise three main channels: *Sushumna, Ida* and *Pingala.* Of these, *Sushumna* is of para-mount importance. This is the central nadi extending from the base or root chakra, Muladhara, via the cerebrospinal axis to the crown chakra, *Sahas-rara* ('*thousand-petalled lotus*' i.e. infinity). The central rod of the caduceus of Hermes represents Sushumna. While vivifying prana always flows through this central canal of the subtle body, empowering the function of the higher chakras, with the spiritual progress of the soul or Self, this flow intensifies and finally as the consciousness of the aspirant becomes more spiritually elevated, the serpent-goddess herself stirs, 'awakens', and begins her ascent along this most blessed of the nadis. As she rises to the insistent call of the quickening Self, her energy successively frees, activates and balances the core chakras, bringing the possibility of ever-higher conscious-ness and enlightenment together with psychic powers appropriate to the soul's spiritual attainment.

Ultimately, Kundalini reaches and pervades the crown chakra preparing the way for Self-realisation and God-consciousness, the highest goal of human life. In this state, the realised soul is capable of attaining *Samadhi* during meditation; a state which defies description, but which can be likened to a condition of undifferentiated 'Beingness', in which the soul experiences ineffable bliss and merges with its own Divinity, the Self. Samadhi, God-realisation, and the ability to 'fly' through higher dimen-sions, which these confer, are symbolised by the outstretched wings at the top of the caduceus.

On either side of the Sushumna, the two major nadis, Ida and Pingala, spiral upwards, coiling round the central energy-column like the snakes of the caduceus; a double helix of vital force ascending from the genitalia and terminating in the hemispheres of the brain and the crown chakra, Sahasrara. As they rise and twist, their figure-eight paths cross at the chakras, imparting energy and spin to these whirling discs of vital force. Ida ('*comfort*') originates in the Muladhara, its serpentine course running from the left side of the vulva or left testicle and ending in the right cerebral cortex. The energy of Ida is Yin and lunar. It has feminine attributes and corresponds to the left side of the body (left somatic) and to the right side of the brain (right cerebral); it is introverted, passive and enigmatic, light-blue of colour, cool in temperature and has negative polarity. Pingala ('*tawny*') is its complement; also originating in the Mulad-hara, its serpentine course starts in the right testicle or right side of the vulva and ends in the left cerebral cortex. The energy of Pingala is Yang and solar. It has masculine attributes and corresponds to the right side of the body (right somatic) and the left side of the brain (left cerebral); it is extrovert, active and overt, red in colour, hot in temperature and has positive polarity. The contrasting qualities of Ida and Pingala do not stand in opposition; they are complementary and synergistic: a marriage of opposites. The caduceus symbolises the balance between the two major energies of the cosmos – the feminine and the masculine principles – a harmony that brings spiritual consummation.

Autonomic nervous system

On a lower level, Ida and Pingala correspond to the parasympathetic and sympathetic nervous systems respectively. Their Sanskrit names denote this correspondence. Ida means 'comfort', which in a word encapsulates the slowing, calming and nurturing effect of parasympathetic action, while Pingala, translated as 'tawny', captures an image of something untamed, clawed, fanged and reactive – well suited to the 'flight or fight' nature of sympathetic stimulation. Significantly and archetypally, anatomical diagrams of the autonomic nervous system invariably portray the parasym-pathetic tracts in blue (cool) and the sympathetic in red (hot). Both limbs of the autonomic nervous system are closely related to the function of all the chakras and any disruption of homeostasis brought about by chakra dysfunction will impact on both these systems and elicit a compensatory response.

Sympathetic nervous system

The sympathetic nervous system is markedly masculine and geared for survival in a hostile world, which it achieves through mediating the neuronal and hormonal stress response. In this respect, it is closely related to the root chakra and the adrenal medulla. *Adrenaline* is its chief neuro-transmitter: a substance that primes the body for action. Characteristically, during stress response, sympathetic stimulation suppresses the functions controlled by the parasympathetic nervous system; by putting these on hold, the body's defensive capabilities are enhanced. The sympathetic nervous system may be powerfully stimulated by stress responses generated from memories stored in the emotional brain: the amygdala. This is particularly seen in post-traumatic stress disorder and panic disorder. Cortisol (hydrocortisone) produced by the adrenal cortex is related to these sympathetic masculine responses. It is known as the 'stress hormone' and is an essential part of the 'flight or fight' reaction to threat, but when someone is exposed to continuous stress and levels of this hormone remain high for extended times, deleterious effects result, and are associated with on-going suppression of parasympathetic action; the equivalent of masculine domination of the feminine; a key factor in human suffering and human psychopathology.

Parasympathetic nervous system

The parasympathetic nervous system is essentially feminine in its effects and synergistically in opposition to the action of the sympathetic system; its chief neurotransmitter is *acetylcholine*. The sympathetic 'flight or fight' action is followed by the parasympathetic 'relax and restore' response, or in military terms: after active service and contact with the enemy comes – R and R – 'rest and rehabilitation.' In archetypal terms, the sympathetic nervous system represents the warrior and the parasympathetic the caring mother, sister, or daughter, who wipes his brow, tends his wounds, nourishes and re-energises him, but also the lover who restores his erection after battle and makes love to him, diverting his mind from the struggles of the day. In homeopathic terms, and remedy correspondence, these roles are exemplified in *Ferrum* (iron), the warrior; *Mag-carb* (magnesium carbonate), the mother/daughter; *Calc-carb* (calcium carbonate), the wife, nurse and housekeeper; and *Cuprum* (copper), the lover and female warrior.

Shakti

These are analogies to be considered in depth later, but if we consider for a moment the image of the warrior in the caring embrace of his lover and exalt this to the highest symbolic level, we enter the first chakra Muladhara where life and the spiritual path begin, and there we find the serpent-goddess of Kundalini, *Shakti*, coiled around her divine lover, the warrior-god *Shiva*, whose 'enemy' that must be destroyed in the ascent of the Sushumna is the 'false-self.' They represent the Divinity within us and their path is our path – the path of individuation. Each of us is cast in the role of hero, or heroine; each of us faces and must overcome the seductive ploys and deceits of our self-absorbed lower-self. As we tread the hero's path, we are enfolded and cherished in the enveloping spiral arms of the loving Cosmos. The force and drive of the universe course through the twin nadis Ida and Pingala and are expressed through their hand-servants the parasympathetic and sympathetic nervous systems. At the first step we take towards self-realisation, the sleeping goddess in Muladhara stirs, another step and she awakens, another and she overshadows us: loving, sustaining and inspiring, but also stern and uncompromising. She is the primary force of the manifest creation, who in her uncompromising, adamant, remorse-lessness is known as *Kali*: the "Black Goddess," also embodied in the Black Madonna of medieval Christian myth.

Primacy of the feminine

The primacy of the female principle is implicit in the *Yin-Yang* symbol, in Kundalini and in the hexagon, and is confirmed at the chemico-physical level of life in the autonomic and endocrine systems. The parasympathetic nervous system, the feminine limb of the autonomic nervous system, chiefly uses acetylcholine as its preganglionic and postganglionic neuro-transmitter, whereas the sympathetic nervous system, which is essentially masculine, only uses adrenaline (masculine) at its postganglionic nerve endings and is dependent on acetylcholine (feminine) for the preganglionic transmission of its effects. Similarly, progesterone, a hormone of paramount importance in the female menstrual cycle and pregnancy, is the precursor of both female and male hormones (androgens) – progesterone is the mother hormone, just as acetylcholine is the mother neurotransmitter.

Great Mother Goddess

In keeping with this evidence, it is significant that the primal, distant and aloof sky-gods, honoured and feared by the hunter-gatherers of the Upper Palaeolithic period, 20,000 to 10,000 BCE, were soon lost to myth, and, with the development of a society centred round agriculture, replaced by a Great Mother Goddess, whose power and presence were witnessed in the seasons and the crops. The earth itself became a feminine epiphany of the Divine and was venerated; the harvest was the fruit of her womb and evidence of her maternal, nurturing nature. She was however, also experi-enced as fierce, implacable and remorseless, often painfully evidenced in times of famine and flood. Throughout Europe, archaeological excavations of the Upper Palaeolithic period have consistently brought to light small, voluptuous stone figurines thought to be statuettes of primordial goddesses, indicative of the matriarchal religion which was dominant in those primitive times. Greek mythology relates the story of the dethronement of the first sky-god, *Ouranos* (Uranus). His downfall was violent and utter. The severed symbols of his masculinity were cast into the ocean and from the union of semen and surf was born the exquisite Goddess of Love, Beauty and Sexual Desire: *Aphrodite* (Venus); her wide domain extending to Creativity and Procreation. From the dethronement of the Sky-God, a powerful goddess emerged to whom all the gods and goddesses, now more human and immediate, were vulnerable.

By the end of the Neolithic period (7000 to 3200 BCE in Greece), with the dawning of the Bronze Age, the old, unifying Mother Goddess religions of the agrarian societies were supplanted by the warlike patriarchies of new city states, which paved the way for the religious divisions and discord of Judaism, Christianity and Islam. Greek mythology provides many instances of this shift from matriarchy to patriarchy and its associated disempowerment of the feminine, but the most significant was the myth of Apollo's slaying of the monstrous she-serpent Python at the very edge of the sacred chasm at Delphi, the most hallowed shrine of ancient Hellas. From that moment, Apollo became the chief deity of the Delphic oracle, and it was believed that the incumbent priestess, still known as the Pythia or Pythoness, owed her gift of prophecy to his inspiration. In a trice, the feminine principle was made religiously and secularly subordinate. The effects are still with us today and are often intrinsic to much of the pain and suffering witnessed in the consulting room.

Despite the Great Goddess' dethronement by the patriarchal hierarchy, her spiritual prominence persisted in the soul of the people and her sacraments were observed every five years at Eleusis in Attica during the most sacred and solemn of all religious ceremonies celebrated by the ancient Greeks. Their eminence was such that they were invariably simply referred to as the *mysteries*. The rites celebrated the eternal cycle of the great polarities, death and rebirth, and were steeped in secrecy and superstition. In Western religion, her memory lives on in the cult of the Divine Mother: the Blessed Virgin Mary of Roman Catholicism. In homeopathy, *the restoration of her power is intrinsic to the healing of the soul*!

Ares and Aphrodite

Mythology takes us further into the mystery of the spiral and its marriage of opposites, the fundamental energy of the root chakra and the symbolism of Kundalini. With the emergence of the Bronze Age warrior, whose ascendancy over the earth-revering, Neolithic farmer created and maintained the rift between the masculine and feminine principles, myth sought to reunite these seemingly conflicting energies, but with the characteristic insight of received wisdom did so in a relationship fraught with passion, jealousy, possessiveness and conflict. Aphrodite, the ultimate personification of the feminine, the quintessential image of sensuality, refinement, beauty and creativity, although married to *Hephaistos* (Vulcan), the primordial god of the volcanic earth, became the on-off lover of *Ares* (Mars), the God of War, the ultimate personification of the crude, carnal, aggressive, swashbuckling male. Their union is clandestine and illicit, yet irresistible, punctuated with recurrent ruptures and reconciliations, and spiced with either rage or rapture. They live out the repulsion and attraction of opposites and the criss-crossing of the nadis on a grand mythical stage. Together, Aphrodite and Ares represent the unconscious, basic drives and instincts of Freud's Id, which, acting according to the so-called 'pleasure principle,' always strives to satisfy the instinctual needs while avoiding pain and displeasure. The basic life instincts are *sex* and *survival*; these are embodied in the Goddess of Love and the God of War respectively, and are seated in the Muladhara.

Masculine and feminine energy

Although humans present as either male or female, they are always bisexual, androgynous beings. Yin and Yang are present in both genders, just as Ida and Pingala and the opposing functions of the autonomic nervous system are common to all; both man and woman produce male and female sex hormones. Men possess a relatively predominant Yang and a recessive female-ness, or background-functioning of Yin; and women possess a relatively predominant Yin and a recessive maleness, or background-functioning of Yang. The predominance in both cases is relative and of varying degree; 'there are feminine or Yin-motivated men and masculine or Yang-motivated women.'[3] Therefore, when we consider the abuse of the feminine, the victim can be either male or female. When the brash bully in a boy's school torments and victimises the gentle, introverted classmate who prefers music to rugby, when a man is raped and sodomised, it is still the feminine that is being dominated and abused by the masculine.

The feminine and masculine principles must be considered from a universal perspective, as are *Yin* and *Yang*. They are not terms for personal sex or gender-linked characteristics, even though feminine traits are obviously more predominant in women and masculine traits in men. *'The symbolism of 'masculine' and 'feminine' is archetypal and therefore transpersonal,*[4] and it is also trans-gender.

References

1 Lilley DJ. *Healing The Soul – Volume one*. Glasgow: Saltire Books, 2014. pp341–343.
2 *Ibid.*, pp418–420.
3 Whitmont, Edward, *The Symbolic Quest: Basic Concepts of Analytical Psychology*. Princeton NJ: Princeton University Press, 1991. p178.
4 Neumann, Erich, *The Origins and History of Consciousness*. Bolongen Series XL11. Princeton, N.J: Princeton University Press, 1993. xxii.

27

ANIMA AND ANIMUS

Contrasexual archetypes

Jung analysed the androgynous nature of the human being and defined the archetypal male and female elements, which are common to the unconscious mind of both genders. He named these elements the *anima* and the *animus* and considered them to be powerful, autonomous and independent complexes or energies within the collective unconscious of humanity. Together, they represent the supreme pair of opposites and are indispensable to the survival of the species. In the personal unconscious of the male, the anima is the feminine element, or the inherited, timeless image, or archetype, personifying all the feminine tendencies in a man's psyche; and conversely, in the personal unconscious of the female, the animus is the masculine element, or the inherited, timeless image, or archetype, personifying all the masculine tendencies in a woman's psyche.

They are termed the archetypes of *contrasexuality* and are usually unconscious. According to the American author, Jungian analyst and one-time Episcopalian priest, John A Sanford (1929–2006):

> A man ordinarily identifies with his masculinity and his feminine side (anima) is unconscious to him, while a woman identifies herself consciously with her femininity and her masculine side (animus) is unconscious to her.[1]

While this is true of the majority of men and women, this identification with the personal qualities that are symbolically masculine or feminine may be inadequately achieved resulting in varying degrees of feminisation in the male and of masculinisation in the female. This is found in many homosexuals and lesbians. The contrasexual archetype is then no longer entirely unconscious and in fact may assume such conscious stature that its qualities become a considerable part of the identity and personality of the ego-self, which may further develop its potentialities. Since androgyny is the natural state of the soul, the varying degrees of contrasexual identification that occur amongst individuals of both genders cannot be considered in any sense abnormal or contrary to natural law; a fact that needs to be acknowledged and respected by the religions of the world. Despite the increased inclination to identify with the qualities and tendencies of the opposite sex, homosexuals and lesbians are just as subject to the problems of lack of integration of the archetypal male and female elements as are heterosexuals.

The contrasexual archetypes must not be confused with the masculine and feminine stereotypes created by society, which arbitrarily prescribes and encourages different emotions, behaviour, responsibilities, attitudes, habits, interests and occupations for men and women.

Projection

The anima and the animus being archetypal are universal and part of the pattern of spiralling energy that pervades and animates the creation. They are consequently *numinous*: charged with great psychic energy, which can overwhelm the emotions. Like the intersecting nadis, Ida and Pingala, with which they are intimately associated, these contrasexual archetypal energies are subject to the attraction and repulsion of opposites. This results in what is termed *projection*. Knowledge of the dynamics of projection is of vital importance in understanding much about the motivation of human behaviour, and particularly, the relationship between the sexes. The man who has identified with personal qualities that are archetypally masculine, fails to recognise qualities that are archetypally feminine as part of his own personality and typically projects his recessive, feminine side onto women. Women similarly project their recessive masculine side onto men when they fully identify with their feminine nature and fail to recognise qualities that are archetypally male as part of their personality. In both instances, the contrasexual archetype has not been integrated into the conscious life of the ego-personality, and the man then typically projects his anima onto women, and the woman typically projects her animus onto men.

The psychic image of the contrasexual archetype that is projected is primarily drawn from the *collective unconscious*, which is the timeless repository of all the images and symbols of the universal and eternal feminine and masculine portrayed down the ages in myth, legend, folklore, tales, art and religion. The predisposition for the personal unconscious to access archetypal images, contrasexual or otherwise, from the collective unconscious in this way, is innate, and is manifested both creatively and in dreaming. These images are further conditioned and modified by the peculiarities of our culture and by our personal experience of important members of the opposite sex, particularly paternal or maternal figures.

Anima projection

All projections are either positive or negative. Through positive projection, the recipient of the projected image will be unrealistically glorified and idealised, even to mythical proportions in the mind's eye of the one who is projecting the image, or conversely, through negative projection, the recipient will be unrealistically belittled and disparaged. In both instances, the true nature and qualities of the recipient are obscured by the romanticised or demonised image that is projected onto them. This is particularly so when the anima or animus are involved because of the intense energy of the nadis that powers them. In the throes of projection, reason, prudence and discernment are swept aside by powerful emotions. The projected image is so compelling that the recipient will either become irresistibly attractive or extremely repulsive to the one projecting the image. Infatuation, an impulsive, immediate, intense attraction for either a man or woman about whom little is known, is one of the signs of positive anima or animus projection, as is intense jealousy and compulsive possessiveness.

In the case of the positive anima projection and its associated infatuation, the man 'falls-in-love' with the projected, idealised, feminine image that he has superimposed on the woman of his dreams. She becomes the object of his erotic fantasies and his sexual yearning, and he imagines that if he can have her emotionally and sexually, he will be happy and fulfilled. He thinks he is in-love, but who is this woman that he 'loves?' In the process of projection, he has lost sight of the real person, the seeming object of his interest, and sees her rather as he wants her to be, the living personification of the perfect woman unconsciously visualised in his inner myth. He dresses her in the raiment of his feminine soul and wants her to live-out and fulfil this image for him. In imposing these unrealistic demands, he robs her of her independence, her self-determination and the right to develop her individual personality beyond the constraints of his anima image. However, flattered and valued she may have felt at being the object of his intense focus, she now finds herself *under his domination*: her choice of clothes, hairstyle and makeup, the music she may listen to, the friends she may have, in fact, every aspect of her life dictated to by her prescriptive, constricting partner. If she resists or should stray from his chosen path, she is exposed to his anger, his resentment and his possessiveness, often expressed through silence, surliness, petulant anger or suspicious and jealous behaviour. Sexually, she may become aware that the dynamic of his passion is compulsive, unrelated to their relationship, or her needs. During the act, it seems as if he were detached from her and fantasising about someone else. He, in turn, has a compulsive need to have sex with the woman who bears his feminine, soul image, but will only feel a measure of togetherness with her during that time. This may lead to an insatiable need devoid of true love and tenderness. This is a prescription for much unhappiness and discord, often centred about the sexual life, which inevitable erodes the health of the couple and disrupts their partnership.

Negative anima projection

Often, when a breakup is inevitable, the positive projection of the anima swiftly changes to a negative projection. This is the spiral path, portrayed by the coiled snakes on the caduceus, which prevails before psychic equilibrium and integration are attained. The woman, previously vested with the idealised image of the feminine, abruptly becomes the target of negative anima projection; she is vilified and transformed from an object of idolatry into the symbol of the witch; an object for hate, not love. The man blames the woman for his dark moods instead of taking responsibility for his own selfishness and immaturity. This is so often the way with men. The moods that descend upon him are from the incompletely consummated, and, thus, frustrated longing for his own unconscious femininity – *his true, beloved soul-mate*; the woman he unrealistically chose to fulfil this goddess-image becomes the scapegoat. As much as she was previously adored, she is now abhorred.

The homeopath will recognise in these fundamentally blighted relationships, constantly being played out in every layer of society, the interweaving, opposite, yet complementary, energies of *Lycopodium* (Club Moss) and *Lachesis* (Bushmaster Pit-viper). *Lycopodium*, the right-sided remedy that projects the anima and seeks to dominate the recipient, and, *Lachesis*, the left-sided remedy that inverts the anima projection and converts love into hate

Animus projection

The same positive or negative projections can be made by women and imaged onto men. When the positive, masculine animus image of a woman is projected this way, the man is seen in the inflated guise of an icon, hero, victor, mentor or spiritual guru. He becomes a charismatic being who mesmerises her and represents the other half of her soul, without whom she feels she cannot be psychically or sexually complete. In the less mature, physical prowess, good looks, suave manners and sexual allure will provide the initial attraction, but in the more sophisticated it will be the command of words and mastery of grand ideas and concepts that elicit the projection of the animus. She is captivated and enthralled by him, vests him with superhuman attributes and places him on a lofty pedestal; in doing so, she surrenders her independence, her individuality, her own creative power and often her morality. Certain magnetic personalities, such as Rudolph Valentino, had the power to attract animus projection on a large scale, and, consequently, in death aroused mass hysteria. As John Sanford points-out in his exceptional book on the subject of the anima and animus, *The Invisible Partners'*– Adolph Hitler received widespread animus projection from the women in Nazi Germany, with devastating effect:

> He (Hitler) had an archetypal quality when he spoke, and a fascinating power with words. I once asked a Jewish woman friend of mine, who had escaped from Nazi Germany just in time, how it was that the German women were so ready to send their sons to Hitler to be destroyed in his war machine, and why it was that they did not object. She answered that they were so fascinated by his words they would have done anything he asked.[2]

It is apparent that the projection of the animus is particularly weakening to the one who is projecting it. It engenders a condition of passive dependency in which the soul is literally offered up to someone else's safekeeping (Pulsatilla, Lac caninum). While some recipients of such canine-like devotion and adoration may feel flattered and empowered, and others more unscrupulous may use it as a springboard to seduction, many men will soon find the relationship with the hero-worshipper uncomfortable, embarrassing and cloying; something to extricate oneself from. Jung described the recipient's condition in lurid terms:

> A real animus projection is murderous, because one becomes the place where the animus is buried exactly like the eggs of a wasp in the body of a caterpillar, and when the young hatch out, they begin to eat one from within, which is very obnoxious.[3]

He describes the animus as having been buried, and this is apt, because the psychological function of the animus on a conscious level is lost through projection. The projector has a weakened ability to think rationally and deliberate and is exposed to making superficial, spontaneous, emotion-based responses to life's challenges.

Negative animus projection

As seen in the case of the projected anima, the negative animus projection can follow hot on the heels of the positive. If the woman's interest or advances are rebuffed, the swing can be rapid and total. 'Hell, hath no fury like a woman scorned.' The curve of the spiral swings away into repulsive mode. In a trice, the hero becomes a despicable villain, responsible for her disappointment and humiliation and unworthy of consideration. Or, through a more gradual process of familiarity with the 'knight in shining armour,' she discovers his feet of clay, her fantasy wanes, and with the withdrawal of the animus, her reason is restored. Unfortunately, all too often in animus projection, the transfer of the projector's power to the recipient is so complete that independent thought and critical barriers are erased. An on-going star-struck state develops. Addicted to his charisma, or parasitically dependent on him, the woman can become clay in the hands of an unscrupulous or egotistic recipient. When religious teachings and a common cult are part of the magnetic pull, tragedy can result as witnessed in the case of David Koresh at Waco and the Reverend Jimmy Jones in Guyana, when so many lost their lives blindly following persuasive, false messiahs.

Pulsatilla (Meadow Anemone) is a homeopathic archetype well suited to a woman suffering from the weakening and dependency producing effect of continuous animus projection. In this respect, it is as typical as *Lycopodium* proves to be in the treatment of persistent anima projection.

Mutual projection

When both a man and woman simultaneously project their positive contrasexual images onto each other, a state of mutual fascination and infatuation results, which intensifies the feeling of being in-love twofold; both will be convinced that they have found the perfect relationship. However, the success of the partnership cannot depend on projection; this provides only the in-love aspect; the vital element of real human love, developed from knowing one another, from shared life experiences and from reciprocal respect and caring, and which endures in spite of frailties, idiosyncrasies and life's vagaries, has yet to be attained.

As John Sanford explains so beautifully:

> To be in love with someone we do not know as a person but are attracted to because they reflect back to us the image of the god or goddess in our souls, is

in a sense, to be in love with oneself, not with the other person ... no human being can match the gods and goddesses in all their shimmer and glory.[4]

Some people move from one relationship to another, repeatedly shifting their projection onto different partners in their search for the perfect relationship. As soon as the intense magic of the projection fades and they fall out-of-love, they move on, like a bee seeking nectar, from flower to flower, never tarrying long enough for true love to take root. As will be discussed later (Healing the Soul volume 3), this tendency is characteristic of people strongly influenced by the *tubercular miasm*.

Projection problems

Since most love relationships commence with projection, its function is essentially good and basic to the survival of the species; it brings people together and provides an initial foundation upon which a shared-life can be constructed, but its pitfalls and limitations need to be understood, and, most importantly, the role it plays in creating so many disastrous relationships founded on delusion. Failed relationships, domestic warfare and broken homes are central to much of the misery that contributes to the development of disease in society. Children exposed to the results of misplaced anima and animus projection are often wounded at soul level even when still in the uterus, resulting in many of the behavioural and learning problems that present in paediatric practice. As Dr Letari stressed during the Second World War, the primary causes of conflict must not be sought in the nation, but rather in the home where life begins and where the warping of the soul too often has its origin.

Integration of the contrasexual archetype

We owe a huge debt of gratitude to Carl Gustav Jung for providing us with a symbolic model of the structure of the psyche and defining its various elements. The concept of the anima and the animus is fundamental to understanding the forces at work in the psyche. His postulates, applied through the techniques of analytical psychology, have proved verifiable and are of inestimable value in the practice of homeopathy, providing insight into the dynamics of human behaviour, the emotional patterning of disease and the symbolism of the homeopathic remedy. In the light of the contrasexual symbols, the dominant sidedness (laterality) of remedies becomes highly significant. By linking the science of the chakra energy system, colour symbolism, Freud's and Jung's structural models of the psyche, classical mythology, miasmatic profiling and homeopathic provings to the psychosomatic picture of the patient, a rich tapestry of correspondences and analogies is revealed, which facilitates the unravelling of the patient's personal mystery, the selection of the appropriate remedy and the induction of healing. *Disease is primarily a consequence of imbalance and lack of integration within the psyche.*

The most important balance that must be achieved in the pursuit of health at the deepest level is *the integration of the contrasexual archetype into consciousness* and to surface the underlying, eternal *androgyny* of the soul, essential to its union with Spirit. By only recognising, valuing and developing those symbolic qualities that pertain to our physical sex, we repress and remain insensitive to a vital part of our human potential; by incorporating those symbolic qualities innate to the contrasexual archetype, we are able to release the otherwise repressed feminine in man and the repressed masculine in women, avoid anima/animus possession (see below) and withdraw our projections.

Healing at soul level necessitates the establishment of the positive attributes of the repressed, contrasexual archetype in the psyche of the man or woman.

In the man, the realised (integrated) energy of the anima opens up the man's psyche to feelings, emotions, tenderness, gentleness, relatedness, empathy, commitment, fidelity, friendship, compassion, imagination, fantasy, romance, inspiration, intuition, aesthetic awareness, artistic creativity, and, above all, unconditional love. These qualities portray a cornucopia of blessings, which must bring fulfilment to the individual, happiness and security to his family and benefit his work and society.

In the woman, the realised (integrated) energy of the animus brings strength to the woman's psyche endowing her with confidence, assertiveness, authority, eloquence, initiative, enterprise, organisational skills, decisiveness, independence, ambition, focus, logic and vitality; all attributes of great value to herself, her family and her community.

Internal projection – *'archetypal possession'*

However, just as the projection of the un-integrated, symbolic contrasexual archetype may be outwards, as previously described, it can also be an internal process in which the unrealised anima or animus, while remaining unconscious, is projected into the personality of the man or woman. The personality is then, at times, *'possessed'* by the qualities of the contrasexual archetype, leading to incongruous behaviour, apparent to others, but not perceived by the one possessed.

The man, who has not consciously integrated the feminine archetypal qualities of emotion and relatedness, when taken over by his anima in this way, may manifest behaviour that is melodramatic, overemotional, childish or selfish. *The repressed, rejected or denied feminine, anima energy is pushed into the Shadow and then escapes in a corrupted form* replacing empathy and sensitivity with moodiness, spitefulness, emotional instability and sentimentality; fidelity with possessiveness and jealousy; aesthetic appreciation with sensuality; tenderness with effeminacy; imagination centres round sexual fantasy; love and romance become a series of turbulent relationships or affairs; and the man withdraws from his wife and family.

The woman, who has not consciously integrated the masculine archetypal qualities of independence, logical thought and leadership, when under the sway of her repressed animus, reveals its warped and negative energy: assertiveness becomes aggressiveness; ambition becomes ruthlessness; rational thinking becomes self-opinionated dogmatism; authority becomes dictatorial; independence becomes arrogance; eloquence becomes verbosity and a very officious, censorious, quarrelsome, dissatisfied and self-centred woman emerges who is a trial to all who come in contact with her.

From this it is clear, that when repressed anima or animus energy surface, they do so in an inferior, inefficient mode, rendering the man less able to relate to others in an emotionally balanced way, and the woman less able to express measured judgement and opinion.

Repression of anima or animus

Like all energies in the psyche, the qualities of the anima and animus, collectively called by Jung the Eros and Logos archetypes respectively, demand expression either internally through their incorporation into the soul/ego-self complex, or externally through our relationship with others. Their expression must enhance the quality of our lives. If they are repressed (quite distinct from the inner-projection/possession already described) the unmodified attributes of our gender identification may become exaggerated and caricatured, producing either a strutting, aggressively competitive and ambitious macho-man (repressed anima), or a vacuous, ineffective, dependent and languid type of female (repressed animus). *The man so affected has lost touch with his emotions, and the woman has lost touch with her strength.*

Healing through integration

One of the benefits of an extended life is the gradual emergence of repressed contrasexual characteristics through the natural involution of dominant gender-related traits. In the post midlife marriage, it is not unusual to see a formerly dominant husband assuming more domestic responsibilities, giving more time to relationships and mellowing into greater capacity for empathy and emotional sensitivity, while his previously dependent wife has become more self-assured and practical and has taken over the managing of their affairs and assumed a leadership role in the community. Life itself is a healing experience.

While the theory and methods of analytical psychology can identify and explain problems in the functioning of the psyche and can provide the analysand with remedial therapy, support and counselling, it is constitutional homeopathic treatment that can restore balance to the psyche in the most simple, elegant and effective way. Selected on the basis of the emotional profile and prescribed in an energy form and potency which permits it to act upon the psyche, the correctly chosen homeopathic remedy can overcome the repression which lies at the root of all psychic imbalance and bring about the integration needed to further the individuation of the soul and simultaneously heal the associated physical consequences of psychic distress.

Integration of the anima or animus is a critical part of the *individuation* process, whereby the emotional consequences of life-experiences, the innate aspects of the personality, and the components of the unfolding psyche, develop positively and creatively, and merge, or integrate, over time into a balanced and advanced being.

An overview of the Anima and Animus (adapted from and added to: *On Jung* by Anthony Stevens).[5]

- They are the contrasexual complexes within all of us.
- The female complex or principle in man is the Anima.
- The male complex or principle in woman is the Animus.
- They possess the power and influence of autonomous complexes or archetypes.
- The Anima is the inherited, timeless image, imprinting, or archetype of the woman in man.
- The Animus is the inherited, timeless image, imprinting, or archetype of the man in woman.
- They are unconscious and are unconsciously projected upon the person of the beloved.

- They are the prime reason for passionate attraction or aversion.
- Together the Anima and the Animus represent a supreme pair of opposites indispensable to the survival of the species.
- Imbalance between these opposites constitutes disease.
- The integration of these opposites is the goal of individuation.

* * * * *

Copper and Iron – the feminine and the masculine metals

The goddess and the god that represent the consciousness of the root chakra, Muladhara – which is at the instinctual animal level of sex and survival and is the primal seat of Ida and Pingala, and the anima and the animus – are Aphrodite, the Goddess of Love, and Ares, the God of War.

The ancients and the alchemists understood that just as the physical body is only a symbol and vehicle of the eternal, animating soul, so, behind all forms moves a higher reality: dynamic, timeless and essential, which informs matter and imbues it with its unique energy and nature. Seeking physical symbols for these powerful and fundamental divine archetypes, they recognised in the radiant beauty and malleable softness of burnished copper the nature and attributes of golden Aphrodite, the most exquisite of all the goddesses, and likewise in iron, the metal of conflict and conquest, they identified the belligerent, aggressive, extrovert nature of Ares, who thirsted for bloodshed and the tumult of battle. Astrologically, these correspondences were extended to the closest heavenly bodies. The beauty of Aphrodite was seen reflected in the splendour of the planet Venus, and the nature of the warlike Ares in the red planet, Mars.

Pursuing the intuition of the alchemists and marrying their conviction to the image given us by the Rishis, which depicts the dormant, fundamental power, Kundalini, as the goddess Shakti coiled serpent-like round the lingam of the god Shiva, we find a confirmatory and very simple, physical symbolic representation of the divine interplay between the feminine and masculine Cosmic energies: the electromechanical solenoid. In this device, a tightly packed copper helix (Shakti/Aphrodite) is wound round an iron armature or core (Shiva/Ares). When an electric current is passed through the copper wire an electromagnetic field is created. The copper coil is shaped so that the iron armature can move back and forth within it, altering the coils inductance and thereby becoming an electromagnet, providing motive force or kinetic energy. The feminine symbol is once more seen as primary; it is the flow of electricity in the copper solenoid, which produces magnetic poles on the masculine, iron armature and induces it to move.

Together, the encompassing feminine spiral solenoid and the masculine phallic armature provide a humble metaphor for a sacred image of the androgynous Divinity within us. The current that awakens the sleeping goddess is the soul's focused and committed desire to walk the path of individuation and spiritual realisation. An energy field is created, and its motive force causes Kundalini to ascend. The rising of the goddess power (female) lifts the focus of consciousness (male) and weakens the power of the ego-self over the soul. The projection and repression of the contrasexual archetypes is reduced; their energies become more integrated and balanced; awareness of synchronicity and Cosmic cues awakens; and dialogue between the unconscious and the conscious, through enlightening dreams and intuitive insight, increases. Thus, the reality of the soul begins to change and unfold!

Within the physical body there is another important symbol, which confirms ancient wisdom: the *corpus luteum* (Latin: yellow body). After the release of an ovum from an ovarian follicle, the empty follicle, which secretes progesterone, the mother hormone, first forms the *corpus haemorrhagicum* (Latin: bloody body), a name that refers to the visible collection of blood left in the follicle after its rupture. From this develops the corpus luteum, a temporary endocrine organ essential for the continuing high levels of progesterone necessary to maintain pregnancy should fertilisation take place. Although it is called the yellow body, it is far more orange than yellow in appearance due to concentrating *carotenoids* from the diet. Enclosed within it remain dark red vestiges of congealed blood, residual from the corpus haemorrhagicum.

Why carotenoids should be concentrated in the corpus luteum remains uncertain. They are pigments occurring in the chloroplasts and chromoplasts of plants and some other photosynthetic organisms like algae, some bacteria and some fungi. A well-known carotenoid is *carotene*, which gives carrots their bright-orange colour. Although the reason for their presence in the corpus luteum has not been explained, we can be sure that it is not by coincidence, or without purpose. What is important to us in unravelling the myth of the corpus luteum is the fact that these unsaturated hydrocarbons are associated with photosynthesis, a process by which solar light energy, water and carbon dioxide are catalysed by the respiratory pigment of plants, *chlorophyll*, to produce the fuel and oxygen essential for the survival of all advanced organisms.

As with all forms projected into the physical world, the corpus luteum presents through its appearance and its functions an epiphany of creative forces otherwise invisible to us. It is not an inconsiderable metaphor for it achieves dimensions quite disproportionate to the size of the ovary from which it develops. In the centre of the corpus luteum, and even more so in its precursor, the corpus haemorrhagicum, we find the deep red of blood – red from the haemoglobin that colours it. Haemoglobin is the respiratory pigment of vertebrates and central to its molecule is the element iron: the element of war, of Ares, and of the red energy pattern of the first chakra, Muladhara, and its basic instincts, the passions of aggression and sex. Iron is also the Yang element, which symbolises the lingam of Shiva. Around this red core, like the coils of Shakti and the copper of the solenoid, lies the quite vivid orange of the corpus luteum: the colour of the second chakra, *Svadhisthana* ("sweetness"). Orange is recognised as feminine-red and Yin, and it is furthermore, the colour of copper, the metal of Aphrodite, who is not only the goddess of the procreative sex of the first chakra, essential to the survival of the species, but also the Goddess of Love in the deeper sense of attraction, desire, sensuality, pleasure and relationship, which pertain to the second chakra. Yet again, the symbolic union of the female and male principles confronts us, now depicted in the organ that produces and sustains the embryo in the uterus.

While the symbolic element of the first chakra is *earth*, the very foundation of the energy spiral or pyramid of life, the element that symbolises the second chakra is *water*, which represents the ebb and flow of our emotions, both conscious and unconscious. The consciousness in rising from a first chakra focus to that of the second chakra evolves from preoccupation with survival, tribe and territory, which is characteristically male, and centres on relationship, receptivity, feelings, emotions and nurturing, which are clearly feminine qualities.

Just as masculine iron, *Ferrum*, epitomises the action of Muladhara, so feminine copper, *Cuprum*, encompasses that of Svadhisthana. Next to silver, copper is the most '*watery*' or fluid of all metals and manifests this quality in its marked ability to conduct electricity and heat, which can be equated with emotional flow, the qualities of responsiveness, receptivity, rapport and sensitivity. However, copper's primordial association with the watery domain and its denizens is most clearly confirmed in its central position as the core atom of *haemocyanin*, the respiratory pigment of the ocean's invertebrates, the molluscs and crustaceans, where it fulfils the same function as iron in haemoglobin, supplying oxygen to the tissues. Even the most advanced cephalopods, the cuttlefish and the octopus, remain dependent on copper, not iron, to sustain their physiology. When the severed genitals of Ouranos impregnated the sea, it was the goddess who rose all-powerful from the waves and made the ocean her own; and copper is her metal.

Both the ovaries and the testes develop embryonically within the sphere and influence of the second chakra, but whereas the ovaries remain second chakra organs, the testes descend into the realm of the first chakra as they leave the pelvic cavity, and the influence of the second chakra is weakened. This explains the usually greater need for bonding and relationship before sexual commitment that exists in women, whereas in the majority of men, especially those who have failed to integrate their contrasexual qualities, the force of the libido reigns supreme.

The carotenoids that colour the corpus luteum orange are associated with photosynthesis, which depends on chlorophyll. Chlorophyll is the respiratory pigment of plants, just as haemocyanin is of invertebrates and haemoglobin of vertebrates. The core atom of chlorophyll is *magnesium*, as copper is of haemocyanin and iron of haemoglobin, each set in a porphyrin frame. There is therefore an evolutionary progression in the respiratory pigments from magnesium to copper and from copper to iron. Yet again, the feminine is revealed as fundamental and primary.

Magnesium, the 'doula of the Universe' is a pivotal archetype, hence, a pivotal remedy! Without magnesium there would be no chlorophyll, no oxygen-rich atmosphere, no protective ozone layer and nature would not be green. Magnesium shares in the metaphorical nature of the colour green, just as copper is related to orange and iron to red. The symbolic essence of green is peace, harmony, renewal, abundance, trust, joy, love and balance. In all cultures, it is the colour of Mother Nature and of womanhood; it is universally associated with plant-life and is symbolic of planet Earth, the only green planet. Magnesium is the mother enzyme central to the homeostasis of all life forms; it is the essential activator or catalyst of the enzymatic reactions that maintain function and life. In its role of catalyst, the archetype initiates, presides-over and conducts reactions, yet remains detached: a characteristic of those who, whilst giving advice and support, maintain an impersonal, objective and unprejudiced stance; those who can mediate and arbitrate without partiality, bringing justice, reconciliation and peace through a Solomon-like wisdom. Without magnesium there can be no harmony, no balance, no homeostasis; she is the great mediator. She is the archetype of the Great Mother Goddess herself, *Demeter* (Ceres), Goddess of the Harvest, who together with her daughter *Persephone*, Goddess of the Underworld, was the central divinity of the Eleusinian Mysteries.

Magnesium, more than any other element, displays the supporting, nurturing and protective, yet objective and uncompromising love of the wise mother. No mother can be wiser and more caring, yet more forbidding, stern and relentless than Mother Nature.

The supreme homeostasis of life is the mediation and balancing of the energies of Ida and Pingala and bringing the anima and the animus together in harmony. Where the evidence of such union is revealed, where the embrace of Shakti (orange) and Shiva (red) finds fruition in the persistence of the corpus luteum, the Great Mother's blessing and grace is represented by the presence of her handmaidens clad in ochre (the carotenoids). She herself wears the mantle of nature's green and the centre of her power is the fourth, or heart chakra, *Anahata*, the chakra of love!

References

1   Sanford JA. *The Invisible Partners: How the Male and Female in Each of Us Affects Our Relationships*. New York NY: Paulist Press, 1980. pp12–13.
2   *Ibid.*, pp15–16.
3   Jung CG, The Vision Seminars, Part Two. Zürich: Spring Publication, 1976. p493.
4   Sanford JA. *The Invisible Partners: How the Male and Female in Each of Us Affects Our Relationships*. New York NY: Paulist Press, 1980. p19.
5   Stevens A. *On Jung*. London: Penguin Books Ltd, 1999. p46.

28

THE PERSONA

The creation of the ego-structure, as a compensation for the inherent lack of basic trust of the soul, leads to the elaboration of two components of the psyche that are of particular importance to the homeopath: the *persona* and the *Shadow*. These are aspects of the patient that the physician will have to contend with throughout the process of healing the soul, for success requires transforming the persona into an authentic semblance of the soul/ego-self complex and bringing the contents of the Shadow from the dark recesses of the unconscious into consciousness. Both tasks are essential for the spiritual progress of the soul, and both are fraught with difficulty, because they constitute a direct challenge to the subterfuges of the ego-self and the rectitude of the superego: they remove its prime defences and bring about a stark encounter with reality.

The persona and the Shadow counterbalance one another and are complementary in their psychic effects, both in the creation of a false-self and in its dissolution. Recognising the characteristic features of the persona in a patient and understanding their function provides insight into the repressed and unrealised contents of the patient's Shadow. By the same token, releasing repressed psychic energy from the Shadow loosens the rigid profile of the persona making it susceptible to beneficial change.

The Persona

The word derives from the Latin word for the mask worn by actors engaged in solemn ritual plays in classical times. Hence, persona refers to the social face, mask or semblance that a person dons when interacting with the outside world. It is designed to impress and influence others, ease social exchange, facilitate relationships and conceal the true nature of the one behind the persona. It hides the mark of Cain![i]

---

i This curse was the result of Cain murdering his brother Abel and lying about the murder to God. (*See Chapter 22.*)

It is also an outer display of identity, often strongly stereotyped by gender, vocation, status, social norms, culture, ideology and stage of life. The persona may be supported by various props, which add to its identity and apparent substance. Most of these are to do with the external appearance and general presentation e.g. adornments, clothes, uniforms, hairstyle, beard, moustache, perfumes, make-up, facial expressions, posture, gestures, mannerisms, diction, vocabulary, language. The tools of the actor are the trappings of the versatile persona. To these may be added all that modern medicine and surgery can do to enhance and change appearance e.g. cosmetic surgery and botox injections. The ego-self that is over-concerned with the good opinion of others, can spend a lifetime devoted to these wrappings and ribbons of the psyche. The persona, pertaining as it does to the outer dressing of the ego-self, is archetypally, symbolically and miasmatically equated with the skin, the external envelope of the body.

Though the persona is based on the rigidity of a deeply rooted ego-personality and may present in a correspondingly fixed and predictable form, the ego-self may possess a chameleon-like skill in adopting various guises suited to circumstances and its objectives. At any one time, it is possible for more than one persona to be combined. The persona required in a particular situation is often dictated by social criteria, hence, an established persona may be masked by secondary personas donned for expediency, conformity and success. Over a lifetime, an individual will wear many personas, but most often these cloak a core personality, which remains constant and familiar to those who are close to them.

The persona is the inevitable, external representation of an underlying archetype. Archetypal patterning produces it, but it is not an archetype. When emotionally distressed, one may inwardly address the archetypes of the psyche, the anima and animus, for insight into images received via dreams or through inner vision, but as Jung remarked, it would be absurd to hold discourse with the persona, which he recognised as merely "a psychological means of relationship."[1]

Persona identification

The persona is not inherently pathological but can assume disease eliciting proportions if a very weak ego-self identifies too closely with it. In contrast, a strong ego-self relates to the outside world through a realistic and flexible persona. When a person is 'all persona', the entire being is orientated towards external things and awareness is confined to the social role that is being played, be it doctor, lawyer, artisan or labourer, or the gender role of mother or father. 'An unreflecting state of mind in which they ... have little or no concept of themselves as beings distinct from what society expects of them.'[2] They are conformists, excessively concerned about what other people think of them. Such an ego-self is blind to internal impressions and promptings and fails to respond to them. This is a form of dissociation and denial.

The ego-self that has identified with its own mask is hidden from itself. It is not conscious of having a persona since the persona has become its very identity. To the soul, the ego-self is now doubly masked, split off and beyond reach. Similarly, the therapist finds the subject unresponsive to counselling. No matter how persuasive, advice seems to go in one ear and out the other; it fails to take root. The ego-self has become what Edward Whitmont terms a '*persona-identified pseudo-ego*' cast in the mould of a social stereotype determined by collective standards, which may be good, bad or indifferent. The individuality that would give to the particular role a personal colour, initiative and direction is barely present or absent. The person is a clone of their occupation, institution or society. This stereotyped condition is reflected in the Kali (potassium) archetypes, especially Kali-carb (potassium carbonate). Potassium is an intracellular electrolyte essential for cell physiology and nerve conduction. The amount of potassium needed for optimal function has very narrow parameters and deviation to either side of the strictly imposed normal values results in serious dysfunction. Too much or too little intracellular potassium can impact on the heart and endanger life. Potassium may not err; it has no latitude for 'individuality'; the 'collective' dictates to it; it must conform, or the heart suffers! The heart along with the arterial system and blood is symbolic of the ego-self and its emotional tides, confirming the close relationship between the potassium archetype with its cardiac affinity and the society-cloned, ultra-conservative pseudo-ego.

Without nourishment from the unconscious from which it has split, the personality of the pseudo-ego is rigidly set, and, hence, psychologically fragile and brittle (Thuja). The lack of synergy between the pseudo-ego and the Id-powered unconscious causes the latter to erupt occasionally into consciousness in an unmanageable way bringing the energy of the repressed individuality to the surface and temporarily fracturing the petrified state of the personality. This experience is frightening because it endangers conformity and threatens the pseudo-identity. But, being Id generated the experience is healing. The person in this state needs the impact of individual feeling, which will move them towards a sense of their own special identity.[3] The conflict is between conforming to the collective or establishing the uniqueness of their individuality.

When the adaptation to reality is insufficiently individual and almost wholly collective, the result may be an inflation of the ego-self. Since identity is now totally vested in the social role and the social order, when success and prominence result, the ego-self feels empowered and superior. This arrogance freezes psychological and moral growth (Platina). They owe their soul to the ideology of the system they represent. Protected by conformity to prescribed values, they abrogate their personal morality and responsibility and without compunction or conscience perpetrate acts dictated by a higher authority: the voice of the elected collective. In Nazi Germany this had disastrous consequences.

Non-conformist persona

At the other extreme are those who fail to develop an adequate collective persona and compensate for this by going against the stream. Such individuals do not wish to conform and tend to tilt against established norms. They reject the collective and wish to flagrantly display their individuality, but often in irresponsible or injudicious ways that clash with order and considered opinion. They are rebellious, provocative and over-defensive, lack good manners and civility and have no concern for propriety of language or dress. Some may take up a cause and become activists. These reactionaries resemble the anal-expulsive Sulphur and the militant Causticum archetypes.

Non-persona

When the ego-self is extremely weak, the sense of identity remains poor or fails to develop. As a result, the persona is colourless, lacking personality and projection, and a very grey, introspective, timid, hesitant, over-diffident individual emerges. There is a paucity of facial expression, the countenance is largely inscrutable, eye contact is avoided, and the voice is inaudible, indistinct or toneless; physical gestures are minimal or awkward and self-conscious. There is a lack of presence and the insipid, inconspicuous image portrayed is really a *non-persona*. This degree of blandness indicates huge repression and the presence of a dense, dark, Shadow aspect, charged with pent-up Id energy.

Alumina: an archetype without identity

Such a *'non-being'* must be compared with the fundamental archetype Alumina, which holds the energy pattern of pure clay (aluminium oxide), an ancient symbol for the crucible into which the soul incarnates: an anonymous receptacle that must be 'fired' by the soul/ego complex to become a distinct individual. In the Alumina archetype, this function is repressed. With the soul in abeyance and the weak ego-self failing to assume office, the archetype is prey to persuasion by others.

To describe someone as being 'like clay in one's hands', pictures perfectly the insubstantial, unformed, impressionable nature of the clay persona. Lacking a sense of identity, vision and focus, the self-effacing, irresolute Alumina is easily influenced by the opinion and behaviour of others and the imprinting persists.

Clay can be moulded and manipulated into any shape when moist and yielding – when fired, it dries and hardens into a rigid, but brittle form. In this, we must compare the Silicea, glass archetype, which is closely related to Alumina; the earth's crust or 'skin' being largely made up of quartz and clay. In contrast to Alumina, Silicea, despite its yielding nature when young and its gentle, unassuming persona, possesses an intrinsic strength and inner conviction that is quite foreign to Alumina, and only the dark Silicea is threatened by a turbulent, brooding Shadow (Isaac Newton). This distinction between the two archetypes can be visually discerned by comparing the clarity and sharply-delineated lines of a quartz crystal with the opaque, formless density of a lump of clay. The former, reaches upwards and outwards, ever adding to its crystalline structure with geometric precision in response to inner patterning (morphic resonance); the latter, remains amorphous and earthbound, unless patterned by external influences. Silicea can act as a prism, it is translucent to light, which it refracts into all the colours of the spectrum, revealing an archetype of great sensitivity, refined consciousness and high aspiration. Aluminium, in contrast, is a metal that reflects 80% of the light that strikes it, making it of value in lighting fixtures; it also reflects heat so effectively that it can be used to protect fire fighters; in addition, it is non-magnetic – all signs of a closed-off, repressed, un-empathetic archetype, lacking presence. Both Silicea and Alumina, being major constituents of the earth's crust are sensitive to the moon's phases. Their symptoms are worse at the full and new moons and both archetypes experience general aggravation from moonlight. This relates both archetypes to the moon, to the feminine principle and to the collective unconscious along with Argentum, Ars-alb, Calc-carb, Cuprum,

Folliculinum, Lac lupinum, Luna, Lycopodium, Phosphorus, Pulsatilla, Raven, Sepia and Sulphur.

Pure aluminium is soft and has little strength. In industry it has to be alloyed with small quantities of other metals (e.g. copper, magnesium, manganese, and zinc) to give it rust-resisting capacity and the strength, hardness and resilience needed for fusing, casting and shaping. This need to acquire strength (identity) from an external source (persons, things) is an archetypal characteristic of the Alumina personality.

The weak sense of self of the Alumina archetype creates the need to model others for identity, drive and direction. This can prove beneficial or detrimental depending on those they model. Outer adornments become substitutes for lack of individuality. Some hide behind sartorial elegance: they dress conservatively and give great attention to their appearance. More commonly a startling assertion of presence is needed to give colour to so pallid a persona. Tattoos, body-piercing, outlandish, gaudy or tattered clothing and weird, colourful, punk hairdos may serve this purpose. Dark glasses add further fortification. It is as if they are wearing armour. Developing a good physique or having cosmetic surgery may provide a synthetic identity and flashy, expensive possessions may serve the same purpose. Others, try to create a macho image by reckless, irresponsible behaviour, antisocial acts and defying authority or social norms. Paradoxically, these shrinking-egos derive confidence from the spotlight effect of the eccentric pseudo-persona they invoke.

The protective screen permits negative Shadow material to surface, adding murky colours to the pseudo-persona's palette and the potential for dire consequences. Violent thoughts and impulses may rise into consciousness and be directed against themselves or others by way of self-mutilation, cruel or homicidal acts. The trigger is often the sight of a sharp instrument such as a knife, razor or screwdriver. When they cut themselves, the welling up of dark, red blood onto the surface temporarily relieves their inner torment. The blood, like the heart, symbolises the ego-self. As it flows, it seems to their unconscious as if their ego-self has at last found expression by venting through the mask of the pseudo-ego; its appearance, though momentary, brings them into reality and gives them a fleeting sense of identity. The associated release of repressed tension, though transient, is so intense it makes the need to inflict self-injury habitual. Because of their destructive impulses, they fear the symbols that provoke them: *fear of knives; fear of sharp pointed things – pins and needles; fear of anything red; fear of losing self-control; fear of their own impulses.* Cannot bear to look at a knife or at blood, because of the thoughts and urges they arouse – *thoughts frightful seeing blood or a knife.*

The lack of a sense of identity, value and personality in the Alumina, clay archetype may result from:

- *No role model as a child*: e.g. a father seldom at home and a mother who is aloof.
- *Lack of love*: as in *Pulsatilla, Nat-mur and Aurum*, lack of love (lack of true, unconditional and consistent love) may lead to a weak identity together with a sense of being unlovable, unimportant and unworthy.
- *Parental contempt*: overbearing, dictatorial, hypercritical and derogatory parents may blight the development of a personal sense of worth, personality and identity – often an aggressive, coarse, intimidating, disparaging, abusive father and a weak, ineffectual or indifferent mother – the mother may also be disparaging, either independently, or echoing the father.
- *Humiliation – intense humiliation; being scorned; ridiculed – humiliation ever-repeated!*
- *Religious discipline*: being brought up in a family with strict religious beliefs in which behaviour is *regimented* by observance and tradition.
- *Psoric environment*: a heavily psoric, poor, lower working-class upbringing – they experience themselves as one of the faceless multitude.
- *Loss of identity*: due to programming (e.g. rigid discipline; army training), imprisonment, various forms of abuse (including rape) and domination – the right to assert an identity is removed – the right to have a choice is denied.
- *Sexual failure*: in the male Alumina, identity and sexuality are closely linked.

Provings of Alumina have disclosed a number of symptoms indicating the archetype's lack of a persona, lack of identity and lack of a sense of self.

- *Confusion of mind: confusion as to his identity:*
  - *As if it were not his own.*
  - *Sensation of duality.*
- *As if in a dream.*
- *Delusions, imaginations:*
  - *Consciousness belongs to another.*
  - *When he sees something, he sees through somebody else's eyes.*
  - *When he says something, somebody else has said it.*
  - *Illusion of hearing: his own voice seems changed.*
  - *Head belongs to another.*
  - *Head separated from the body.*
  - *Mind outside his body.*

- ○ *Being numb.*
- ○ *Everything is unreal.*
- ○ *Sees thieves and robbers.*
- **Dreams of robbers.*

The *dream of robbers* is noted in highest grade and coming from the unconscious it is symbolic of the loss or theft of the ego-self (identity) and its persona.

Outer envelope

The persona is the 'skin' or outer raiment of the ego-self and the psyche, and the skin is the seat of the first disease that beset humanity: *Psora*. In perfect accord with this symbolism and the history of disease, *Alumina, representing the archetype without an identity, is also a major anti-psoric and a leading remedy for diseases of the skin.* The absence of persona is reflected in the condition of the skin. The skin is impoverished, it is terribly dry, lacking oil and fails to sweat even in hot weather. Skin symptoms are worse in winter when more clothing (more persona) is needed and better in summer.

The death of Herakles: the stereotype super-hero

The connection between the development of a persona-identified pseudo-ego, the 'clothing' (persona) of the ego-self and the skin is illustrated in a myth about the death of the great Greek hero and demigod Herakles (Hercules).

Jung remarked that public or professional individuals, who have stereotyped behaviour forced upon them by the world and try to meet these expectations become identical with their persona, and, in doing so, pull on a poisoned shirt that will slowly and surely kill them psychologically. He likened this to the myth of Deianeira, who unwittingly killed her husband Herakles with the poisoned 'tunic of Nessos'.

Deianeira was an exquisitely beautiful young woman and much prized by her husband, Herakles, who had fought and overcome the mighty river god Achelous to win her. Unfortunately, the highly-sexed Herakles found it impossible to remain faithful to her. His amorous liaisons were legion, as were his illegitimate progeny, and marriage, much to Deianeira's grief, did not change his erotic compulsion.

One day, while journeying to Thessaly, the couple came to the river Eunos, which was in full spate. Herakles, always eager for exercise, elected to swim across, but paid the local ferryman, the centaur, Nessos, to carry Deianeira across the river on his small craft. Once in mid-stream, the lecherous creature, in character with most of his kind, attempted to violate his lovely charge. Struggling desperately against his lustful strength, Deianeira managed to thwart him and with loud screams alerted Herakles to her plight. He, still on the bank making ready to swim, swiftly took up his bow and from afar shot Nessos with a poisoned arrow. The penetrating impact of the arrow brought the intensely aroused centaur to orgasm. As he lay bleeding to death, and the poison coursed through his body, in a gesture of hateful vengeance, Nessos told Deianeira that if she should mix his spilt semen with blood from his wound, add olive oil, and secretly anoint her husband's shirt with the mixture, it would act as a powerful love potion and she would never again have to fear his unfaithfulness. Knowing that centaurs were custodians of diabolical arts and thinking his words a last act of contrition, the gullible Deianeira hurriedly collected the unsavoury ingredients in a small jar, sealed it, and unknown to her husband kept it by her. It did not occur to her that the centaur's blood would be tainted with the deadly Hydra's venom that tipped her husband's arrows.

The years passed, they set up home in Trachis and Herakles continued to enjoy the many dalliances that came his way. Deianeira, older now, grew more resigned to his infidelity and the ghastly mixture remained in the jar, but not forgotten. Something stayed her hand, possibly the unwholesome nature of the 'love' potion or some inner premonition of disaster. The parade of young lovelies did not threaten her position, she was the great hero's wife, and her husband's potency was such that her own diminished desires were not neglected. And, so it might have continued, had Herakles, away on a campaign of conquest, not taken captive the princess Iole, daughter of King Eurytos, whose fatal beauty had driven him to slay her father, her entire family and destroy their city, Oechalia. Although a prisoner, the princess bravely rejected the advances of her father's murderer. Her stubborn resistance, keened Herakles's desire to a point of obsession, and with no thought for Deianeira, he resolved to install her in his palace at Trachis.

On his voyage home, he stopped off at the Cape Kenaion headland to make a thanksgiving sacrifice to his father Zeus for the capture of Oechalia. This was a very solemn ritual and required the correct vestments. With this in mind, he had earlier sent his herald, Lichas, to Trachis to fetch the necessary ceremonial robes. Foolishly, while about this task, the loose-tongued, dim-witted herald told Deianeira that his master was bringing home a girl of great beauty to live at the palace, and that, by all accounts, he was smitten with her. Deianeira was distraught at the unwelcome news for she knew she could not hope to compete with a younger woman under the same roof. Only the dread potion seemed to stand between her and utter rejection. Closing her mind to any misgivings, with trembling hands and pounding heart, Deianeira rubbed the loathsome oil into the material of Herakles's tunic before giving the vestments to Lichas.

No sooner had Herakles arrived at Kenaion, than he set about conducting the sacrifices. Once the fires were prepared, he pulled on his tunic and then his ceremonial robes and took up the sacrificial knife. As he approached the altar to make the initial offering, the heat of the flames melted the oil in the tunic and activated the Hydra's poison in Nessos's blood. A sudden, intense burning of his skin brought him to a halt and caused him to cry out in pain, but this was nothing compared to the unendurable agony that immediately followed as the poison oozed over his body and began to eat into his flesh. Bellowing in anguish and rage, he overturned the altars, uprooted trees and then in the throes of his extremity, believing that Lichas was to blame for his sufferings, he seized him, swung him about his head three times and hurled him over the cliff into the sea that seethed below. Mad with pain, he threw off his robes and tried to rip off the tunic, but it had become part of him, fused to his skin, and as he frantically tore at the fabric, he ripped strips of flesh away with it, laying bare the bones. Writhing and screaming in agony as the virulent poison corroded his body, Herakles was carried to his ship and conveyed back to Trachis. On hearing the news of her husband's torment, overcome with grief and guilt, Deianeira hanged herself.

Knowing that only death would bring him relief, Herakles ordered a funeral pyre to be erected and had himself laid upon it. He then commanded those attending him to set it alight, but no one dared obey. Finally, a passing Aeolian shepherd, Poias by name, taking pity on him, ordered his son Philoktetes to light the pyre. Out of gratitude, Herakles ordered his bow, quiver and arrows to be given to the youth; weapons he would use to good account many years later at the siege of Troy, for it was an arrow from the bow of Philoktetes that would kill Paris, the Trojan prince whose abduction of Helen of Sparta had caused the war. Before the flames could reach Herakles's tortured body, lightning bolts shot down from the black and brooding sky above and reduced the pyre to a smouldering heap of ashes. Zeus, the sky god, had claimed his favourite son and raised him to Olympus.

The study of the psyche takes us yet again into the wonderland of myth and dream. Herakles was the greatest hero of classical mythology: a stereotyped, masculine figure characterised by extraordinary strength, fearlessness, practical ingenuity and astounding sexual prowess. His nature was intensely passionate and emotional. His image is recreated in the modern action-men of fiction and film. His death is less well known, and, as with Oedipus, a tale worth telling to give emphasis to the insights it contains. The ancients were intuitively keened to the peculiarities of human nature. They wove this knowledge and wisdom into the fabric of their fables and legends, producing works of human psychology that have inspired artists, sculptors, composers, authors and students of the mind ever since they were first told.

The myth describing the death of the foremost hero of the ancient world must contain symbolic wisdom. Carl Jung recognised this and related the myth to a psychic state in which identity and persona are fused as one, as was the skin and tunic of Herakles: producing the persona-identified pseudo-ego of Whitmont. The frightful image of Herakles attempting to tear the deadly tunic from his back, graphically portrays the jeopardy of the soul trapped in the armour of a persona grafted to the ego-self. It is a pathological 'stuck' state of mind, symbolised in the myth by destruction of the tissues, even to the bone, indicating the underlying syphilitic miasm that has built up on the foundation of *Psora*. This psychic encumbrance may conjure dreams of being unable to divest oneself of garments, wearing tight, restrictive or heavy clothing (Lachesis), being overdressed or clad in gaudy, conspicuous attire (Lycosa); or the dreams may focus on the skin itself, which is experienced as being tight, thick, hard, rough or coarse (Sulphur). At the other extreme, failure or refusal to incorporate the collective image held in the conformist persona may be expressed in dreams of being naked in public – 'discovering suddenly while walking in the street that one has on a transparent gown; of appearing in filthy rags at a reception; of being an oyster without a shell or a flabby mass of jelly.[3]

The persona and the skin

Knowing of the prime role the psyche plays in disease causation, it is to be expected that problems seated in the society-persona-ego axis are often reflected in conditions of the skin. When the persona is fused to the identity of the ego-self, there is no distinction between the individual 'skin' (ego-self) and the collective 'clothes' (persona). It is as if the skin cannot breathe and an actual skin disease may coincide with this state.[3] Eczema or urticaria will often be its expression. Deepening of the 'stuck' condition may lead to auto-immune conditions (*sycosis*) of the skin such as scleroderma and psoriasis. Miasmatic progress to a syphilitic level will lead to destructive ulcerative lesions extending even to the bone (as with Herakles).

The opposite state, a weak persona, will be similarly mirrored on the skin, but in the form of some infectious state be it parasitic (e.g. scabies), fungal (e.g. ringworm), or bacterial (e.g. impetigo). The lack of emotional resistance to the stressors of life becomes lack of skin resistance to infection.

Collectivity and individuality are seen to be a pair of polar opposites. Whereas collectivity pertains to the persona and its interaction with society, individuality relates to the Shadow and the repressed qualities of the psyche. There is an oppositional and compensatory relationship between the persona and the Shadow. *The brighter the persona, the darker the Shadow.*[3] Being over-focused on the persona means denial of the Shadow. The more the identity is seated in the persona, its role in society, external appearance and attractiveness to others, the more the individuality, the genuine inner being, is neglected and repressed. In consequence, the Shadow becomes darker and more negative.

By bringing the individuality and the persona together in a mutualism that adapts to both the needs of the psyche and the requirements of social engagement, in a wholesome, unselfish and authentic manner, healing of the soul is promoted.

Attributes of the persona

Adding to material gleaned and adapted from Anthony Steven's, *On Jung*[4], the following attributes can be given to the persona.

- The Persona is not an Archetype.
- The Persona is a compensatory creation of the ego-self.
- We adapt to society through the Persona.
- The Persona is part of the Personality.
- It is not the Individuality.
- It is a mask [affectation, semblance].
- It is a functional complex.
- It is used for purposes of adaptation.
- It is used for reasons of convenience, strategy, expedience and compromise.
- It represents the role we play; the face we don when relating to others.
- The Persona oils the wheels of social intercourse.
- Social success depends on the quality and efficiency of the Persona.
- To be efficient it needs to adapt flexibly.
- A supple Persona can be a vehicle for deception and duplicity.
- The better the Persona reflects the Ego-qualities behind it:
  - The better adjusted the Personality.

- ○ The more authentic the Personality.
- ○ The more confident the Ego-self.
- A personality that is 'all Persona' has excessive concern for what other people think.
- The Persona is packaged to please.
- Traits thought to be desirable are built into it.
- It is the tool of the actor, the politician and the lawyer.

References

1 Jung CJ. Two Essays on Analytical Psychology. *The Collected Works of CG Jung* Vol 7: London: Routledge & Keegan Paul, 1953. p199.
2 Dawson T, in Young-Eisendrath and Dawson T ed. *The Cambridge Companion to Jung.* Cambridge. 1977. p267.
3 Whitmont EC. *The Symbolic Quest – Basic Concepts of Analytical Psychology.* Princeton NJ: Princeton University Press, 1991. pp157–159.
4 Stevens A. *On Jung.* London: Penguin Books Ltd., 1999. p42.

29

THE SHADOW

The Shadow

Within the unconscious of the psyche lies the dark, denied part of ourselves: our personal Shadow, a repository of everything we have no wish to be and a cornucopia of infinite riches: the jewels that constitute what we should be, will be and actually are.

The Shadow is an unconscious aspect of the personality of which the conscious ego-self is unaware and with which it cannot spontaneously identify. Its formation starts early in life as we discern the difference between what we innately feel is 'good' and what we innately feel is 'bad'. This differentiation is complemented by the judgement and values of our caregivers and role models, who in turn have been informed by their culture, religious belief or philosophy of life. From about 6 years of age, at the start of the latency stage of psychosexual development, the super-ego or ego-conscience develops. Though it is mainly unconscious, the super-ego influences conscious thought and decision making. It develops from identification with the 'father' – the masculine principle intuited in a parental or significant authority figure – and from the incorporation of society's norms and values. The union of these influences creates the template for an *'ideal-self'* with which we try to conform. Failure to comply with the standards represented by the ideal-self, produces feelings of guilt, which help to keep us on the straight and narrow road of correct behaviour and make us socially acceptable. To this interplay within the ego-self must be added the conscience of the soul; the sometimes-small voice of the higher-self, which is pure and unconditional in its promptings towards authenticity and sublimation.

From the combination of these influences, a personal moral code emerges and those feelings and qualities that we deem bad, unacceptable, harmful, inferior or primitive are rejected by the ego-self and repressed into the Shadow, which becomes the hidden, negative side of the personality: a part of our being that we deny. The disowning and rejection of the 'bad' is captured in the saying: 'get thee behind me Satan'. What is retained in the ego-self and what is consigned to the Shadow will vary, not only from person to person, but also between families and cultures. Since the defining process begins so early in life, upbringing and conditioning are major influences, dictating whether or not free expression may be given to fear, tears, vulnerability, needs, anger, aggression, sexuality and strong emotions. A child's background may even discourage religious or spiritual aspiration, artistic expression, intellectual development or financial ambition, qualities that are usually regarded as virtues. More consistently, however, it is those traits that are deprecated socially and religiously that are denied and repressed into the unconscious, such as sexual lust, depravity, greed, laziness, selfishness, egotism, prejudice, envy, anger, resentment, hatred, cruelty and revenge. Stripped of their human connotation, i.e. their warped presentation, these traits represent the basic instincts of the Id, sex and aggression. Their repression is in defiance of the uncompromising and persistent Id; an opposition that elicits the psychic conflict intrinsic to the hidden cause of disease. To maintain this morbid psychic-split, the ego-self, consciously and unconsciously, builds opposing traits into the persona. *Hence, the Shadow and the persona stand in counterpoint to one another.*

The chronic miasms and the Shadow

Miasmatic influences play an important role in determining what is expressed and what is repressed culturally, domestically and personally. Miasms, like morphic fields, extend their formative influence over cultures, nations, cities, suburbs, families and individuals.

Psora

The psoric miasm encourages diffidence, respect, modesty, stoicism, frugality, temperance, abstinence, industry, conservatism and religious devotion: a list of 'virtues' that necessitates significant and often severe repression within the dynamics of the psyche and imposes a heavy burden of anxiety and guilt. Psoric repression bears all the trappings of ultra-Calvinism. At its core, is the denial and repression of the primitive aspects of the psyche: the immense power of the basic instincts of the Id: *sex and aggression*. To achieve this requires tenacious identification with a *moralistic persona* that embodies, amongst other archetypal forms, the personality traits of the self-righteous puritan; the religious fundamentalist; the naïve, self-sacrificial humanitarian; and the perennial, self-effacing, passive victim. The intensity and rigidity of the persona indicates a proportionate intensity and density of the unrealised Shadow. *It reflects a state of psychic petrification.*

Sycosis

The sycotic miasm, though more insular in its effect, can similarly permeate communities, neighbourhoods and families. Whereas, *Psora* is repressive and impoverished, *Sycosis* is expressive and profligate. The influence of *Sycosis* is insidious and when flagrant is capable of causing a steady degradation of the normal goodness, integrity and moral rectitude of a family. Those who succumb are cold, cunning and calculating. Their ways are devious, underhand, seductive, manipulative and amoral. Self-gratification and selfishness are central to their interactions with one another and society. Alcohol, drugs and sex, play a destructive role in the family dynamics. Children are exposed to all forms of abuse and corrupting influences and brought up to experience deceit, crime, incest, promiscuity, alcohol and recreational drug abuse as the norm. Unless they resist, they too will be inexorably drawn into a similar life and perpetuate it to the downfall of others. It is evident that in a sycotic milieu much that would be exiled into the Shadow of the unconscious in a psoric household, may see the light of day and that those born into such an environment are consciously faced with the innate duality of the human state: the conflict between light and dark. Yet, for all its quick sands, the sycotic state is fluid; the persona wears two faces, not one; and *more of the Shadow is incorporated in the conscious life: a state essential to individuation.*

Syphilis

Syphilis is more circumscribed in its range than *Sycosis,* except in times of anarchy, revolution and war; starkly evidenced in the human rights abuse, ethnic cleansing and war crimes perpetrated by the so-called Islamic State in Iraq and Syria. Here, the dark, menacing stranger of the unconscious has emerged in all *his* destructive hatefulness and the qualities of light have been consigned to the Shadow. In *Syphilis,* it is the feelings and values that are decent and noble, which are repressed; *the Shadow becomes the hidden, positive side of the personality.* The contention between good and bad intrinsic to the duality of sycosis has been subsumed and relegated to a minor dynamic as archetypal evil gains ascendency within the psyche.

Tuberculosis

In the psychological profile of the combined miasms, *Tuberculosis* and *Carcinosis,* a process of sublimation is evident. *Sublimation necessitates the emergence of repressed energy from the Shadow.* In the tubercular miasm, the psoric element in the miasmatic mix has again taken centre stage and the syphilitic element has receded, but remains hugely influential, its passion and fire permitting the Shadow to break through the cold, rigid reserve of

Id = unconscious instincts

the psoric persona, igniting the artistic and creative aspiration of the psyche and firing its drive for freedom and expression. The romantics knew that the price of artistic genius is often melancholia. The tubercular creative spirit is subject to *bipolar swings between manic ecstasy and morbid depression.* During a phase of intense, artistic creativity, inspiration from the Shadow bursts forth charged with the irrepressible libido-vitality of the Id. As the creative tide loses momentum and ebbs away, the miasmatic morass sucks the ego/soul complex once more into the fathomless abyss of the Shadow. Its syphilitic fires quenched, the animated, vivacious, dazzling presentation of the persona is eclipsed and replaced by a psoric visage heavy with despondency and suicidal despair.

Carcinosis

Carcinosis, which is a combination of the psoric, sycotic, syphilitic and tubercular miasms adds to the creative and revolutionary fervour of *Tuberculosis*, a refined aesthetic awareness, a great love of nature and the arts and a deep concern for the welfare of others, expressed through acts of selfless service. But the price of altruism may be malignancy. The aggression and reproductive power of the Id attempts to resolve severe repression and emotional control by establishing a physical lesion potent with aggressive and proliferative energy. By this means, Shadow energy is externalised, and malignant disease reveals its soul-healing power.

The Shadow is dynamic and functional

Shadow

Though rejected, repressed and denied, the contents of the Shadow are dynamically alive and active within the personal unconscious. Emotions, feelings, urges and impulses, that are repressed rather than resolved or sublimated, gain potential energy, augmented by the relentless outflow of the Id. *Shadow contents possesses powerful centrifugal force.* They are obsessional, compulsive and autonomous and are marked by *affect*: the capacity for latent emotions and feelings to break through into consciousness, invade the individuality and temporarily overwhelm the self-contained ego-self. This eruption occurs when events incrementally or abruptly challenge the adaptability of the ego-self. The pose of the persona is ruptured, and Shadow contents burst forth with an intensity that shocks the ego-self and others. The exposed Shadow reveals a psychic wound and the cause and nature of the emotional paroxysm provide invaluable insight regarding the nature of the wound and the associated weakness (inability to adapt) of the ego-self. This holds true when the outburst has been facilitated by alcohol. *When the pose of the persona is breached, and the control of the ego-self weakened by imbibing any substance, the spontaneous surfacing of otherwise unseen traits provides vital information about the content of the Shadow and the pretences of the persona.*

Although repressed and beyond ego-self-awareness, *Shadow qualities and drives remain functional* and capable of impinging on conscious behaviour. *Because they are out of sight, they remain uncensored and unmodified and hold disruptive potential.* Their intrusive presence produces eccentricities and contradictions in behaviour that are clearly visible to others, but largely lost to the one possessing them. Shadow qualities are often in striking contrast to the values, principles and behaviour we hold dear. Acknowledging that within us all lurks an inferior, primitive, unprincipled being, Goethe declared that the longer he lived the more certain he was that there was no act that had ever been perpetrated by mankind of which he too was not capable. It takes a clever person to perceive this truth, a brave one to own it and a wiser one to confront the Shadow that embodies it. By admitting its presence and identifying its traits and idiosyncrasies, it becomes possible to break its compulsive influence.

Jung, writing of the Shadow said:

> Unfortunately, there can be no doubt that man is, on the whole, less good than he imagines himself or wants to be. Everyone carries a Shadow, and the less it is embodied in the individual's conscious life, the blacker and denser it is.[1]

> The Shadow is a moral problem that challenges the whole ego-personality, for no one can become conscious of the Shadow without considerable moral effort. To become conscious of it involves recognising the dark aspects of the personality as present and real. This act is the essential condition for any kind of self-knowledge.[2]

Most telling was his observation:

> Filling the conscious mind with ideal conceptions is a characteristic of Western theosophy, but not the confrontation with the Shadow and the world of darkness. *One does not become enlightened by imagining figures of light, but by making the darkness conscious.*[3]

The struggle between the ego-self and the soul can be measured in the balance existing between the covertness of the persona and the overtness of the Shadow. The more the Shadow is brought into consciousness, the more transparent and authentic the persona becomes: a transition that progressively frees the soul from the domination of the ego-self and facilitates individuation. The more the ego-self identifies with the persona, the less the Shadow is assimilated and the more dense, dark and powerful it becomes. By assimilation, the Shadow imparts power and strength to the psyche. For example, when a depressed person is made conscious of the repressed rage underlying their depression and becomes familiar with its content, the depression lifts and they become invigorated. Conversely, denial, repression and rejection empower the Shadow and deplete the psyche. These dynamics are wholly consistent with Hering's Law of the Direction of Healing!

Shadow possession and enslavement

The Shadow is compulsive, obsessive and autonomous by nature and when it becomes empowered, instead of the conscious personality incorporating the Shadow, a process essential to individuation, the opposite is possible: *the Shadow may possesses and enslave the personality.*

Dr Jekyll and Mr Hyde

This reversal is brilliantly and intuitively portrayed by Robert Louis Stevenson in his novella: *The Strange Case of Dr Jekyll and Mr Hyde*: a story of such impact that the expression Jekyll and Hyde has come to mean an individual bedevilled by a dual personality given to swinging between the extremes of good and evil.

One night in 1885, the plot came to Stevenson in a dream from which his wife urgently wakened him. In its throes, he had cried out in such distress that she thought he was in the grip of a terrifying nightmare. Angry rather than relieved, Stevenson asked: 'Why did you wake me? I was dreaming a fine bogey tale.'[4] He had witnessed the ghastly transformation that he would later portray as that of Jekyll metamorphosing into Hyde. The experience precipitated him into a frantic fever of writing. Within a week, the draft was complete.

The story is remarkable for its insights into the duality of human nature and the psychic turmoil it can induce. Dr Henry Jekyll, a man of good professional and social standing is troubled by the contention of good and evil within him. Stevenson describes him as a 'large, well made, smooth-faced man with something of a slyish cast perhaps, but every mark of capacity and kindness.' The 'slyish cast' betrays the fact that hidden beneath the guise of a kindly gentleman, lurks a less-principled personality, subject to urges unbefitting a man of Jekyll's background. Jekyll admits himself to be 'fond of the respect of the wise and good among my fellow-men,' revealing his need for the approbation, respect and good opinion of his peers. We can be sure that he adopts a charming persona to win these. He later confesses that he assumes a 'more than commonly grave countenance

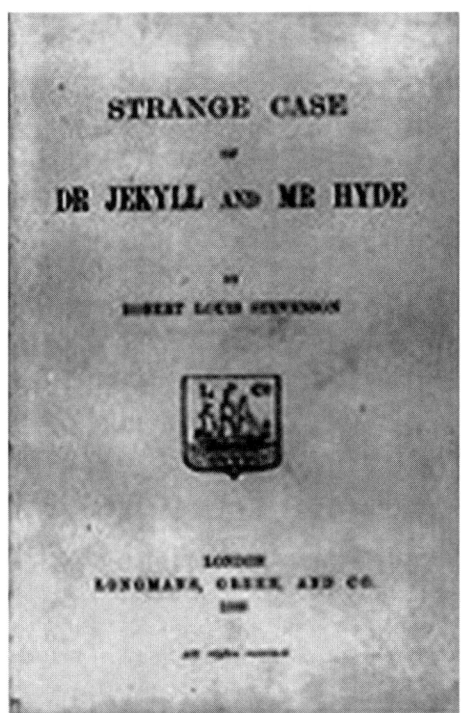

Figure 29.1 *Title page of the first London edition (1886)*
(Wikipedia)

before the public masking 'a certain impatient gaiety of disposition,' which leads him to all manner of pleasures and indulgences, which the Victorian Stevenson leaves to our imagination, but which causes Jekyll to feel 'a morbid sense of shame.' Unable to overcome his secret vices, he resigns himself to a life of 'profound duplicity,' but constantly dreads exposure and rejection by society.

In his laboratory, he devises a potion that will so transform him that he will be unrecognisable – free to revel in depravity without fear of discovery. The being that emerges from his Shadow into the light of consciousness is Edward Hyde: a smaller, younger man filled with devilish vigour – cruel, hateful, cold and pitiless, the very personification of evil. He is in some way misshapen and warped, the mere sight of him sufficient to evoke repugnance and hatred. A moral leper, he is devoid of human feeling, conscience or guilt and committed to a path of debauchery, corruption and violence. His youth and diabolical vitality derive from his being the Shadow personality of Jekyll, suffused with all the repressed energy not lived out in Jekyll's external, everyday life. *To touch the Shadow personality, either by possession or assimilation, is to be charged with new or youthful energy*. His small, deformed appearance points to his origin within the dark, compressed confines of the rejected-self. Hyde is cold and utterly detached. In breaking free from the bonds of ego-repression, the Shadow casts aside the hypocritical veil of the persona, abandons morality to the ego-self and focuses its drive on living-out the forbidden and taboo without restraint.

Jekyll, always conscious of his own intemperance, discovers that he is far more evil than he ever supposed himself to be. Once possessed, he delves beyond the personal Shadow of Jekyll into a deeper, darker realm and touches collective or archetypal evil: an evil that is utterly selfish and devoid of all humanity: an evil of satanic dimensions.

John Sanford, a Jungian analyst, commenting on Jekyll's predicament warns about the dangers of living out the darkest impulses of the Shadow:

> CG Jung once wrote that we become what we do. This helps us to understand . . . the reason for Jekyll's demise. Once he decided to *be* Hyde, even if only for a while, he tends to *become* Hyde. The deliberate decision to do evil leads to our becoming evil. This is why living out the darkest impulses of the Shadow cannot be the answer to the shadow-problem, for we can easily become possessed by or absorbed into evil. . . . This attests to the archetypal nature of evil, for it is one of the qualities of the archetypes that they can possess the ego, which is like being devoured by or made identical with the archetype.[5]

Stevenson details the inexorable possession and devouring of Jekyll by Hyde with masterly skill and a remarkable grasp of morbid psychic processes. Initially, Jekyll is confident that he will be able to transform from Jekyll to Hyde and back again at will, but each change imparts more power to Hyde. Eventually Jekyll can no longer control Hyde, who is able to spontaneously assert his demonic presence, taking over Jekyll involuntarily in his sleep. Horrified by the dreadful implications, Jekyll vows before God that he will never invoke Hyde again and to this end commits himself to religion – a common ploy of the delinquent ego-self – seeking by devotion to fortify himself against the seductive influence of Hyde.

For a while, he keeps Hyde at bay, but that which we resist persists and grows stronger. One night, the urge overwhelms Jekyll, and, a Hyde, primed with repressed energy, is let loose on the city. No sooner has the transformation been achieved than Hyde rushes out with savage, lustful intent and within moments commits a violent and vicious murder. Jekyll is appalled and his determination to stop the transformations becomes more adamant. In an effort to purify himself, he engages in philanthropic endeavours. But he has gone one step too far. While sitting in a park congratulating himself on his recent altruism and how it will redeem him, he looks down and to his horror sees his hands changing into those of Hyde; the first time such a spontaneous metamorphosis has taken place whilst he is awake. With the police hunting Hyde as a murderer; the transformations taking place ever more frequently; and larger and larger doses of the potion being required to reverse them; Jekyll is trapped and faces the reality that he will soon become Hyde permanently. Finally, the last of the restorative potion has been used and lacking a vital ingredient to make more, Jekyll faces the terrifying reality that the final metamorphosis is imminent. Whilst waiting for the monstrous change to occur, Jekyll writes a letter of confession detailing the awful truth. His last words are: 'I bring the life of that unhappy Henry Jekyll to an end.' Rather than face death by execution, Hyde in a final syphilitic act, commits suicide.

Jekyll's attempt to neutralise the threatening presence of Hyde by formalised religion and charitable works are methods common to those caught in a conscious and unconscious struggle with their Shadow-self. Seeking support from an external source that promises redemption to the faithful and paying for it from the purse rather than the heart,. is a poor substitute for addressing the lack of basic trust that produces the struggle. Rarely does such self-serving reverence stem from a true change of morality, which would be the most positive move towards unification of the psyche. As with Jekyll, it is fear rather than love that motivates them: fear of the pain of the internal struggle, fear of the split disintegrating their sanity and fear of spiritual damnation. When habituation has rendered the dark side stronger than the ego-self, lip service to religion serves only as window-dressing; beneath the surface the unresolved desires and impulses persist and gain strength. Duality holds sway. Religion pulls the wool over the eyes of the gullible ego-self making it self-righteous and complacent. As Jekyll experienced in the park: when you believe you have no Shadow, the Shadow has you!

Jekyll failed to accept and honour the tension of opposites within him. To incarnate is to step into duality; hence, duality is essential to the spiritual path of the soul and it is the tension of opposites, as with electricity, which provides the energy and drive needed for transcendence. To refuse the 'pain' of the tension is to refuse to live out life with trust and positivity. It is the masculine aspect of the ego-self that objects to and shies away from the birth pains of the soul, attempts to avoid them, and plunges the psyche into greater misery and travail. The masculine strategises, manoeuvres and compartmentalises – the feminine accepts, embraces and incorporates; the masculine is innate to division and diversification – the feminine is innate to union and wholeness. It is the masculine in Jekyll that devises a potion to escape the tension of opposites. In doing so he polarises the Shadow, identifies with it and causes psychological disaster. Repression of the

Shadow is similarly futile; it is equivalent to waging war with the implacable Id, which will project what is repressed onto others, the world and even God.

The answer must lie in surrender and acceptance not opposition and contention. These are qualities of the soul, not of the ego-self. Only the feminine soul can embrace light and dark, positive and negative, Shadow and personality, anima and animus and bring about synthesis within the psyche. To the ego-self, represented by the logical, pragmatic masculine mind, the union of opposites is irrational – a conclusion that obviates resolution. In truth, it is the soul and the ego-self that represent the real opponents. Trying to solve the pain of opposites through the machinations of the masculine ego-self is doomed to failure for it is the equivalent of setting a thief to catch a thief. Surrender, the watchword of the feminine soul, is active, positive, creative, loving participation in whatever is unfolding in the 'Now.' The 'Now', being true, perfect, wise and loving, is the grace of the Supreme Consciousness charged with the unifying force of the Cosmos. In the state of ego-suspension essential to surrender (the acceptance of opposites), the Divine Grace is able to operate within us, subsuming all opposites and moving us towards Self-realisation – the healing of the soul!

Sanford points out that it is worth noting that in Stevenson's story the feminine figures are few and far between and when they do occur they are seen in an exclusively negative light.[i] Our first sight of Hyde is of him in the act of viciously trampling on a little girl. The women consorting with Hyde were 'wild as harpies.' The maid who opens the door of Jekyll's house to the narrator Utterson on the final night is 'hysterically whimpering.' In the laboratory on that final night, even Hyde himself is described as 'weeping like a woman or a lost soul.' Throughout the book, the feminine principle is depicted as victimised, weak and ineffective, or witchlike. Stevenson consciously or unconsciously touches upon one of the deepest truths for . . .

> . . . when psychological consciousness is refused, as Jekyll had refused it, the feminine part of us, our very souls, weakens and languishes and falls into despair, a tragedy, for it is this very feminine power that can help find a way around what is otherwise an insoluble problem.[5]

Even archetypal evil is never 'pure', unadulterated, absolute evil as embodied in the mythical figure of Satan; it is always relative to good and therefore dependent on its opposite for existence.

> No sooner was Jekyll completely possessed by Hyde than Hyde himself died by suicide. This too is instructive, for it tells us that evil eventually overreaches itself

and brings about its own destruction. Evidently evil cannot live on its own but can exist only when there is something good upon which it can feed.[5]

From a miasmatic perspective, the strange story of Jekyll and Hyde portrays a predictable miasmatic decline from *Sycosis* to *Syphilis*: from profligacy to destruction. At the opening of the story, we find the outwardly respectable Jekyll wrestling with his demons of lust whilst trying to preserve an irreproachable reputation. This is the state of Thuja, the arch-sycotic and analogue of the Tree of Knowledge of Good and Evil; an archetype that wears a false front masking all-manner of deviousness and duplicity. When he turns to religion and philanthropy to curb his urge to wallow in the evils of Hyde, he moves into the world of Anacardium: an archetype that sits with an angel on one shoulder and a devil on the other, each whispering in his ear conflicting instructions of admonishment or seduction. Ever-diminishing internal duality draws him inexorably towards another archetypal form as personality and Shadow merge in a diabolic liaison: Mercurius, the arch-syphilitic – a brutal archetype without empathy, conscience or guilt. Jekyll and evil have become one!

The story demonstrates how archetypes are juxtaposed in the matrix of the collective unconscious and how the resident archetype can change, though never arbitrarily, always in accord with universal patterning.

Stevenson leaves us in no doubt about the dangers of recreational drug abuse, for though Jekyll's 'potion' has no name, it could well be cannabis, ecstasy, LSD, cocaine, methamphetamine or an opiate. It could also be alcohol. The strange story holds particular relevance and a dire warning for the youth of today.

* * * * *

The Cornucopia of the Shadow

In Greek mythology, the realm of souls was known as Hades and the god who ruled this dark domain bore the same name: Hades, God of the Underworld. In psychological terms, Hades, the shadowy dimension, equates not only with the afterlife, but also with the unconscious, both collective and personal *and particularly the Shadow*. Hades, the death-god, is by his very authority and function, grim, uncompromising, pitiless, stern and irrevocable in his decrees, yet just and unbiased. Although he presides over the dark, troubled, turbulent and painful aspects of our emotional lives, he must not be confused with either Satan or Lucifer; he is not the enemy of humanity, nor does he tempt us towards the 'fall'. Significantly, he bears another name, Pluto, which throws a different light on his nature. Though given to him by the Romans, the name is derived from the Greek *Ploutōn*, a later name for Hades, often conflated with *Ploutos*, who was God of Wealth. The conflation is apt and far from accidental, because even a god has a light and a dark side. Hades represented the dark aspect of the infernal godhead: the violent abductor and violator of Kore, who, as Persephone, became Queen of the Underworld. Pluto, his light, positive alter-ego, was venerated as a stern ruler, but also as the loving husband of Persephone, and, like the dragon of old, the guardian of treasures beyond measure, including the boundless riches of the earth – the bountiful crops upon its surface and the incalculable wealth of minerals hidden within it. To distinguish him from the gloomier Hades and denote his function as Lord of Abundance and Riches, Pluto is symbolised in art bearing a cornucopia or *'horn of plenty'* overflowing with fruits, jewels, gold and silver.

In contemplating the central myths of the world, as ever, we are confronted by the wisdom of the ages. The story of Hades/Pluto and Kore/Persephone and her mother Demeter, stands at the heart of the Eleusinian Mysteries, the most hallowed and secret religious rites of ancient Greece and it stands at the heart of esoteric homeopathy. The Mysteries were intended *'to elevate man above the human sphere into the Divine* and to assure his redemption by making him a god and so conferring immortality on him"* (my italics).[6] However worded, this is the very purpose of life and of homeopathic therapy.

Pluto is God of the Shadow and also the God of Wealth! The Shadow is not only the abode of Lucifer and Hyde, but also the repository of spiritual treasures beyond imagination.

Spiritual development necessitates making the unconscious conscious. The contents of the Shadow must be brought up from the depths of Hades and sublimated. Through this unfolding, the soul achieves wholeness and Oneness with the Immortal Divinity that is its Essence: the very object of the Mysteries!

The contents of the unconscious are the fruits and jewels contained in Pluto's cornucopia. Charging all is the Id, the centrifugal, driving force of the psyche, like the ocean's tides and waves, ever working towards throwing out the psychic flotsam and jetsam of life onto the shores of consciousness. It is an energy field bearing the basic instincts and all the fundamental qualities and attributes laid down in the constitution from conception. The Id bears the imprint of all that seeks expression from the collective unconscious; all that is rejected or repressed from the conscious mind by the ego-self (at the injunction of the super-ego); and all that has never reached consciousness: the instinctual drives and the fantasies and urges related to them. The Shadow also contains all the unresolved emotions of the ego-self, dating from pre-natal life to the present: emotions that could not be processed or coped with at the time due to their enormity and which were repressed into the unconscious, often with their related memories. To achieve psychic equilibrium (soul-healing), these emotions, and their attendant memories, need to be brought to consciousness, resolved and dissipated.

Concealed beneath these unconscious elements that form the deepest levels of the personality, the Shadow harbours a hidden wealth compared with which even these jewels pale: the fundamental consciousness of our souls – our divine heritage – our spirituality – our Essence or True Nature. Although Essence is one, it comprises different qualities that we can term Essential Aspects! Amongst these can be numbered the '*Virtues of the Godly*' (see Spirit – Chapter 20 pgs 276–277) and the seven classic virtues: *charity, faith, fortitude, hope, justice, prudence and temperance*. Qualities such as *confidence, courage, strength, reliability, integrity, peace, joy, serenity, caring, nurturing, empathy and wisdom* are all part of this spiritual treasure-trove and are true to our Essence. Although we have access to these qualities, and may, at times, display them according to our disposition and circumstances, due to the interposition of the morally-deficient, self-centred ego-self, their expression is invariably fitful, qualified and conditional. Nonetheless, the archetypal Idea or Form of each virtue exists within us as an unsullied, immutable and eternal principle: *the finest jewels of the Shadow*!

We bring this immaculate, spiritual heritage, this Essence, with us onto the earth plane, embodied in the unblemished innocence of a babe. It would seem that these soul qualities charged with their infinite power and exquisite perfection, should prevail over all negativity and adversity, but belying appearances, from conception, our core perfection and truth are already veiled by karmic, miasmatic and constitutional inheritance: all factors that distort the infant and child's perception of self and reality. To this will be added the influence of body identification, differentiation between pain and pleasure, striving for pleasure and avoidance of pain, the sense of self and of the 'other', and the unnerving experience of perceiving oneself to be discrete, isolated, separate and cut-off from the rest of reality: all factors that impose ever-deepening duality upon the developing soul/ego complex.

Associated with these deviations from wholeness come the various inadequacies and disruptions of the holding environment that occur in all early life experience. Abuse, deprivation, neglect, abandonment and other forms of severe impingement are particularly damaging, but even in the absence of serious traumatic experience, the inevitable inconsistencies in the dependability and nurturing of the holding environment and the singular nature of the child will collude towards undermining the continuity of soul-consciousness on which basic trust depends.

Finally, the influence of the mother (or significant mother figure) is critical to the personality of the unfolding soul/ego complex. During the first months of life, the child's consciousness is symbiotically merged with that of its mother and what she perceives herself to be, and what she perceives the child to be, become what the child will perceive itself to be. On this initial, precariously subjective foundation, the worldview of the parents is built to create the child's worldview. Almost without exception, the assumptions of the parents do not reflect the soul dimension, but a materialistic or convoluted and prejudiced religious interpretation of the meaning of life. Since the deeper dimension of Reality is not mirrored back to the child, either in the quality of the holding environment, or, in the assumptions, nature or behaviour of the parents, this wondrous dimension becomes peripheral and blurs out of focus as the child incrementally loses contact with its own True Nature, or Essence.

Shadow projection

According to Jung:

> Projections change the world into the replica of one's own unknown face.[7]

> A man who is unconscious of himself acts in a blind, instinctive way and is in addition fooled by all the illusions that arise when he sees everything that he is not conscious of in himself coming to meet him from outside as projections upon his neighbour.[7]

Other than through emotional paroxysms and the intrusion of Shadow characteristics into customary behaviour, the Shadow most clearly reveals its contents through projection. Projection is one of the most important psychological defence mechanisms recognised by Freud and it is invariably employed by the ego-self in its attempts to deny the existence of the Shadow and to avoid confrontation with it. Repressed Shadow qualities are unconsciously projected away from the ego-self and fixed upon the personality and habits of others.

It is an interesting exercise to ask anyone to detail what characteristics in other people they find most intolerable, objectionable, irritating and unacceptable. The 'despicable' traits they enumerate provide a résumé of their own repressed and unresolved characteristics.

These qualities in others are unacceptable precisely because they represent the very qualities they have rejected and repressed in themselves. That which they cannot accept in themselves, they find impossible to tolerate in others. By the same token, negative qualities that do not trouble us excessively, and for which we are ready to find extenuating circumstances, generally do not pertain to our Shadow.

As Dr Edward Whitmont (1912–1988), a founding member of the CG Jung Institute of New York, tells us:

> There is always an archetypal urge for a scapegoat, someone to blame and attack in order to vindicate oneself and be justified.[8]

The 'other' is always potentially *the archetypal enemy*, the one who is blameworthy when compared with our own pretentious 'innocence'. To the extent that we need to proclaim our virtue, the 'other' must be stained with all the vices we fail to acknowledge in ourselves.

The projection of the Shadow onto others is a psychological stratagem not limited to individuals, it can be engaged in by groups, cults, religions and entire nations. The collective energy and drive behind such projection creates a powerful morphic field permeated by bigotry, contempt and hatred. Where there is resonance, the projection will have a pervasive and perverse effect, bringing about terrible consequences. Every minority and every dissenting group carries the Shadow projection of the majority,[9] be it black, white, Jew, Christian, Muslim, Irish, Palestinian, Russian or Chinese. At times of conflict that create intense polarisation of patriotism and/or religious faith, the enemy is scapegoated, dehumanised and demonised. Shadow projection is reciprocal, each side perceiving the other as the incarnation of evil and not deserving of humane consideration. This collective paranoia and scapegoating underlies all kinds of prejudice and is responsible for discrimination, persecution, genocide and civil war.

The compulsive need to project the Shadow is everywhere about us. When people come together socially, and alcohol loosens tongues, conversation often gravitates to gossip about those who are not present: their misfortunes and misguided behaviour being paraded with relish. Often the voice of the projector will drop to a conspiratorial level as if some unseen eavesdropper might hear the reprehensible information being divulged. Censure is implicit in their hushed tones and pained facial expression, as is the desire to convince their audience of their own strength of character contrasted with the shortcomings of the one being discussed. The degree of criticism and consternation evinced give good indication of the intensity of the projection, both on the part of the gossiper and the responsive listeners. Hypocrisy and gossip are happy bedfellows.

The rubric *gossiping* yields few remedies: Ars-alb; Borago; Calc-carb; Causticum; *Hyoscyamus*; Lachesis; Pareira: Stramonium; Veratrum.

Given the prevalence of gossip in everyday life and its use as a vehicle for projection, this meagre rubric exemplifies how certain rubrics fail to represent the full spectrum of implicated archetypes. It is necessary to go to the stronger, more malicious, rubric – *slander* – to gain a better idea of the archetypes eager to undermine the reputation of others. The rubric indicates a psyche burdened by repression and strenuously attempting to compensate through harsh projection.

Slander: disposition to slander.
*Veratrum; *Nux-vom*; Amm-carb; Anacardium; Ars-alb; Belladonna; Borax; Causticum; Coral-rub; Germanium; Guaiacum; Helonias; Hyoscyamus; Ipecacuanha; Lachesis; Lycopodium; Mercurius; Nat-carb; Nat-mur; Nit-ac; Pareira; Petroleum; Phosphorus; Sepia; Spigelia; Stramonium.

Archetypes that slander

Nasty rubrics, like this one, confirm the unpleasant characteristics of certain key archetypes and often provide unexpected insights about those we thought innocent. It is a useful exercise to try and guess which archetypes would find a home in such a rubric and to compare their nastiness and the reasons for it. A cursory look at the outstanding remedies in the rubric brings it alive and makes it accessible to memory. We should expect the three members of the toxic *Solanaceae* to be present – Belladonna (deadly nightshade), Stramonium (poison apple) and Hyoscyamus (black henbane) – for they are central to the structure of the ego-self and to the tension between the conscious and unconscious minds – as also, the closely associated Veratrum-alb (white hellebore), a remedy for the ego-self that is inflated with pride, self-righteousness, religious fanaticism and contempt for others.

The bitter, twisted and vengeful 'nitrogen remedies', Nitric acid and Ammonium carbonate, have to be in this rubric along with the fundamental, snake-archetype, Lachesis, whose venom is saturated with nitrogen in the form of ammonia salts and whose tongue is often too loose and spiteful. Some pairings and groupings are evident: the cowardly Lycopodium and its degraded look-alike Petroleum, always deprecating others to better their image; Causticum and Phosphorus, so alike that they are therapeutically incompatible – so empathetic and compassionate, yet capable of being so very dark; Borax, Nat-carb and Nat-mur, like all sodiums, controlled and deeply repressed; Sepia (cuttlefish) and Coral-rub

(red coral), creatures of the ocean and thus related to the deep, dark unconscious; Ars-alb and Mercurius, the arch syphilitics, and another important
anti-syphilitic, Guaiacum.

Nux-vom will use any means to rise to prominence, success and power,
including besmirching the good name of others. Anacardium (marking nut)
consigns the 'good' of his nature to the Shadow and protects himself
against the hostility of the world with his 'badness'. In his weakness, Anacardium seeks power through meanness and cruelty.

Helonias dioica (unicorn-root) is a woman's remedy and must be compared with Sepia. It is of value when feminine energy is depleted by
domestic responsibilities and childbirth, or effete from self-indulgence and
luxury. As feminine power recedes, the repressed masculine contents of the
Shadow impinge, more and more, on consciousness, threatening the self-
image of the persona making them extremely sensitive to the least contradiction or criticism and averse to consolation; all of which focus attention
on their weakness. Socialising and physical activity temporarily relieve their
emotional and physical symptoms, as does projecting their shadow onto
others: *sits the whole day, finding fault with everyone.*

Significantly, four of the fixated *'pins and needles'* archetypes are to be
found in the rubric: Ars-alb, Mercurius, Nat-mur and Spigelia and to these
must be added Nit-ac, whose pains are stitching as if inflicted by a pin or
needle. Gossip-mongering and slander may well be likened to sticking pins
into a voodoo doll (Lac lupinum), personifying the one being maligned,
with vindictive relish. We can anticipate that the pins and needles archetypes are much-inclined to project Shadow characteristics onto others –
even Silicea!

The nature of the Shadow

Adding to material gleaned and adapted from Anthony Steven's, *On Jung,*[10]
the following attributes can be given to the Shadow.

- The Shadow is unconscious, but dynamically alive and active.
- Shadow qualities and drives can impinge on conscious behaviour.
- Driven by the Id, the Shadow always seeks expression.
- It is an aspect of the soul/ego-self complex relegated to a twilight zone
  in the personal unconscious.
- Qualities deemed undesirable, unacceptable or reprehensible by the
  ego/superego complex are denied, disowned and repressed or hidden
  from view in the Shadow.
- These are the rejected aspects of the ego-self.

- Therefore, when the Shadow impinges on awareness it brings feelings of guilt, shame and unworthiness and fear of rejection.
- The Shadow contains all the unresolved emotions of the ego-self.
- It is the repository of the unrealised Essential aspects of the soul.
- The Shadow possesses qualities opposite to those of the persona.
- The Shadow compensates for the pretensions of the Shadow.
- The persona compensates for the antisocial propensities of the Shadow.
- To face and own one's Shadow is potentially terrifying.
- We therefore unconsciously deny its existence and unconsciously project it onto others.
- We can then hold others responsible for our own 'badness'.
- This scapegoating underlies our prejudices and is responsible for discrimination, persecution, pogroms and wars.
- Through projection, the enemy can be demonised and dehumanised: made unworthy of humane consideration.
- Qualities and traits, we most dislike in others are the qualities and traits we harbour in the Shadow.
- The last Shadow is archetypal e.g. the Shadow warrior.

* * * * *

References

1 Jung CJ. *Psychology and religion*. Collected Works 11: Psychology and religion: West and East. 1938. p131.

2 Jung CJ. *Aion*. Collected Works 9. Part 11. 1951. p14.

3 Jung CJ. *The Philosophical Tree*. Collected Works 13: Alchemical Studies. London: Routledge, 1945. p335.

4 Balfour G. *The Life of Robert Louis Stevenson*. New York NY: Charles Scribner's Sons, 1912 pp15–16.

5 Sanford J. *Dr Jekyll and Mr Hyde*. Meeting the Shadow – The Hidden Power of the Dark Side of Human Nature (edited Zweigg C and Abrams J.) New York NY: Penguin Putnam, 1990. pp30–34.

6 Nilsson MP. *Greek Popular Religion the Religion of Eleusis*. New York NY: Columbia University Press, 1947. pp42–64.

7 Jung CJ. *Aion*. Collected Works 14. 1955. p17.

8 Whitmont EC. *The Symbolic Quest – Basic Concepts of Analytical Psychology*. Princeton NJ: Princeton University Press, 1991. p162.

9 *Ibid.*, p168.

10 Stevens A. *On Jung*. London: Penguin Books Ltd, 1999. pp43–45.

With the concept of the archetype completed and the typography of the psyche considered from both a Freudian and Jungian perspective, the narrative of Healing the Soul is poised to proceed to the evolution of disease in the human race. In volume 3 of *Healing the Soul*, the most precious jewel in the splendid crown of homeopathic philosophy – Hahnemann's theory of the chronic miasms – will be considered in depth. Commencing with the emergence of the ego-self as a disruptive force in the life of the immature soul, the process of disease evolution will be traced in the light of European history from the Dark Ages after the fall of the Roman Empire, through Medieval times, the Renaissance, the Age of Enlightenment, the Romantic period into the Modern Era, when, despite the advance of conventional medicine, the ravages of disease have become more complex, destructive and malignant. Against this ominous background of disease progression, *Healing the Soul* volume 3 will array the homeopathic archetypes that a loving, sentient Cosmos has designed to combat and thwart the seeming inexorable advance of chronic, ego-based disease: archetypes that empower the soul in its perennial struggle with the ego-self.

INDEX